Chapters from
Psychiatric Treatment: Crisis, Clinic, and Consultation

Psychiatrist John Beebe has taught analytical psychotherapy at such institutions as Stanford Medical Center, the California Pacific Medical Center, the University of California San Francisco Medical School, and Pacifica Graduate Institute as well as at universities and training centers in China. A Distinguished Life Fellow of the American Psychiatric Association, Dr. Beebe is a past President of the C. G. Jung Institute of San Francisco. He was Founding Editor of *The San Francisco Jung Institute Library Journal* (now called *Jung Journal: Culture and Psyche*), and American co-editor of the *Journal of Analytical Psychology*. He is the author of *Integrity in Depth* and *Energies and Patterns in Psychological Type* as well as more than 200 book chapters, journal articles, reviews, and other publications.

Chapters from
Psychiatric Treatment
Crisis, Clinic, and Consultation

C. PETER ROSENBAUM, M.D.
Associate Professor
Department of Psychiatry
Stanford University School of Medicine

JOHN E. BEEBE III, M.D.
Department of Psychological and Social Medicine
Pacific Medical Center
University o f the Pacific

CHIRON PUBLICATIONS •
ASHEVILLE, NORTH CAROLINA

JUNGIANEUM
RE-COVERED CLASSICS
IN ANALYTICAL PSYCHOLOGY
SERIES EDITOR STEFANO CARPANI

www.ChironPublications.com

Cover design by Niko Crnčević
Printed primarily in the United States of America.

ISBN 978-1-68503-565-5 paperback
ISBN 978-1-68503-566-2 hardcover
ISBN 978-1-68503-567-9 electronic
ISBN 978-1-68503-568-6 limited edition paperback
ISBN 978-1-68503-569-3 limited edition hardcover

Library of Congress Cataloging-in-Publication Data Pending

Series Editor's Introduction

John Beebe's *Psychiatric Treatment: Crisis, Clinic, and Consultation* (coauthored with C. Peter Rosenbaum, M.D.) was first published by McGraw-Hill in 1975. Since then, it has served as a handbook for many generations of students, psychiatrists, and therapists, interested in looking at the psyche from a depth-psychology-informed point of view. This book, as underlined at the beginning of the original preface, was and is intended "to guide therapists as they enter into therapeutic work." In fact, it is dedicated to those "in training," hence, those who are taking their first steps into the therapeutic profession.

This book—and this is its innovative aspect—addresses the range of situations beginners will have to face (an issue that no other book addressed back in 1975), and presents enough different theories and suggestions for treatment to allow new therapists to get started. It supplies *the needed keys* to understand—as an MD in residence put it—when, "we need a theory to tell us when to use which theory," and to realize that "relying on tradition is not enough" nor "is practice explained because it fulfills the promise of a single theory."

I am thrilled that John accepted my invitation to publish parts of the original book within this series titled *Re-Covered Classics in Analytical Psychology.* I am equally grateful to Chiron's Steve Buser who decided to support this initiative and to make this series possible.

The aim of this series, *Re-Covered Classics in Analytical Psychology,* is to (re)publish masterpieces in analytical psychology that, for different reasons, are out of the market and that find difficulty in getting (re)published.

Re-Covered Classics in Analytical Psychology is an initiative for (re)publishing high standard and academic work in the field of analytical psychology (with a strong interdisciplinary flavor focusing on psychoanalysis at large). This initiative is driven by necessity, as the publishing market has changed in recent years due to the digitalization of the publishing industry, the fact that online shops increased in market dominance and aggressively lowered the profitability of traditional publishing houses. As a result, there are very few companies continuing to survive on the old model of large print runs, warehousing books, and full upfront "good faith" investment upon acceptance of a manuscript for publication. Also, historical Jungian publishers are rapidly shutting down, or are no longer accepting titles. This situation has left a gaping hole whereby up-and-coming and forward-thinking scholars of the Jungian, analytical field lack access to a wider audience and the means to contribute to the greater intellectual and psycho-social/mental health readership communities.

Therefore, I developed this series to preserve the work of our ancestors and to make them available again to the public. I doubt this series will be a profitable experience. For sure it will be a romantic one, whose aim is to preserve culture!

This is one of many initiatives by *Jungianeum: Contemporary Initiatives for Analytical Psychology and Neo-Jungian Studies.* Under this umbrella, since 2022, I am developing a series of initiatives called:

JUNGIANEUM/Books Series: "Re-Covered Classics in Analytical Psychology" and "Neo-Jungian Studies"; JUNGIANEUM/Talks: "Psychosocial Wednesday"; JUNGIANEUM/Yearbook for Contemporary neo-Jungian Studies; JUNGIANEUM/Masterclasses (in collaboration with Pacifica Graduate Institute, USA); JUNGIANEUM/Cultivating the Souls in the Supersociety (interview series on doppiozero.it);

JUNGIANEUM/Biennale (an online conference titled "Democracy on the Couch").

Collection

- Verena Kast, *Father-Daughter, Mother-Son* (2022)
- Polly Young-Eisendrath, *Women and Desire: Beyond Wanting to Be Wanted* (2023)
- Mary Watkins, *Opening to the Imaginal: Waking Dreams and Invisible Guests* (2024)
- Pia Skogemann, *Waxing Femininity: Adult Female Development from the Perspective of C. G. Jung's Psychology* (2024)
- Verena Kast, *The Association Experiment in Therapeutic Practice* (2025)
- John Beebe, *Crisis, Clinic, and Consultation* (2025)
- Mario Jacoby, Verena Kast, Ingrid Riedel, *Witches, Ogres, and the Devil's Daughter: Encounters With Evil in Fairy Tales* (Forthcoming, 2025)
- Thomas Singer & Stuart Copans, *Who's the Patient Here? Portraits of the Young Psychotherapist* (Forthcoming, 2025)

Stefano Carpani, Berlin/Trieste
February 2025

Foreword to the Current Edition

It is amazing to think that John Beebe's and C. Peter Rosenbaum's *Psychiatric Treatment: Crisis, Clinic, and Consultation* was published almost fifty years ago. To some that may seem like yesterday. To others, it may seem like ancient history. And to a few of us, it will seem like both—just yesterday and ancient history. I would like to write something in this preface about the cultural context in which this book appeared, something about the content and structure of the book, and finally some words about its unique value.

Cultural Context

The 1970s was a most interesting time in the development of modern psychiatry. The strong grip that the Freudian psychoanalytic tradition had on the theory and practice of psychiatry in the United States was loosening as evidenced by the fact that many medical schools and university-affiliated hospitals were beginning to explore other modalities of psychiatric treatment and the Chairmanships of the Departments of Psychiatry were no longer controlled exclusively by psychoanalysts. This phenomenon was at least partially ushered in by the discovery of the antipsychotic properties of the phenothiazines in the 1950s which marked the beginning of a psychopharmacological revolution in psychiatry. It led to a much greater interest in biological causation and treatment rather than psychological aspects of psychiatric illness. The phenothiazines led to a much greater ability to control the symptoms of chronic psychotic illnesses and, as result, state hospitals literally started emptying out and closing down. With the closing of large state hospitals, there was emerging hope for the development of community mental health centers to treat psychiatric patients. The emptying of state hospitals, the shift to biological and psychopharmacological treatments of mental illness, and the rise of community mental health centers contributed to the increasing emphasis on crisis intervention and management of psychiatric illness. The 1970s were the heyday of the coming together of these different trends and it is in that context that John Beebe and C. Peter Rosenbaum published their book. Their books reflects all of these trends coming together, although they certainly did not jettison the accumulated wisdom of the psychodynamic traditions that preceded these developments.

Content and Structure of Book

I began my psychiatric training in 1970 and several months of my first year were spent at the Mt. Zion Crisis Clinic in San Francisco. It was a heady time as the new psychiatric treatment modality of crisis intervention was being developed. The management of the acutely ill psychiatric patient was both challenging and exciting. I remember one especially dramatic case when a huge, 6' 5" tall man came into our clinic in a stage of acute psychotic excitement, exclaiming that he was going to bottle all the sperm on earth and send it to the moon. He didn't like our approach to him and bolted out the door. Three of us ended up chasing him down the streets of San Francisco to no avail and, as far as I know, he may have ended up on the moon. In learning how to manage acutely ill psychiatric patients who presented with suicidal, homicidal, psychotic, drug intoxicated, and every other form of emergency condition, we needed all the help we could get and we didn't have Beebe's and Rosenbaum's book. Many of us felt like the cartoon character that I later developed with a colleague, Stu Copans, which we published in *Who's The Patient Here?* around the same time John Beebe published his book.

In a way, Rosenbaum's and Beebe's book was the perfect answer to the dilemma of the cartoon character who of course, was "us." It is a truly rare and wonderful blend of different elements. It breaks the treatment of patients into the categories of the symptoms with which they present: suicidality, addictions, psychosis. It defines the various treatment facilities available to patients at different stages of their illness: psychiatric crisis clinics, inpatient treatment, and outpatient treatment. It explores different treatment modalities from psychopharmacological approaches to individual therapy to couples therapy to group therapy to the uses of dreams and even the uses of the telephone (no internet then). It is a comprehensive textbook. But, in rereading it, I found it was far more than that in the way in which it integrates all the different pieces of modern clinical psychiatry. There is a fine use of clinical examples that are interspersed with thoughtful analysis of the strengths and weaknesses of how a case was approached. There is wonderfully practical clinical wisdom in the detailed management of different situations, whether it is with a suicidal patient, an addicted patient or a psychotic patient. And grounding the careful clinical detail of how people present and are managed are a variety of theoretical perspectives that honor the values of many different approaches.

Conclusion: Enduring Value

What makes the book so unique and valuable in my mind is the way in which Beebe and the other contributors seamlessly blended theory, practice, and case material. Usually such text books are rather one sided in the emphasis of theory or practice or too wedded to one tradition of psychiatry or psychotherapy—biological or psychoanalytical, for example. Jungian books in particular—as John Beebe went on to become one of the finest contributors to the Jungian tradition—are often quite thin when it comes to practical management. In fact, many Jungians take pride in not focusing on technique. But Beebe is not afraid of getting into detail about the techniques of interviewing, of managing, of navigating most difficult situations involving patients, their "ecology" of family and friends or the difficulties of complicated relationships between helping professionals in both inpatient and outpatient settings. In that sense, this book reminds me of my own far more primitive efforts to learn as a medical student when we carried around little black books in which we wrote down the "pearls" that experienced clinicians would pass on to us. John's book is full of so many pearls of wisdom about dealing with so many difficult situations that it makes me feel like a student all over again in the presence of a wise clinician. I wish I'd had his book fifty years ago and what is even more amazing is that I find it is still quite relevant and timely fifty years later because the insights about human behavior, motivation, and suffering seem to transcend time.

Thomas Singer, MD
San Francisco

Introduction to the Current Edition

To revisit my authored and co-authored chapters from *Psychiatric Treatment: Crisis, Clinic, and Consultation* returns me to the person I was 50 years ago, two years after graduating from the psychiatric residency program at Stanford University Medical Center. At that time, I was teaching emergency psychiatry to both psychiatrists and psychologists in training at Pacific Presbyterian Medical Center in San Francisco and supervising psychiatric residents at the Langley Porter Psychiatric Institute of the University California. I was also completing my third year of analytic training at the C. G. Jung Institute of San Francisco, trying to transcend my resume. It was wonderful to undertake to capture in writing what I had learned by becoming a psychiatrist—a practical education in the medical application of psychological principles, analogous to C. G. Jung's fortunate experience when he worked under Eugen Bleuler at the Burghölzli. This practical proficiency has always shined through Jung's writing for me, and the reader will see that I have tried to re-create for an American readership consisting of psychiatrists, psychologists, and psychiatric social workers in training what "medical psychology" could still teach them.

I suspect this was the last moment in the history of American psychiatry that a book like this could still have come into being. The field was rapidly becoming far more neuropsychiatric and, to a mind steeped in what Jung meant by medical psychology, accordingly less psychological. The book had a measure of success in its time, becoming the main selection of the Behavioral Science Book Service a few months after its appearance in 1975, and mental health professionals in training, including psychiatric nurses, discovered or were assigned it. Returning to it now, I can see why: it is grounded in actual situations that have to be dealt with, and is unafraid to turn to any source of clinical wisdom. The senior author of the book, C. Peter Rosenbaum, shared my vision for the text, and despite the fact that the medical psychology he'd encountered in his own psychiatric training had been delivered by doctors trained in a Freudian psychoanalytic tradition, he welcomed what I had learned from the Jungian psychiatrists I had sought out for therapy, supervision, and analytic training. That Jung's name crops up frequently is not just an artifact of my own bent, but reflects Pete Rosenbaum's generosity and openness, and the atmosphere created at Stanford by many of the doctors in the department assembled by David Hamburg, which included, importantly, people influenced by Harry Stack Sullivan. The degree to which these early teachers of mine understood how pragmatic psychological thinking is a medicine, to be deployed with discrimination and care, and that this much intelligence is not merely a poultice, but part of the point of meeting the expectation that people bring to a psychiatrically trained professional when asking that person to see them through the tough time that a mental or emotional crisis can be, resonated with the part of me that appreciated that this was the mindset with which Jung had started. It remains the underbelly of the gut sense with which I still practice daily as a Jungian analyst.

John Beebe
San Francisco

Table of Contents

Note: In this publication, text from the original book is reproduced photographically. The original chapter numbers are retained so that references to chapters, figures, examples, and tables will be correct.

SECTION 1
Crisis

Principles of Crisis Intervention

The following example has been adapted from a first-year psychiatric resident's case description written her first day on the emergency service. The example will be cited repeatedly throughout this chapter because it is typical of the kinds of situations with which the emergency therapist is faced.*

Example 1-1, Anna. Anna, a 24-year-old single, black mother of two, was brought to the emergency room by her cousin, Betty, with whom she had been living since she lost custody of her children to her mother-in-law six weeks before. Betty demanded "total psychiatric" care for Anna: "You have got to put her in the hospital!"

Until Anna moved in with Betty, she had lived in a foster home in a neighboring community. She had been there since early adolescence. Her parents were dead, and she had no family in the area. She had been in continual trouble with the law, mostly in connection with heroin addiction.

Cousin Betty was 25, rigid, and a disciplinarian. She saw herself as a reformed sinner;

vis-à-vis Anna her role was that of the strict mother. She found herself rapidly running out of patience with Anna's behavior, which she viewed as irresponsible and bad. On this particular evening she had become furious at Anna for lying, and in the midst of their argument had made the threat of "total psychiatric care" and forced her to come to the emergency room.

When the emergency therapist first saw her, Anna was tearful and upset, frightened, and angry with her cousin. She was oriented and reasonably cooperative, and her feelings and behavior were within a socially acceptable range. She was able to think rationally. The therapist learned that at Betty's insistence Anna had seen another therapist, Dr. Jones, at the neighborhood health center, and that Anna had an appointment there the next day. The emergency therapist also learned that Dr. Jones was Betty's regular therapist.

This case is typical of the kinds of emergency situations the emergency therapist will be called upon to solve. The reader may wish to ask himself before proceeding how he would have approached the crisis of Betty and Anna. Later in this chapter we shall discuss how the case was actually handled by the emergency therapist.

---

*In this, as in all other case material presented in this book, data that might identify patients and their families have been changed to ensure privacy.

A CRISIS AS A PLAY IN FOUR ACTS

C.G. Jung[1] has suggested that a typical dream is like a play in four acts, an idea we shall develop in our chapter on dreams (Chapter 22). A dream is a sort of miniature, nocturnal emergency in which there is a libidinal upset and a rallying of coping mechanisms to deal with the disturbance and to provide resolution. A typical crisis also has four acts. This four-act model can be used as an aid in collecting and sorting the clinical data in crisis intervention. In the first act the setting is defined and the protagonists are shown; we observe their lifestyles. In the second act a situation develops: a new character appears, or an action or event produces change, with its attendant uncertainty and tension. In the third act the development culminates in a peak of tension. In the fourth act a solution is reached.

These same four stages are present in the evolution of an emergency. The emergency therapist should train himself to identify (1) the protagonists and their natural setting; (2) the development, or that which emerged before the emergency required professional attention; (3) the point at which the greatest stress or tension was felt; and (4) the solution that is anticipated or expected by each of the participants.

The job of the emergency therapist is to help the protagonists find the solution that has the most capacity for benefit and safety in all their lives. Until, however, he has taken all aspects of the crisis into account, including the principals' own ideas about what a good solution would be, he is in a poor position to achieve this goal. Even if he is wise enough to see what the optimal resolution should be, he still has to assess what portion of this hypothetical best solution is likely to be acceptable to the individuals involved.

The emergency therapist is advised, therefore, to proceed cautiously, gather information about the crisis methodically, and not let himself be drawn too quickly into the drama. If he follows the four-stage model, he is unlikely to lose his professional head. As he gains experience he can go faster, but at first he should take his time.

ASSUMING THE NECESSARY ROLE

To function effectively the therapist should be in a setting that is comfortable and in which he feels adequately supported by the law and by expert consultants to whom he can turn in obscure situations. Most emergency room and training situations do provide such a structure. If he has these resources at his command, the therapist should recognize the extent of his power. However insecure he feels about his abilities, the participants in the crisis see him as the person who has the authority to resolve the situation. He can ask individual family members to leave or to remain in the office while he talks with the "identified patient." He can recommend for or against hospitalization. He is the one who calls the police in if the situation requires legal restraint.

He also incarnates an ancient role, that of the village wise man who knows the way to end distress and is justified in using whatever procedures he believes will achieve his end. The patients expect to have expectations made of them, and the emergency therapist is in a position to define the situation. He should not shirk this responsibility. It is this role that gives him the edge over the participants in the emergency, many of whom may actually understand the emotions involved and the total situation far better than he.

The model described here can serve as a point of departure for each therapist to work out a system that best fits his own needs and talents. Many of the ideas presented can serve as a first approximation for therapists who are in process of letting their own styles evolve. The central task is the same however it is approached: to assess the emergency situation, analyze its components, search for possible outcomes, and assist with the resolution.

A MODEL OF CRISIS INTERVENTION

Step 1—Basic Information Gathering

Using paper and a pencil to record the answers, the therapist must ask basic questions of the people involved: the names, addresses, and phone numbers of the identified patient and of the people with whom he lives or most frequently interacts. The therapist is asking, in effect, who are the protagonists? Often at this point vital details are omitted, including mention of the existence of some of the most significant actors in the crisis. Only later do they appear, and often only after detailed questioning. Such dramatic forgetting is characteristic of emotional stress, and the therapist has a good clue to the most charged issues by the omissions made at this point that later come to light. It is helpful therefore to record what is said at first. The purpose in listening for omissions is not to trap the patient but to understand his conflicts.

The therapist can grasp the ego functioning of the participants by the manner in which they answer basic initial questions. Their ability to communicate, remember, and organize basic information about their lives reveals a good deal about their mental states.

History taking is also therapeutic. Frequently it lets people in crisis know that the particular situation which seems so hopeless or out-of-hand began at some point in time and presumably will end at some point in time, and that in spite of the current investment in the traumatic peak of stress and tension, the persons involved have more of a history and future together than they momentarily believe. Harry Stack Sullivan[2] has said:

> Severe anxiety probably contributes no information. The effect of severe anxiety reminds one in some ways of a blow on the head, in that it simply wipes out what is immediate proximal to its occurence. If you have a severe blow on the head, you are quite apt later to have an incurable, absolute amnesia covering the few moments before your head was struck. Anxiety has a similar effect . . . .

In a psychiatric emergency, the participants are often quite anxious. The therapist's job is to help uncover the events and feelings about which the participants are partially amnesic so the emergency can be placed more rationally into the context of the past that led up to the anxiety. In this manner the future can be ordered to help diminish the effect of the crisis.

At this point the therapist should also ask everything he must know to place the participants in a social context he can understand. Where do they work? What do they do? Where do they live? What religion, if any, do they practice? In general, where do they exist in society? Unless the therapist makes this conscious effort, it is easy to make projections that are unwarranted in terms of the protagonists' actual standards, attitudes, and experiences.

One trap in gathering information is that one of the principals may want to bind the therapist with *pseudoconfidentiality* by asking him to promise not to reveal some particular "family secret" to the others. Agreement to such a request is almost inevitably detrimental to successful intervention for several reasons. First, it sets up a special alliance of "we have a secret" between the therapist and informant that estranges the therapist from the others. Second, it ties the therapist's hands because he cannot utilize information valuable in seeking a resolution. Third, a family secret is almost always a pseudosecret; everyone has known it all along and has pretended ignorance. In fact, everyone else may breathe sighs of relief when a member's drinking, incestuous advances to a child, bizarre thinking, murderous or suicidal impulses, and so on are brought into the open and discussed as a problem that needs to be dealt with instead of buried.

When a participant in a crisis situation approaches the therapist with "Promise you won't tell the others, but . . . ," it is best for the therapist to take the position that although he is interested in hearing what everyone has to say, he needs to be free to use that information in as helpful a way as he can. He *can* promise that he will make every effort not to use the information in an embarrasing or hurtful manner. He explains that to intervene effectively he needs to know what the informant can offer, even though he cannot promise confidentiality. Usually this explanation convinces the informant to give the necessary information. If not, the therapist may inquire about what the informant fears will happen if he divulges the information. If it becomes apparent that his fears are illusory, such as divulging a family secret that is already known or suspected by the others, the informant will usually provide the information. Often anxiety about keeping a secret betrays a real desire to be unburdened of it.

Step 2—Understanding the Development of the Crisis

There are three main considerations in step 2: (1) finding the sequence of events; (2) structuring the interview; and (3) avoiding the dangers of premature catharsis.

The emergency therapist must determine the *sequence of events* preceding the crisis. Patients usually are eager to focus on the peak of stress, but the therapist is interested in firmly understanding how the situation developed.

Thus the emergency therapist wanted to know how Anna lost custody of her children and came to live with her cousin. She wanted to hear how the two women had been getting along during the six weeks they had been living together. At first Betty maintained that the situation had been terrible the whole time. Nevertheless, they had been under the same roof for six weeks, and the therapist reasoned that they must have faced difficulties in living together before and had found ways of resolving them.

Learning about their first weeks together was part of learning about the development of the situation that brought them to the emergency room. By being forced to accept this focus, Betty and Anna obtained some perspective on the crisis they were facing. In turn, they gave the emergency therapist valuable information concerning the coping options they were likely to exercise in dealing with the present crisis.

Usually a therapist is more successful in having patients accept a solution already in their repertoire than he is in having them try a new solution. Many patients have a solid repertoire of healthy coping strategies, but in the development of the crisis events occur that cause the actors to disqualify or discard them. In learning about the development of the crisis, the therapist can frequently identify a strategy that had been effective previously. The discarding of it can be identified and called into question. "Why did you give that up since it was working for you?" the therapist may ask.

Orderly history taking is itself a treatment modality. The patient benefits by watching the emergency therapist bring logical order to what seemed a chaotic situation. The therapist's ability to cope comes through too; there is a great deal of modeling or *ego borrowing* at this phase of the interview.

It is obvious that the emergency therapist will have to be firm in *structuring the interview* if he is to succeed in having patients explain the development of the crisis. The patient may want to jump ahead or avoid elements of clarification because of an overinvestment in the dramatic, insoluble tension. It seems to be human nature to perseverate on traumatic points of anxiety or anger. This tendency of the patient's must be firmly countered or the crisis intervention will become crisis amplification, with the therapist becoming a passionate advocate for the patient's sense of injury.

Premature catharsis can be dangerous. A common error made by beginning therapists is to identify with the patient and to precipitate injudicious catharsis. With homicidal patients, as we shall see in Chapter 4, this can be a dangerous procedure. Freud's[3] famous dictum, "Where id was, there shall ego be," is especially pertinent in emergency work. The emergency therapist strives to give the patient two ways of protecting himself from his overwhelming emotion: structure and distance. This is not to say that the therapist is uninterested in letting the patient express emotion, but that he must strive to create a situation which can contain the emotion expressed. Indeed, the creation of an ego structure large and solid enough to hold the emotion of the patient is a task of the therapist at all times during all forms of therapy.

If he has been successful in creating structure, the therapist can proceed safely to the next stage of understanding the crisis: reliving with the patient the experience of peak stress or tension.

Step 3—Re-experiencing the Peak of Tension in the Crisis

In this step the emergency therapist has four tasks to attend to, namely, (1) approaching the emotion, (2) using special interview techniques, (3) hearing each person out, and (4) mediating catharsis.

When the emergency therapist has been able to slow down the participants enough to find out who they are and how the present turmoil developed, he is ready to *approach the underlying emotion* by asking them to recount the issue that brought them before him, and relive the peak of stress or tension. It is surprising how many patients do not know what it is that set them off, what the last straw was, what hurt most. Here the therapist uses all the skills of the empathetic, open-ended, emotion-releasing questioning and commenting that he has been taught.

Certain *special interviewing techniques* may be helpful. Carl Rogers[4] described the reflection of feeling as a therapeutic method. To release emotion the therapist reflects back to the patient the affective quality of what he has just said, restating the feeling and emotional meaning rather than details of content.

Attention to content can also work. For instance, note taking can be a powerful stimulus for the patient to open up more. It is all right for the therapist to continue to satisfy his own desire for accurate information by note taking, provided he communicates that his main interest is in grasping the feelings of the patient.

Other therapists will prefer to put their pencils down at this point and to emphasize by direct, wordless eye contact that a critical point in the interview has been reached and feelings are now more necessary than facts.

Whatever technique the therapist uses, it is important that *each person has his say*, that each is heard. Again, the therapist offers treatment by listening. To paraphrase John Perry:[5] There is no anger quite like the anger of the person who is not being heard. One reduces anger by listening fully. Relatives must not be allowed to interrupt each other, and each participant may have to be interviewed separately if each is to have his say. It is important that each person feel the therapist has understood his particular stress and has taken in the news of his suffering.

The therapist must *mediate catharsis* for some patients. Certain patients in crisis offer, instead of anger, a blank, dazed, depressed, or retarded affect. The therapist may have to mediate catharsis by making statements such as, "I can imagine with the amount of confusion you have described to me that you must have felt terribly upset just then," or, "I'm positive that being alone for so many weeks after the loss of your wife made you feel tremendously lonely and grieved." With schizophrenic and very depressed patients, the therapist's putting into words what the normal human feeling would be can have a profoundly releasing effect. The schizophrenic patient may suddenly talk sense; the silent, depressed patient may burst into tears.

Anna (cont'd.). When the emergency therapist tried to learn from Anna what she had been lying about, cousin Betty interrupted persistently. It took considerable persuasion to establish Anna's right to speak for herself, but the therapist elected to let Betty remain in the room. It turned out that Anna had lied to her cousin about the time of her appointment with Dr. Jones and that Betty knew she was lying because she had called Dr. Jones earlier in the day to ascertain the exact time.

As soon as this fact emerged, Betty began to

weep. Sensing that an important feeling of a private nature was emerging, the therapist asked Anna to wait outside. Alone with the therapist, Betty said, "I guess you realize I don't like sharing Dr. Jones with Anna." She then related how much it meant that Dr. Jones held her in high regard and how much she feared Anna's telling him things that might make him think less of her. Betty's father, like Anna's, had run off with a woman when she was a little girl, and this point of empathic identification had suddenly become a source of competition.

The emergency therapist asked to see Anna alone while Betty waited outside. From Anna the therapist learned that she had known all along it "wouldn't work" if she saw Dr. Jones, but that Betty kept insisting she go. Anna had even suggested seeing a Dr. Gregg, who had more experience with heroin users, at the same clinic, but Betty had not allowed her to make the arrangements. Finally, sure that Betty was going to be jealous, Anna lied about the appointment time. She planned to miss the appointment and pretend she had the time wrong.

Anna's main emotion centered around the impossibility of doing anything to please Betty.

With knowledge of the background, the therapist found it much easier to understand the impasse that had developed between Betty and Anna and was ready to make plans for them. Betty and Anna were united in trusting the therapist, who had heard both their points of view, and they were noticeably less antagonistic toward each other as the therapist proceeded to help them find a practical solution to the problem of Anna's therapy.

In this third stage the therapist must use all his skill to elicit the peak of stress or tension from the patients, either by hearing it from them or saying it to them. If he has done this job well, he will have the patient's confidence and will be in a

strong position to search for the solution to the crisis.

Step 4—Finding the Solution

The solution lies within the system, not within the therapist. Implicit in all that has been said so far is that the emergency therapist has been working toward a solution to the crisis. If he has conducted the interview properly up to this point, he will already have done much about resolving the problem. There needs to be, however, a specific resolution by the participants, who will now be called upon to do a major share of the work. The therapist should remember he is a consultant to a system, not its savior. Even when he hospitalizes, refers, or prescribes, he should be carrying out solutions that have emerged logically from his consultation with all the participants and for which they are willing to take their share of the responsibility.

The following five tasks are to be accomplished in step 4: (1) bringing the participants together to redefine the situation; (2) gathering from all participants their expectations about the outcome; (3) enhancing the emergence of previously omitted information; (4) suggesting possible solutions to the principals to solicit their reactions; and (5) carrying through with the resolution that seems most likely to work.

Each member of the system in crisis must fully understand the crisis intervention. After the therapist has learned about the development and peak of tension, it often helps to *bring the participants together* and *redescribe the situation* in understandable human terms.

One of his responsibilities is to make explicit certain issues that had been treated as unknowns or secrets. For instance, an alcoholic patient, trying to bind the therapist with pseudo-confidentiality, may say, "I've been drinking heavily, but don't tell anyone." As with other pseudosecrets, the problem is closed communication: everyone knows the patient has been drinking, but he has been unable to say so directly to the people around him. When the group is gathered together the therapist can open the communication channels by saying, "Mr. Williams has been drinking quite heavily in the past week and has been making a number of problems for himself and for all of you, and he is well aware of this." A statement like this can relieve a bind of several days' duration, in which Mr. Williams has steadfastly refused to acknowledge verbally to his concerned relatives the obvious fact that he has been drinking. The emergency therapist frequently has to mediate important self-disclosures in this way.

When gathering *expectations about outcome,* the participants (and outside therapists) should be asked what they think the outcome should be. Preadolescent children may see with clearer vision than older people. Outside therapists, as the case of Anna will show, may possess information unavailable to the emergency therapist that will drastically change his view of the situation.

The participants may have withheld information for fear it would result in moral or legal problems, and the emergency therapist should seek to *enhance disclosure.* He can do so by saying, "I think I have a fair understanding of the situation which brought you here, but it may be that there are some important things I don't yet know. Is there anything that's been left out or anything you think I should know about before we try to make a decision?" If Anna's emergency therapist had been successful in such an attempt, she might have saved herself some embarrassment.

The emergency therapist should *suggest possible solutions* to the patient and the others to see what their reactions will be. Sometimes a shake of the head or a reavealing look will show that one of the participants has qualms about an apparently reasonable solution. These qualms should be aired. The therapist may say, for instance, "I get the feeling, Mrs. Green, that there is something about that idea which doesn't sit well with you." The therapist should seek a solution that is reasonable and that the patient and his social system can

make work. The solution need not meet with the approval of all concerned; it should have a good chance of working and of not being undermined. This principle is especially helpful when *involuntary hospitalization* is indicated. Then everyone has to hear the reason for internment but need not necessarily agree with it. There will usually be no lasting grudge against the decision, despite temporary anger, if the therapist has proceeded responsibly and explained the reasons for his actions.

Finally, the emergency therapist, after having assessed the situation as completely as possible, should *carry through with the solution* that seems best. He should do so simply and unambivalently. This clarity of intent is especially important if the solution involves doing something the patient or others oppose or are highly ambivalent about, e.g., injecting a tranquilizing medication or forcing an involuntary hospitalization. If others are ambivalent, the therapist must not be; he should carry through expeditiously with what needs to be done. An insecure family will often voice doubt over a wise decision mainly to *test* the therapist.

Anna (cont'd.). At this point the emergency therapist called the outside therapist, Dr. Jones, and told him about the cousin's pressure, what its possible origins were, and what the effects had been on Anna. Being new to emergency consultation, she even suggested a referral to Dr. Gregg.

Dr. Jones surprised her by saying, "Aren't you going to hospitalize her there?" When the therapist started to explain that Anna seemed quite rational, Dr. Jones said angrily, "I think you had better evaluate her more carefully," and abruptly ended the call by saying he was in the middle of an appointment and could not talk more for another hour.

The emergency therapist was angry but realized she must not have all the facts. After all, both Betty and Dr. Jones had said that Anna belonged in the hospital, even though the therapist assumed Anna felt coerced by this possible solution.

The therapist asked Betty what her idea of a solution was. Betty said, "I still think Anna needs to go into the hospital."

She asked Anna what she thought, and to her surprise Anna said, "I know I should be there." Anna then revealed that one of her children was with her and that she had come at the little girl with a knife earlier that day. Because she had thought she was going to be admitted, she had not told the therapist about this part of her dilemma; she had assumed controls would be instituted and had talked only about the part of the trouble with Betty that was making her so angry.

It turned out that Betty had withheld all information about the presence of the little girl in their home and about the assault because she feared getting Anna into further trouble with the law and that Dr. Jones (who was black) had gone along because he thought that the emergency therapist's agency could not understand the problems of minority group patients. Betty had told Dr. Jones all the facts, and it was he who had suggested she bring Anna to the emergency room for admission.

If she had gathered expectations about hospitalization from all the participants before she jumped to a solution (referral to Dr. Gregg) based on her preliminary formulation of the case, the therapist could have spared herself embarrassment and avoided the danger of an inadequate crisis resolution. However, her ultimate willingness to listen to the participants saved the day.

Anna was hospitalized, and the emergency therapist called Dr. Jones to inform him. Dr. Jones said that he would have Dr. Gregg visit Anna in the hospital and take over the case when she was ready for discharge. He had not appreciated the depth of Betty's jealousy over him. He even thanked the emergency therapist for calling this fact to his attention. It helped him to understand some angry silences in his recent hours with Betty.

SEVERAL ASPECTS OF CRISIS INTERVENTION

Theories of the Nature of Crisis

A full replaying of the literature on crisis and crisis intervention will not be attempted here. Excellent reviews and reformulations of the current views are provided by Rapoport,[6] Darbonne,[7] Bartolucci and Drayer,[8] and Hirschowitz.[9] Crisis has been seen and studied as the change in an *individual undergoing transition,* as the cumulative toll of major *life-change events,* and as the signal of *strain in a social system.* Strategies of intervention follow naturally from the aspect of crisis that is emphasized, but a complete approach must deal with the individual, the event, and the social system. Some theoretical comments about each of these aspects will be offered as a guide to the overlapping viewpoints in this expanding field.

In the *individual undergoing transition,* crisis is often viewed as disequilibrium, an "upset in a steady state"[10] of the reacting individual who finds himself in a hazardous situation. Lydia Rapoport[6] has written that there are three sets of interrelated factors which can produce a state of crisis: (1) a hazardous event that poses some threat; (2) a threat (to an instinctual need) which is symbolically linked to earlier threats that have resulted in vulnerability to conflict; and (3) an inability to respond with adequate coping mechanisms. Generally the term *crisis* is preferred to the older term *stress* because it offers the idea of a positive turning point rather than the image of a burden or load under which a person either survives or breaks.

The *crisis state* has been carefully studied in light of Erich Lindemann's classic observations of the *acute grief reaction* following the 1943 Coconut Grove nightclub fire, which left many Boston families suddenly and unexpectedly bereaved.

Lindemann[11] identified five points which establish the diagnosis of grief:

1. Somatic distress, including sighing respiration, lack of strength and exhaustion, and loss of appetite and digestive function

2. A sense of unreality about everyday surroundings coupled with a preoccupation with the image of the deceased, which may lead to copying the appearance or behavior of the deceased

3. Guilt

4. Hostile reactions

5. Loss of patterns of conduct

He went on to discuss the *grief work*, which he defined as "emancipation from the bondage to the deceased, readjustment to the environment in which the deceased is missing, and the formation of new relationships." He showed how the therapist could play a constructive role in helping the patient overcome the major resistance to this grief work, the tendency "to avoid both the intense distress connected with the grief experience and the necessary expression of emotion."

If grief work were not accomplished, the following manifestations of an *inadequate grief* were noted:

1. Overactivity without a sense of purpose or loss

2. The acquisition of symptoms belonging to the last illness of the deceased

3. A recognized medical disease such as ulcerative colitis, rheumatoid arthritis, or asthma

4. Alteration of relationships with friends and relatives

5. Furious hostility against specific persons

6. Absence of emotional display, to a schizoid level

7. Lasting loss of patterns of social interaction

8. Unwise social, business, and professional decisions

9. Agitated depression

Lindemann's conclusion was that "sharing the patient's grief work" at the time of normal bereavement could completely prevent the appearance of such late, highly damaging "distorted reactions."

This classic study became the paradigm of much later work in crisis intervention; even the time period for working through normal grief (four to six weeks) became the standard for brief, crisis-oriented psychotherapy. Much literature on the crisis state betrays the origins in the grief state. For example, Caplan[12] defines crisis as

> . . . a state provoked when a person faces an obstacle to important life goals that is, for a time, insurmountable through the utilization of customary methods of problem-solving. A period of disorganization ensues, a period of upset, during which many abortive attempts at solution are made. Eventually some kind of adaptation is achieved which may or may not be in the best interest of that person and his fellows.

Others have tried to define the *phases* of the period of upset that constitutes the state of crisis. Tyhurst[13] identified the period of impact, period of recoil, and the posttraumatic period. Bowlby[14] noted three distinct phases of the separation trauma of a young child entering the hospital: protest, despair, and denial. Kubler-Ross[15] notes that the usual response to news of a fatal illness is a sequence of personality states: shock, denial, anger, bargaining, depression, and acceptance.

Based on these and other important studies, Hirschowitz[16] has provided a useful "crisis sequence." He sees the crisis as proceeding through the phases of impact (lasting hours), recoil-turmoil (lasting days), adjustment (lasting weeks), and reconstruction (lasting months). Each phase is characterized by its own time perspective, emotions, thoughts, goal orientation, and behavior.

Thus far the crisis states we have described have been precipitated by life "hazards," which Caplan[17] points out involve a sudden *loss,* a *threat* of loss, or a *challenge* to new adaptation. Erikson[18] calls these crises "accidental crises," and he distinguishes them from his well-known "developmental crises," which are periods of disorganization marking the transition from one developmental phase in the life cycle to another.

Crisis as an opportunity has been stressed by Tyhurst[19] and Rapoport,[20] and Dabrowski[21] has postulated a developmental instinct that operates by means of a "positive disintegration" of existing personality structures. Crisis thus becomes a normal and to-be-expected transition state at nodal points in development.

Certainly crisis can serve as a catalyst to growth by disturbing old habits and evoking new responses.[22] But against the idea of crisis as a "call to new action,"[6] we have to recall that it can also be a major chance for failure, a "mess," or just another turn of a "maladaptive cycle." Part of the confusion lies in the use of the word "crisis."

Bartolucci and Drayer[23] have observed:

> The use of the term "crisis" to mean periods of acute emotional distress is now well established in the literature. "Crisis" is defined in the Oxford English Dictionary, however, as a "vitally important or decisive stage in the progress of anything, a turning point." Erikson's[24] use of the word in his discussion of developmental phases is therefore correct. On the other hand, the word "predicament" is defined as "a state of being, condition, situation, position, especially an unpleasant, trying, or dangerous situation." It may be presumed that a person going through the stresses of a developmental crisis may be more predicament-prone than at other times. However, initial intervention, as in an emergency room, is obviously aimed more at the presenting predicament than at the possible developmental crisis in the background.

The idea of predicament helps to avoid some of the overtones of an intense, cataclysmic disaster, which seems to be the connotation of the term crisis. The emergency therapist may be called upon to offer *routine service* and to spot *pseudocrises* as part of his emergency duty. He should recognize these predicaments as a valid part of his emergency room caseload.

Routine service for all medical complaints is now sought at all emergency rooms by patients who cannot leave their work or children to come at routine hours. Their predicament is the problem of entry into the health care system. They know they must be seen if they come to the emergency room and choose this way of calling attention to their needs. Persons ambivalent about applying for psychiatric help are notorious in adopting this method of seeking help, and the emergency therapist's primary responsibility is to help the patient clarify his own need and to accept referral to the regular clinic. The emergency therapist should not demand that his patient be "in crisis" before he offers this simple and helpful service.

Alternatively, some people can ask for help only by manufacturing a crisis. Often the style of an entire family may be histrionic; they will appear together in a pseudocrisis that is easily resolved. One of the tasks of crisis intervention is to help such individuals develop a repertoire of less dramatic, more effective ways of communicating their distress.

The life events that lead to crisis have been studied by Holmes and Rahe,[25] who have adopted the interesting approach of establishing a mean value for the stress potential of each of these events. As the score of mean values mounts, the likelihood of crisis increases. When the score is higher than 300,[26] a major depression or physical illness is likely within a year. An adaptation of their scale is presented in Table 1-1.

Crisis as a response to life events leads naturally to the idea that crisis strikes not just a single individual, but a unit of interacting individuals. The unit most studied, of course, is the family, and Parad and Caplan[27] have offered the concept of "family lifestyle" to describe the repertoire of solutions that are available to a family unit in crisis. The crisis intervention must work within the family style if it is to succeed.

Table 1 - 1 Social Readjustment Rating Scale

Rank	Life Event	Mean Value
1	Death of spouse	100
2	Divorce	73
3	Marital separation	65
4	Jail term	63
5	Death of close family member	63
6	Personal injury or illness	53
7	Marriage	50
8	Fired at work	47
9	Marital reconciliation	45
10	Retirement	45
11	Change in health of family member	44
12	Pregnancy	40
13	Sex difficulties	39
14	Gain of new family member	39
15	Business readjustment	39
16	Change in financial state	38
17	Death of close friend	37
18	Change to different line of work	36
19	Change in number of arguments with spouse	35
20	Mortgage over $10,000	31
21	Foreclosure of mortgage or loan	30
22	Change in responsibilities at work	29
23	Son or daughter leaving home	29
24	Trouble with in-laws	29
25	Outstanding personal achievement	28
26	Wife begins or stops work	26
27	Begin or end school	26
28	Change in living conditions	25
29	Revision of personal habits	24
30	Trouble with boss	23
31	Change in work hours or conditions	20
32	Change in residence	20
33	Change in schools	20
34	Change in recreation	19
35	Change in church activities	19
36	Change in social activities	18
37	Mortgage or loan less than $10,000	17
38	Change in sleeping habits	16
39	Change in number of family get-togethers	15
40	Change in eating habits	15
41	Vacation	13
42	Christmas	12
43	Minor violations of the law	11

Recently, Gregory Bateson[28] has argued that all mental life is really an ecological event, the individual's way of experiencing the circuit of interdependence he shares with his environment and other individuals in it. The experience in the mind of the single individual is always, he argues, "news of a difference" traveling through an entire ecological circuit, and the difference is in the circuit, not the individual. Seen this way, the individual in crisis is carrying news of a difference in an ecological system, and logically we should look for signs of strain not only in the single individual who comes in upset, but also throughout his social system. Bateson's ecological view helps to explain some otherwise puzzling crisis phenomena, such as related crises occurring at nearly the same time in the lives of persons who live or work within the same social system.

An elegant study by Yoshiko Ikeda[29] describes a wave of emotional disturbance in a leprosarium in Japan during the spring of 1960, when eleven nurses required psychiatric hospitalization and many other staff members and patients were upset. Much of the turmoil seemed to be a reaction to a new general head nurse who was insensitive in her attempts to bring more modern nursing values to a traditional setting, but the tensions between the old and new ways within the leprosarium also reflected tensions in the larger Japanese culture of that time. Indeed, the staff situation became for a time a national political scandal.

In the smaller unit of the family, a single member's heart attack may coincide with developments in the lives of other members, for instance, elopement, unwanted pregnancy, unemployment, and so on. Most families can recall "one hard year" in which everything seemed to go wrong. Occasionally an emotionally sensitive family member may *anticipate* a period of family crisis with a personal crisis of his own. Acute schizophrenia may appear in a sensitive adolescent who senses the incipient fragmentation of his parents' marriage even before they have faced their incompatibility.

Warren Miller[30] has advanced a theoretical bridge useful to the understanding of such data:

> It is important to consider the patient and the social environment playing a role together in making a psychiatric emergency. In order to facilitate this point of view, I have introduced a concept called the *ecological group,* which refers to the patient and those people in the social environment with whom he has major dynamic relationships. It may include people in the family environment, the work environment, or the medical environment. In short, it cuts across various social systems to include all those people who currently provide sources of gratification and control for the patient and for whom he does the same.

We can now take Bateson's philosophic view and Miller's clinical concept to advance a final statement on the nature of crisis. *Crisis is news of a difference affecting the pattern of relationships within an ecological group.* Thus a single individual's anxiety will be mirrored in physical distress, marital discord, vocational disruption, or social dislocation in the lives of other individuals in the ecological group. The wise therapist will look for signs of strain in other members of the group, as did Anna's when she found strain in Betty, Betty's therapist, and herself before the crisis resolution was completed.

Crisis Intervention as Consultation

In essence, the emergency therapist serves as a consultant to a system in crisis; he must therefore be familiar with the theory of psychiatric consultation, as described in Chapter 31 ("Psychiatric Consultation in the General Hospital"). In practice, certain role obligations fall upon the psychiatric consultant, whether he functions in the emergency room, on the medical ward, or in a community mental health agency.

The Consultant Defines His Role. It is incumbent upon the emergency therapist to identify himself. He must know in his own mind and make clear to the persons he treats whose agent he is. If he is working in a county emergency room, he is the agent of that county, and his primary duty is to promote the mental health and safety of the citizens of that particular county. If he is working in a private capacity, he defines himself as a consultant to the *situation* rather than as the personal advocate of any of the *participants.*

As a consultant, the emergency therapist listens for a *theme* in the information during his work-up of a crisis situation. The feelings of other professionals—police officers, hospital staffs, and secretaries—bear the imprint of the emotion generated by the crisis itself. If he takes these feelings into account, he will gain valuable insight into the specific character of the crisis. A crisis often has a kind of theme that can be recognized only if each new piece of information is viewed as an emotional communication.

In Anna's and Betty's crisis, the theme was competition. Only when the therapist could resist the temptation to compete with Dr. Jones for control of the case could she break through the competitive atmosphere that had grown up between Betty and Anna. This change from competition to cooperation allowed new information about Anna's competition with her mother-in-law over control of the children to emerge, permitting a real resolution to the crisis.

If the beginner can learn to adopt a *consultative set,* he will be able to deal effectively with many of the contingencies that arise. In the example, the emergency therapist decided, as part of the solution, to phone the regular therapist. This is a recommended procedure when a patient is already in therapy. Such a call is more than a courtesy or means to a quick "disposition"; it is part of the intervention.

In this call the outside therapist must be listened to consultatively. It is easy to make one of two false assumptions: that the outside therapist is more competent, or that because he works for a different agency he is suspect. It is better to regard the outside professional as a participant who is intimately involved in the crisis. His identity and role in the development of the crisis and his own experience of the tension must be listened to and evaluated just as the other participants are. He has a unique contribution to make and is a potential strength in resolving the crisis. And he is a member of the ecological group, not a consultant to it.

If the outside therapist sounds angry or rejecting, it is better to listen consultatively than moralistically, to keep from competing with him. The competitive consultant wins a Pyrrhic victory in which he establishes the other professional's lesser competence only to find that that person is now unwilling to cooperate in any plan to help the patient.

Knowing Disposition Resources

The emergency therapist should know what options are available *before* he discusses them with the patient. It is fruitless to discuss brief hospitalization with a patient when the nearest psychiatric facility is a distant state hospital with a reputation for stays of three to six months. Therefore the therapist will have to give himself time away from the patient to think and to check. For the therapist who is unfamiliar with community resources, telephone consultation with a knowledgeable mental health professional can prove invaluable. (A psychiatric social worker is often helpful.) Indeed, it is wise for someone starting a tour of emergency room duty to review and have with him a list of the local resources before he sees his first patient. When the list proves inadequate to handle a given situation, a phone call will often

reveal additional resources. Such calls or consultations should be made with the patient *out* of the room, leaving the therapist free to discuss various options. (Once the referral *decision* is made, the therapist may wish to contact the referral sources with the patient *in* the room so the patient can hear how and why he is being referred and have a sense of what the next person to treat him expects.)

The emergency therapist should be able to effect recommendations to patients *immediately*. For instance, if Anna needs hospitalization, the therapist should already have ascertained that a bed is available and that Anna or a social agency can pay for it. He should not suggest the improbable or impossible, only to then have to betray the patient's expectations. A suicide attempt may occur when a therapist suggests hospitalization and then cannot arrange a bed, vacillates and reverses himself, schedules an outpatient appointment, and sends the patient home more frightened than before.

A good principle for the disposition phase is *never leave the patient in midair.* When you refer him, make sure he knows where he is going, when, and why. Be sure he knows how to contact you if the initial plan proves unworkable.

The use of the telephone has become such an important part of contemporary psychiatry that we have devoted a separate chapter to it (Chapter 24). It is good to become as flexible as possible in using the telephone so that absent members of an interacting social system can talk with each other. Frequently the therapist finds himself handing the phone to the patient so he can talk with another therapist or with a family member who is not present but who has potential to resolve the situation.

Phoning can be a helpful way to make referrals, particularly with patients who are marginally motivated or fearful of rejection. When treating an alcoholic patient, some therapists make it a rule to call the referral resource in his presence, describe his problem to the resource person, and hand the phone to the patient for him to make the rest of the arrangements. With considerate referral, the percentage of alcoholic patients following through will be extremely high, as Chafetz, Blane, and Hill[31] have shown.

Strategies of Crisis Intervention

In crisis intervention, as in many other areas of psychiatry, process is as important as content in conveying implicit messages to the participants. The act of bringing the participants in a crisis together in the same room (or by phone) implies that they can interact to create a successful solution. In his official role as a representative of psychiatry, the emergency therapist refuses to condemn people for having created a system that failed but instead gives them permission to try again to find a common, acceptable solution.

In each case the consulting therapist should do everything possible to help the system find its own solution. It is all right to use therapy or hospitalization to aid the system in finding its own solution, but it is unfortunate when members of the system come to believe that the initiative is no longer theirs and that only their passive compliance with medical orders can make the difference. Medical paternalism quickly extinguishes many of the healthy coping strategies that even marginal patients and families can bring into operation.

The *extended emergency contact*[32] allows the system to find a solution over a period of several days or weeks if one cannot be formulated the first evening. Knowing that there is an interested person who, by acting as a consultant to the ecological group, is assisting it in finding its own solution can be the necessary catalyst. If the system is unable to find a solution, the emergency therapist can offer the alternative of hospitalization at any time.

In general it is more effective to appeal to the strengths of people rather than to underscore their weaknesses. Even when hospitalization is used, the interacting members of the ecological group should be encouraged to stay involved; the ulti-mate burden of finding a solution remains with them. If the hospitalization is effected in the proper manner (see Chapter 10, "Acute Inpatient Intervention"), *discharge planning* begins the minute the patient enters the hospital.

The emergency therapist has several *important prerogatives* in dramatic situations and can exploit the element of drama in a therapeutic way. Because he is working in an emergency context, he has a right to call anyone, however far away, and make unusual demands, such as that the person participate in family interviews or communicate with others in the ecological group. No one is going to blame the emergency therapist for doing everything he can do to respond to the emergency.

Exploiting the drama that has been used by patients to make the situation seem more drastic than it is is an effective means of encouraging the members of the ecological group to interact in a healthier manner. At a time of crisis, long-standing defenses can be dropped because the situation is exceptional. At such a time individuals can communicate openly, cry in each other's presence, make admissions of a personal nature that in another context would be too damaging, and not suffer unduly.

The reason for these changes is that everything occurs under the aegis of "the emergency"; to some extent the emergency therapist can bear the onus for what is revealed. Such revelations, he implies, are part of resolving this particular crisis; they do not mean that from now on life will be a series of endless confessions. Nevertheless, steps taken now by the therapist and by the system that he is influencing may have a long-lasting effect.

Often intervention is best done *near the original setting* of the crisis by a team of mental health professionals who can share the tasks of working with the participants. Often the team is based in a regional mental health center.[33] The "social network intervention" of Speck and Attneave[34] extends further into the community to visit the homes of families in crisis and is capable of assembling as many as forty friends and neighbors for a *network meeting* to help in the emergency. (Some other ways of organizing emergency work are discussed in Chapter 11.)

Patients often remember emergencies with respect. If it is properly handled, the emergency can provide a new model to an ecological group, one in which problem solving becomes more important than winning or losing hateful confrontations.

REFERENCES

1. Jung, C. G.: "On The Nature of Dreams," in *The Structure and Dynamics of the Psyche, Collected Works,* Pantheon, New York, 1960, vol. 8, pp. 294–295.

2. Sullivan, Harry Stack: *The Interpersonal Theory of Psychiatry,* Norton, New York, 1953, pp. 151–152.

3. Freud, Sigmund: *New Introductory Lectures in Psychoanalysis,* Norton, New York, 1933, p. 112.

4. Rogers, Carl: *Client-Centered Therapy,* Houghton Mifflin, Boston, 1951.

5. Perry, John W.: Personal communication, 1970.

6. Rapoport, Lydia: "The State of Crisis: Some Theoretical Considerations," in Howard J. Parad (ed.), *Crisis Intervention,* Family Service Association, New York, 1965, chap. 2.

7. Darbonne, Allen R.: "Crisis: A Review of Theory, Practice and Research," *Psychotherapy: Theory, Research and Practice,* **4**(2): 49–56 (1967).

8. Bartolucci, Giampiero, and Calvin S. Drayer: "An Overview of Crisis Intervention in the Emergency Rooms of General Hospitals," *Am. J. Psychiat.,* **130**(9):953–959, September 1973. Copyright 1973, The American Psychiatric Association.

9. Hirschowitz, Ralph G.: "Crisis Theory: A Formulation," *Psychiat. Ann.,* **3**(12):33–47, 1973.

10. Lindemann, Erich, and Gerald Caplan: "A Conceptual Framework for Preventive Psychiatry," unpublished paper cited in Rapoport, loc. cit.

11. Lindemann, Erich: "Symptomatology and Management of Acute Grief," *Am. J. Psychiat.,* **101**:141–148, September 1944.

12. Caplan, Gerald: *An Approach To Community Mental Health,* Grune & Stratton, New York, 1961, p. 18. By permission.

13. Tyhurst, James C.: "The Role of Transition States–Including Disasters–in Mental Illness," *Symposium on Preventive and Social Psychiatry,* Walter Reed Army Institute of Research, Washington, D.C., 1970, p. 150.

14. Bowlby, John: "Separation Anxiety," *Internat. J. Psychoanal.,* **41**:89–113, 1960.

15. Kubler-Ross, Ellsbeth: *On Death and Dying,* Macmillan, New York, 1969.

16. Hirschowitz: op. cit., p. 38.

17. Caplan, Gerald: *Principles of Preventive Psychiatry,* Basic Books, New York, 1964, p. 35.

18. Erikson, Erik H. *Childhood and Society,* Norton, New York, 1963.

19. Tyhurst: loc cit.

20. Rapoport: loc. cit.

21. Dabrowski, Kazimierz: *Positive Disintegration,* Little, Brown, Boston, 1964.

22. Thomas, W. I.: *Social Behavior and Personality Contributions of W. I. Thomas to Theory and Social Research,* E. Volk (ed.), Social Science Research Council, New York, 1951, pp. 12–14, cited in Rapoport, loc. cit.

23. Bartolucci and Drayer: op. cit., p. 954.

24. Erikson, Erik H.: "Growth and Crises of the Healthy Personality," *Psychol. Issues,* **1**:1–171, 1959.

25. Holmes, Thomas H., and Richard H. Rahe: "The Social Readjustment Rating Scale," *J. Psychosom. Res.,* **11**:213–218, 1967.

26. Holmes, Thomas H., and Minoru Masuda: "Life Change and Illness Susceptibility," in John P. Scott and Edward C. Senay (eds.), *Separation and Depression,* American Asso-

ciation for the Advancement of Science, Washington, D.C., 1973, pp. 161–186.

27. Parad, Howard J., and Gerald Caplan: "A Framework for Studying Families in Crisis," in Howard J. Parad (ed.), *Crisis Intervention*, Family Service Association, New York, 1965, chap. 4, pp. 53–74.

28. Bateson, Gregory: *Steps to an Ecology of Mind*, Ballantine Books, Inc., New York, 1973, p. 454.

29. Ikeda, Yoshiko: "An Epidemic of Emotional Disturbance among Leprosarium Nurses in a Setting of Low Morale and Social Change," *Psychiatry*, 29:152–164, May 1966.

30. Miller, Warren: "A Psychiatric Emergency Service and Some Treatment Concepts," *Am. J. Psychiat.*, 124:924–933, 1968. Copyright 1968, the American Psychiatric Association.

31. Chafetz, Morris, Howard T. Blane, and Marjorie J. Hill: "Engaging the Alcoholic to Enter into Treatment," *Frontiers of Alcoholism*, Science House, New York, 1970, chap. 2.

32. Miller: op. cit., p. 931.

33. Lieb, Julian, Ian Lipsitch, and Andrew Slaby: *The Crisis Team: A Handbook for the Mental Health Professional*, Harper & Row, New York, 1973.

34. Speck, Ross V., and Carolyn L. Attneave: "Social Network Intervention," in Clifford L. Sager and Helen S. Kaplan (eds.), *Progress in Group and Family Therapy*, Brunner/Mazel, New York, 1973, pp. 312–332.

Evaluation of the Suicidal Patient

... The sociologists and clinical psychiatrists, in particular, have been peculiarly unstoppable. Yet it is possible—in fact, easy—to plow through any of their innumerable books and articles without once realizing that they deal with that shabby, confused, agonized crisis which is the common reality of suicide.

A. Alvarez, THE SAVAGE GOD[1]

EVALUATION

Evaluation is emphasized because it is critical to all psychiatric work. Evaluation implies judgment, and judgment implies *feeling*, a function of consciousness,[2] without which the gathering and logical ordering of factual data remain as preliminary as catgut knots tied in orange skins by surgeons studying to do a procedure. Psychotherapists must be in touch with their own and their patients' feelings if they are to make reasoned judgments. And they *do* make judgments (feeling-decisions) constantly, despite stereotypes to the contrary; what they strive to avoid making are stupid, impulsive, or moralistic judgments.

Evaluation is especially important in working with suicidal patients because the wish to kill one's self is almost always the end state of feeling-confusion, of being in the *closed world*[1] of ambivalence about whether to live one's own feelings or the internalized feelings of others. Suicide may not represent a clear-cut decision to die, but rather the end of a tortured inability to find one's own life to live. If he is to be helped at all, the suicidal person must find someone who can guide him in the process of evaluating his own life.

The current literature on "suicidology" (as this mechanical name implies) often deals in statistics and sociology. Facts and theories are important in understanding suicidal crises in general but neglect the emotional impasse of the individual patient. Exceptional books by Hillman[3] and Alvarez deal directly with suicidal emotion. This chapter too will present some statistics and sociology to be used as a background against which feeling-understanding can be brought to individual situations.

This chapter does *not* assume that under all circumstances suicide is to be prevented, although prevention is an obvious and usual medical goal. To postulate a dogma of prevention is to deny the individual nature of evaluation. We do not wish to bypass the slow, even painful, feeling-decisions. What suicide must be prevented by involuntary hospitalization? What choice rests with the patient? What suicide is justified? Resolving these questions takes time, for feeling as a process is slower than thinking; the impression develops rather like a photographic negative, by saturation.

There is no substitute. The argument against an

automatic policy of prevention belongs not so much to civil liberties as to therapy itself. Unless the emergency therapist has worked faithfully to evaluate the patient, he cannot counsel survival convincingly. He will be just another stranger telling the patient how to feel. If he has come honestly by a feeling-judgment that alternatives to suicide exist, his patient will surely hear him. If he knows no more than he wants to work with the patient and share the pain of the ongoing feeling-struggle, the care exercised in evaluation will rarely have been in vain. Usually the patient's closed world will have opened.

THE SCIENTIFIC STUDY OF SUICIDE

Introduction

Suicidal behavior has received enormous scrutiny during this century. A unique summary of the literature available in English up to 1970 is provided by Lester.[4] This is a definitive presentation of research findings and major theoretical perspectives, and it is well worth the careful study of workers in the field. Available books on suicide that introduce the emergency therapist to current suicidology are Farberow and Shneidman's[5] *The Cry for Help* and Stengel's[6] *Suicide and Attempted Suicide.* The following section provides a summary of this broad field.

Theories of Suicide

Many theories have been advanced to explain suicide, but four major types of theory are noteworthy[4]: (1) suicide seen as a disturbance in the individual's relation to society (Durkheim)[7]; (2) suicide seen as an expression of the individual's struggle with aggressive impulses (Freud)[8]; (3) suicide seen as the attempt to manipulate others in the environment (Adler)[9]; and (4) suicide seen as concretizing the symbolic process of death and rebirth (Hillman).[10]

Suicide as a Sociological Disruption. Durkheim postulated two characteristics of the societal group, each of which has a role in determining the suicidal behavior of its members. These were the degree of *integration* of the societal group, and the degree of *social regulation* it imposed upon its members.

Integration of the society means that its members possess shared beliefs and sentiments, interest in one another, and a sense of devotion to common goals. If integration is high, *altruistic suicide* is common, as for example by kamikaze pilots loyal to the Japanese Emperor in World War II. If integration is low, *egoistic suicide* is common, as for example in modern Hungary, where a Durkheimian explains the high rate by the lack of political ties that allows excessive individualism to develop.

Social regulation is the control exercised over members. Where social regulation is high, *fatalistic suicide* is common, as was the case on many slave ships. Where social regulation is low, *anomic suicide* is common, as President Eisenhower mistakenly assumed was the case in Sweden, where he felt social welfare made life too easy for its inhabitants.

Suicide as a Struggle with Aggression.[4] Litman[11] in reviewing Freud's writing on suicide, has shown that by 1910:

> Freud had recognized many clinical features of suicidal behavior: guilt over death wishes toward others, identification with a suicidal parent, refusal to accept loss of libidinal gratification, suicide as an act of revenge, escape from humiliation, or as a communication, and the connection between death and sexuality.

In *Mourning and Melancholia*, Freud[8] cited his first theory of suicide. He argued that suicide was the outcome of the ego's struggle to deal with loss. When an ambivalently loved object is lost, the energy that has been bound up in the loved one is relocated in the ego; the *identification* with the lost loved one is equally ambivalently perceived, and mourning takes a pathological turn and becomes melancholia because the hostile feelings once directed toward the loved one are now being turned against a part of the self. Ambivalence is particularly likely to occur after a death because a primitive anger at being abandoned collides with guilt that attends the expression of negative feelings toward the loved one. This guilt is sustained by tradition: "Speak no ill of the dead." Litman notes that *ego splitting* is an inevitable consequence of loss, even if there is no ambivalence, because room must be made in the ego to restore the lost object. Thus a complexity of emotion comes to be directed toward a part of the ego, and an intense inner dialogue may be set in motion by loss: now love, now hate, now *ambivalence*, the conscious pain of feeling-confusion. Such dialogue contributes to the pathological introspectiveness, the exhaustion, and the paralysis of melancholic individuals who often cannot stop it. Sylvia Plath's[12] poem "Daddy" is a vivid example of this internal dialogue that splits and exhausts the ego. Plath's father died when she was 9, and she spent years preoccupied with him and his fate. Her poem, addressed to him, shows her intense desire to be "finally through" with him and his introject, "the vampire who said he was you."

Suicidal people often struggle with an intense preoccupation with dead parents. Presumably this is based on inadequate grief, following the Lindemann observations in Chapter 1. If grief work is not accomplished, as in a dazed, denying family, *perseveration* of aspects of grief goes on. One of these aspects of normal grief is desire for reunion with a lost loved one, and it feels to the patient whose grief was blocked as if the loved one is somehow forever pulling him into death, where they can be together. This obsessive idea feels morbid and annoying to the suicidal person, who is kept back from progress in his own life, but until he has accomplished the grief work, death

absolutely will not go away, and the patient is locked in ambivalent combat with the emotional claims the dead person has on him.

In *Beyond the Pleasure Principle*, Freud[13] explored his later idea of a primary drive toward death. This theme was too metaphysical for most of Freud's followers, but it was adopted by Melanie Klein and Karl Menninger, who view it as a primary aggressive drive, the source of aggressive energy. Their observations relate suicide to *ambivalence* and *variations* in the directing of this aggressive energy, the death-dealing part of the personality.

Melanie Klein relates the development of ambivalence to the internalization of the death instinct, or aggressive drive. Klein[14] feels this instinct is originally identified in projection onto the mother whose "bad breast" is felt to be the cause of the child's hunger and pain. The baby feels at one with the "good breast," which is responsible for his feelings of satisfaction and relief. The bad breast is outside him, split off and dreaded: this is the paranoid-schizoid position of earliest infancy, with its intense *persecutory anxiety*. Only at a later stage does the infant learn that "when he loves and hates his mother, it is one and the same person whom he desires and attacks."[15] Then he has to weigh his pain when hungry against her pain when attacked, and the conflict of ambivalence starts. Ambivalence is the core of the infantile depressive position. Furthermore, the infant's belief in the power of his destructive impulses is greater than his belief in the power of his loving impulses, and he suffers intense fear that his negative feelings will destroy his mother or her love for him. This is *depressive anxiety*. Only gradually is it outgrown, and only if the mother establishes that the infant's negative feelings do not in reality destroy her.

Hendin[16] has applied psychoanalytic findings in his study of the effects of different national styles of child-rearing on the way adult suicidal patterns appear in three Scandinavian countries. In Denmark, a long period of dependency is encouraged, and aggression against the parents is severely checked to ensure "proper" dependency gratification. The child is disciplined by arousing his guilt. Suicide rates are high. In men, suicide follows the loss of a mother or wife; in women it follows the birth of the children, thus reflecting the frustration of their own dependency needs. The depressive pattern is a classic retarded involutional depression with ambivalence and guilt over repressed hostility.

In Sweden, separation from the mother comes early. Direct expression of both anger and dependency is discouraged, and the major anxiety is intense self-blame over performance failure. The resultant depression is anxious and agitated, connected with shame and a striving to improve a failing performance. The suicide rate is high. Men kill themselves in the grip of self-hatred over job failures, women from a sense of failure in their heterosexual relationships.

In Norway, both aggression and dependency are encouraged by a mother who centers her emotional life on her child. Neither guilt nor shame are invoked in child-rearing. Rather, the culture instills fear of envy rather than fear of failure, and a national style of injustice collecting and nursing grudges develops because blame for failure is projected onto others. The suicide rate is low.

It would seem that depression and suicide are least likely to occur if the mother is able to *accept* the projection onto her of the withholding bad breast and most likely if the mother has to present herself as *only giving*, thus forcing her child to experience his aggression as a threat to his dependent needs. The implications are obvious for a country like the United States, where the "positive mother" is glorified in holidays such as Mother's Day, and the "negative mother" is not admitted to exist.

The death instinct has been most specifically explored by Karl Menninger[17] in *Man against Himself.* In all suicidal motivation, Menninger discovers three strands: a wish to kill, a wish to be killed, and a wish to die. Each relates to the use of the aggressive drive.

A practical application of these dynamics is made in referral decisions. Successful psychotherapy of suicidal patients usually involves a strong recapitulation of attitudes toward the original mothering figure and of the wish to kill, the wish to be killed, and the wish to die. It is a good idea to establish early in evaluation the nature and strength of these attitudes and drives to determine whether treatment is best conducted in a private practice setting, where dependency, anger, and guilt are likely to be more focused and intense (because there is only one mothering figure), or in a clinic setting, where the institution shares some of the mothering function and receives some of the anger and blame. Often the "Swedes" (patients with anxiety about performance failure) do better in private settings, and the "Danes" (patients with guilt over hostile dependency) do better in clinic settings. Very hostile patients do best in clinic settings.

Suicide as the Attempt to Manipulate Others. One motive of many suicidal fantasies and acts is the suicidal individual's knowledge that he can attain from or do to others in suicide what he cannot easily attain or do in life. The suicidal patient may assume that his death attempts will attract the desired attention and devotion; provide a real or symbolic reunion with loved ones; cause anguish, grief, and guilt in those who have "let him down," overburdened him, or treated him unjustly.[18] Or as Adler[9] argued, death may be perceived as finally establishing a validation of his worthlessness and proof that he is not worth caring about. (For patients with long-standing inferiority feelings, with rage and envy at "healthy" others, suicide is the ultimate vengeful victory of the *inferiority complex.*)

These complex and often contradictory emotions may result in a paradox: although the suicide attempter may wish to establish that he cannot be loved, the successful suicide often acts as if he will be around to receive the love and attention which will come to him posthumously.[19] The paradox obtrudes into both evaluation and treatment.

When the manipulative intent is transparently obvious to the harrassed therapist or internist (although it may not be obvious to the patient), there is a strong temptation to speak disparagingly of a "suicide gesture" and dismiss the patient as a "hysteric" who should, in effect, go home, grow up, and learn how to express conflict in a more mature manner. What may not be obvious in such an incident is the intensity of feeling which precipitated the "gesture" and the realization that at least in this stage of the patient's life a gesture may be the closest he can come to expressing how he feels.

Indeed, the patient may present his "childish" behavior in such a way (or at such a time, 4 A.M. being one of the favorites) that he elicits punishment for it. If the therapist is led into becoming an angry parent figure, the patient has succeeded in bringing a child he cannot control to a father who will give him a scolding. Occasionally such scoldings help. More often they succeed only in further alienating the patient from his own infantile parts that, like a real infant's, find it necessary to act up still more to regain attention. When the therapist takes the infantile signal for attention seriously, he interrupts this vicious cycle and allows the "infant" in the patient to enter treatment along with the bewildered adult.

This split between more and less mature portions of the personality is found frequently in suicidal people, who are notorious for neglecting their dependent needs because they are ashamed of them. When they begin to overcome their antipathy to the less mature parts of themselves, they can be taught to take care of their own dependent needs, and the need to manipulate others into doing so lessens. This is sometimes spoken as *learning to take care of the child within* and is a critical step in the psychotherapy of hysterical patients.

Suicide in the Evolution of Identity. There are certain life crises of identification in which people find themselves hopelessly locked into a lifestyle which is no longer successful; yet they do not know how to aid themselves in their evolution to the next phase of life. It is as if both personal and cultural rites of passage or initiation were not available to them. The person perceives suicide as the only means of shedding an outworn identity state, as a snake must shed its skin, for the new self to emerge magically after death.[20]

One common complex of this sort found in gifted young adults is called by Jungians the *puer aeternus*, a particularly "inflated" offshoot of the familiar Wunderkind.[21] *Puer aeternus* means eternal boy and is exemplified by the myth of Icarus, who flew too close to the sun on wax wings built by his father, and plunged to his death in the sea. Many young people who show promise are extravagantly praised for being gifted. Influenced by an older generation's aspirations for them, they are reluctant to become adults by confronting the issue of how to develop their gifts and idealism into realistic productivity.[22] Some resolve the dilemma by becoming dilettanti, others by becoming perpetual graduate students who style themselves Renaissance men. A few refuse any compromise (as did Zelda Fitzgerald) and find that their inability to relinquish the godlike prerogatives of eternal youth leads to a psychiatric crisis of catastrophic proportions.[23]

A more common resolution of "puer inflation" is a suicidal crisis. Alvarez[24] describes his own unsuccessful suicide attempt at age 31, in the midst of great precocious success as a critic, in terms which suggest it was a death-of-the-puer experience.

Active suicidal fantasies develop in this extreme form, often without relation to major setbacks in the outer world; it feels to the patient like an attack from within. If this *death experience*[25] is allowed to occur symbolically, a giving up of the puer adaptation and a maturing of the personality often ensues. If the death experience is blocked by well-meaning friends and therapists who attempt to help the young person retain his airy imperviousness to life, it may assert itself in a suicide attempt. Alvarez describes his own experience as follows:[24]

The truth is, in some way I *had* died. The overintensity, the tiresome excess of sensitivity and self-consciousness, of arrogance and idealism, which came in adolescence and stayed on and on beyond their due time, like some visiting bore, had not survived the coma. It was as though I had finally, and sadly late in the day, lost my innocence.

... Certainly, nothing has been quite the same since I discovered for myself, in my own body and on my own nerves, that death is simply an end, a dead end, no more, no less.

... Before the pills was another life, another person altogether, whom I scarcely recognize and don't much like—although I suspect that he was, in his priggish way, far more likeable than I could ever be. Meanwhile, his fury and despair seem improbable now, sad and oddly diminished.

Thus suicidal phenomenology becomes an unconscious way out of the ego impasse. The therapist tries to make the process at least somewhat more conscious, to locate which part of the patient needs to be sacrificed to make way for new growth. His goal is to lead the patient to a voluntary sacrifice of old, no longer viable attitudes so that life itself may be preserved.*

Classification of Suicide

Classifications of suicide are more helpful to sociologists than to therapists in evaluating patients.[27] Furthermore, each classification introduces its own bias as to what will and will not be considered suicidal behavior. Nevertheless, each system helps identify individuals who seem consciously or unconsciously headed toward self-destruction. The English coroner system distinguishes these four classes of death: natural, accidental, suicidal, and homicidal (giving rise to the acronym NASH). It is an imperfect system: the chronic drinker, frequently warned by doctors, dies a "natural" death of cirrhosis; the soldier, no longer wishing to live, volunteers for and is killed on a dangerous mission, dying an "accidental" death, which makes him a posthumous hero; the actress unwittingly takes a lethal overdose, thinking it sublethal, and dies a "suicide," even though her death was unintentional.

Shneidman[28] introduces the concept of intentionality into the classification of deaths and distinguishes between *unintentioned, subintentioned, intentioned,* and *contraintentioned.* The drinker's death was subintentioned; the soldier's, intentioned; the actress', contraintentioned. It is the therapist's job to see if individuals whose words and acts suggest subintentioned and intentioned self-destruction can be swayed from their lethal paths and if those flirting with death can find safer ways to express themselves. At times fate itself appears to deny the intention to die.

Example 2-1. A 29-year-old man crashed two small planes without injury and was captured by a policeman who shot to kill and missed. The policeman reported, "He begged me to go ahead and kill him. He said he wished my aim had been a little better." The man's wife had announced her intention to leave him. He went for a flying lesson and forced his pilot-instructor to crash the airplane nose first onto the ground. The policeman's first shot, aimed at his head, missed, and the second shot succeeded only in knocking the rifle out of this hijacker's hand. Despite the two crashes and two shots, he remained unharmed.[29]

Lester[30] has argued that it makes sense to recognize that all acts of suicide fall on a continuum of lethality from thoughts through threats, attempts, and completed deaths. A particularly difficult problem for the emergency therapist is evaluating the lethal intent of a suicide threat,

---

*Nevertheless, patients are encountered for whom the solution of total physical death subbornly insists upon itself. It is the only solution the patient finds satisfactory, no matter how many alternatives are explored. Hillman[26] has argued that we must respect the choice of suicide when it is made responsibly. Jung emphasizes that death is part of nature: it has a place in the ecology of a healthy personality and on occasion is the only way an unhealthy personality can bring its sickness to an end.

whether it is made verbally or through "gesture." He must first dismiss the popular idea that those who threaten suicide rarely attempt it. In fact, most patients who make serious or successful attempts at suicide have threatened to do so in the preceding days and weeks. Likewise, many persons whose blatantly nonlethal attempts have been dismissed as "hysterical gestures" may later make lethal ones. For every seven attempts at suicide, one succeeds. [31-33]

Some [34-39] have attempted to discriminate between suicidal acts that are lethal and nonlethal in intent. This work is preliminary, and we prefer this principle: *anyone who threatens suicide or makes a suicidal gesture needs to be taken seriously and evaluated carefully.*

Suicide Statistics

Official statistics underreport suicides. [38] In recent years in the United States, approximately 22,000 persons will have been adjudged suicides each year; another 5,000 to 8,000 are assumed to have killed themselves but have not been adjudged suicides by a coroner's jury. Officially, more than 11 of each 100,000 people in this country take their own lives each year. Compared to other countries studied by the World Health Organization, the United States is about midway in incidence. Greece, Northern Ireland, and Italy have official rates below 6.0 per 100,000; West Germany, Austria, and Hungary above 20.0 per 100,000; and West Berlin 41.3 per 100,000.

Data from attempted suicides allow sociologists to define characteristics of groups that have the highest and the lowest risks for suicide. From these data, suicide danger-rating scales have been constructed. From knowledge of these risks, predictions can be made about suicidal behavior for a class of people, but it is always the individual and members of his immediate group with whom the emergency therapist is concerned. To date, no danger-rating scale discriminates absolutely between the person who will probably not make a suicide attempt and the one who probably will.

The data in Table 2-1 demonstrate sociological factors in the United States correlated with low and high risk for suicidal behavior. Whenever a patient falls in several of the high-risk categories, the emergency therapist's index of suspicion about suicide potential should be high and his evaluation more careful. [40-43]

Even though a patient may fall primarily in the lower-risk categories of Table 2-1, he is not immune from suicidal risk.

> *Example 2-2.* A young black engineer with a devoted fiancée, a good work record, and no problem with alcohol had little known present stress, no known physical problems, and excellent interpersonal resources. On most suicide-rating scales he would seem to be a low risk. However, he had a past history of an LSD trip on which he "learned" the insignificance of life, and he had made several serious attempts at suicide. Moreover, this time he had a plan of action for completing suicide. His doctor wisely hospitalized him.

It would have been easy for this man to disguise his distress in an interview conducted to screen him and to agree to psychotherapy on an outpatient basis. His deep preoccupation with death would have been missed.

The studies from which Table 2-1 was derived suggest that emotion isolation is an important factor. Sociology confirms common sense: lack of participation in the human group drives people to suicide. Also, recent studies point to anger, energy depletion, and difficulties in adaptation to rapid changes as contributors. In some cases the collection of better suicide data from a population follows new understanding of its problems [44]: witness studies of black suicide undertaken only at the end of the decade of James Baldwin, Eldridge Cleaver, and the Watts riot. [41]

A few aspects of Table 2-1 deserve amplification. Suicide increases with age, showing, as Alvarez [45] notes, the fallacy of the serenity of old age. The steady rise is shown in Figure 2-1, based on the work of Choron. [46] The low suicide rates for

Table 2-1 Sociological Factors and Suicide Risk in the United States

Factor	Lower Risk	Higher Risk
Age	Childhood, adolescence (see Figure 2–1)	Middle, older age (see Figure 2–1)
Sex	Women (30%)	Men (70%)
Family status	Over 24 years old, married with children Over 35 years old and never married	Separated, divorced, widowed
Race	Black*, Oriental	White, American Indian
Religion	Jewish, Catholic	Protestant
Profession	Noncompetitive and/or low demand for interpersonal giving, e.g., white-collar workers, craftsmen, taxi drivers, machine assemblers	Competitive and/or demanding of interpersonal giving, e.g., doctors, lawyers, policemen, housekeepers, nurses
Employment status	Employed at job or at home	Unemployed
Geographic		
1. Local	Stable areas and neighborhoods; suburbs; homeowners	Transitional and slum urban areas; renters
2. National	East coast, midwest	West coast (especially San Francisco)
Health	Good; no history of chronic depression or alcohol abuse	Poor, and/or chronic depression or alcohol abuse
Political	Wartime; political or religious persecution	Peacetime; little persecution

*However, see Hendin[41] for possible change in this trend.

married people may reflect not only the companionship of marriage but also its outlet for aggression; one wonders what would have happened to George and Martha in Albee's *Who's Afraid of Virginia Woolf?* had they not had each other to fight. Rates are lower during times of war and religious persecution, when an external enemy increases group solidarity and provides a focus for aggression.

Personal Factors

We move from the anonymity of statistics to the feeling-uncertainty of the individual patient; the case of Alice will be cited often as an example. This chapter focuses on understanding why Alice behaved suicidally; the next chapter describes the treatment of Alice and other suicidal patients.

Example 2-3, Alice. Alice, a 45-year-old divorced woman, was brought into the emergency room by the police, whom she had called earlier that evening to report that her husband was threatening to kill her. In response to the call, the police met Bradley, a 50-year-old man who had been living with Alice and with whom she had just taken a year-long business tour of the United States.

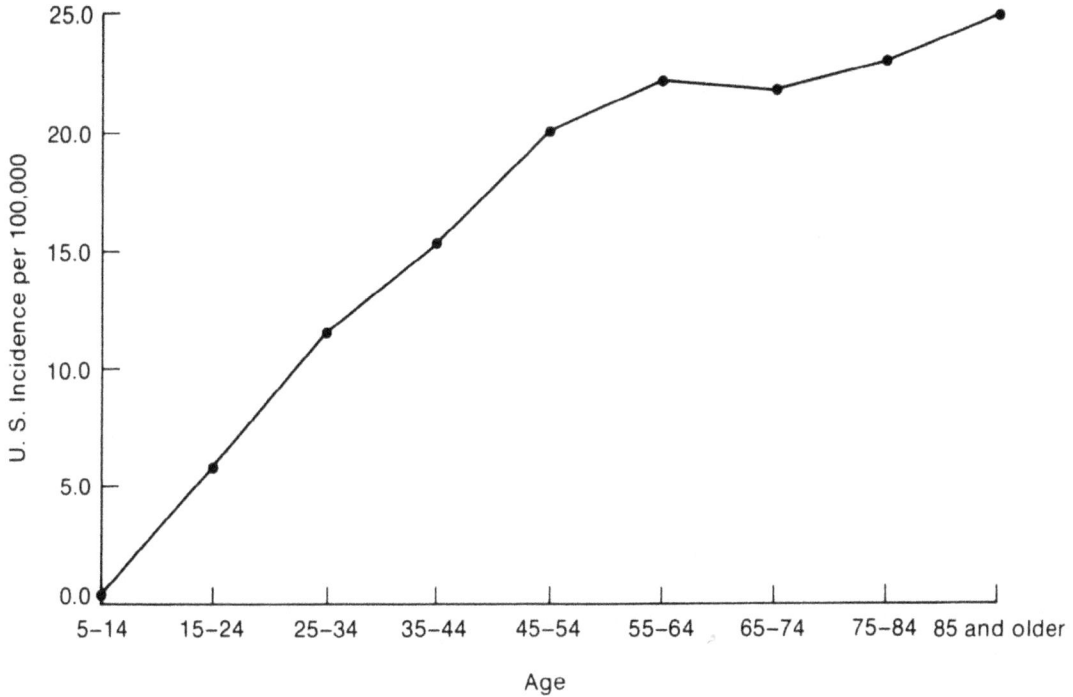

Figure 2–1   Incidence of suicide by age. [Based on [46] .]

This tour had included a visit to her son in jail. Bradley and Alice had been drinking and quarreling, but Bradley agreed to the policeman's suggestion that he leave for the night. After he left, Alice called a taxi to take her to "some motel, it doesn't matter where," spent her last $10 on a room, swallowed a bottle of Sominex, called the police, and said, "You'd better come and get me, I just took something."

In the emergency room she was given ipecac. Later, when the first-year psychiatric resident saw her, she insisted tiredly she could take care of herself. The record showed similar attempts three and four years before; both times she had been released from the emergency room without follow-up plans.

This time the psychiatrist, noting she had no resources and would not return to Bradley, recommended hospitalization and threatened to sign a seventy-two-hour hold until the situation was clarified. Alice finally agreed to enter voluntarily at county expense. The admitting diagnosis was "depressive reaction in a passive-aggressive personality, possible alcoholism." She insisted on returning to the hotel to get her things, so the resident drove her there in his car. When she was admitted to the psychiatric unit she said, "I didn't know anything this nice was here," and prepared to go to bed.

The resident felt that Alice might attempt suicide again in spite of the impulsiveness of her previous gesture and her request for help. He was willing to impose the seventy-two-hour involuntary hospitalization to obtain time for further evaluation and because he knew that the risk of a repeat attempt is highest in the three days after a suicide attempt.

From a sociological point of view, this patient was high risk. She was outside society, in transit, divorced, jobless, restless, and she drank. But her first suicide attempts belonged to the period before her present rootlessness began. Old records revealed that her husband had held a managerial position in a munitions firm. What lay behind her immediate problems?

Chronic Predisposing Factors. Usually even a sudden, impulsive suicidal act has an extensive background. Often there is evidence of a *death trend,* in which deaths of family members, deaths of aborted or live-born children, and so on are prominent in the patient's history. Such losses, often under dramatic and tragic circumstances, were found in nearly all fifty suicidal patients in one study,[47] and three-quarters of the losses had occurred by the patient's adolescence. Again we recall Sylvia Plath's adult preoccupation with her father, who died when she was 9.

The link between past loss and present depression may be the *anniversary reaction* described by Hilgard and Newman.[48] This reaction surfaces at a time that evokes the memory of the loss—on the anniversary of suffering. Obvious reminders are the actual dates of loss, such as the yearly anniversary of a spouse's death.[49] Less obvious reminders come when a patient reaches the same age as a parent who died or when the patient's child becomes as old as the patient when a parent was killed. Seasons can bring on reactions: one woman became depressed every March, when the first warm days reminded her of her contact with an abortionist. Frequently women who lose babies, whether by therapeutic, illegal, or spontaneous abortion, find themselves unaccountably depressed and even suicidal on the day the baby would have been born.

> *Alice (cont'd.).* The day after admission, Alice willingly told the resident about her life. Her father had left home when she was 14; her mother raised her and her brother, who had become a policeman. Alice was unable to give up her father, however, and when she was 17 followed him after work and discovered that he lived with another woman. Shortly after

this incident her father was killed in a fire. Talking about this event, the patient suddenly burst into tears and was surprised at the intensity of her feelings.

Shortly after her father's death, Alice met Fred. He was a handsome, charming man, and they quickly married. She became pregnant with Don, and while she was carrying him she learned that Fred had escaped from prison in Missouri. Fred became brutal and began to drink heavily and was physically cruel and frequently unfaithful to her. She left Fred soon after their second child was born. The day before she attempted suicide Alice had visited her son Don in prison. Until the age of 17 he had been an outstanding student. On his seventeenth birthday he was in a car accident in which three people were killed; he was sentenced by an outraged court to five years in prison, in spite of the fact that Alice tried vainly to have the sentence commuted. Two years after Don went to prison, Alice made her first suicide attempt.

Don was 17 when he was sentenced; Alice was 17 when she learned of her father's infidelity. Alice was 19 when her father died in the fire; when Don reached 19, Alice made her first suicide attempt. Delinquency and death have their eerie anniversaries. Alice appeared to be reacting to Don's imprisonment as she had to her father's disappearance and death: by following him into exile and punishing herself for his loss.

Although distant or recent loss is not prominent, most suicidal patients, even if their attempts appear impulsive, have been thinking about death for some time. Alvarez, while intoxicated on Christmas Eve, took an overdose of sleeping pills after a marital squabble. He too had "been incubating this death for longer than I recognized." When things went badly for him as a youth, he recited a litany to himself, "Iwishlwere-dead . . . Iwishlweredead." One day, he writes, ". . . suddenly I heard the phrase as though for the first time. . . . I repeated the words slowly, listening. And realized that I meant it. It seemed so obvious, an answer I had known for years and never allowed myself to acknowledge."[50]

In addition to hearing about the current distress, the emergency therapist must learn about old losses, anniversary reactions, previous suicide attempts, and other long-term incubations of the wish to die. Often the lethal risk is clarified only after the chronic background is revealed.

Personality Styles. *Predisposing personality styles* for suicide are the (1) impulsive, (2) compulsive, and (3) risk-taking. Some patients cannot control *impulses*, such as reactions to minor stress, and become suicidal. A San Francisco man became frustrated in the midst of a traffic jam, left his car, and jumped off the Golden Gate Bridge; a housewife stabbed herself with an ice pick when her children refused to do the dishes. Such people are usually more prone to attempt than to complete suicide.

The impulsivity of persons who make dramatic life decisions to communicate feelings they cannot put into words is more lethal. Alice's dramatic search for her father and her impulsive marriage show the beginnings of a stubborn, impulsive streak that surfaced in her conflicts with men. Such impulsivity combines willfulness with an inability to put the same feelings into words.

Alice (cont'd.). The day after Alice was admitted, Bradley called her therapist to confide that she was "kind of peculiar." Alice habitually called the police when she was angry with Bradley and had had him locked up twice. This made Bradley "sore," even though he "liked her spunk." He compared her to Don, who a few hours after her visit had made an impulsive attempt to escape from prison. He had been caught immediately and sentenced to solitary confinement with a loss of parole, all of which Alice had read about in the newspaper. That night she had started the quarrel with Bradley which ended with two calls to the police and a suicide attempt.

Alice admitted to feeling anger toward the policemen who responded to her first call, because they did not do more to protect her. She said she called the police right after taking the pills because she was still angry with them. The fact that calling them led to her life being saved seemed less important to her than that she had taught them a lesson about how to treat people in trouble.

Compulsive personalities are high-achieving and perfectionistic. They have difficulty adjusting their needs and goals to changing circumstances and are inflexible in their habits. In middle and later life they are predisposed to involutional depression. They may for a short time become acutely and dangerously suicidal. When this personality pattern is recognized in a depressed person past the middle of life, the clinician must be alert to the high lethal risk. To some extent compulsive defenses appear with age, and the ability to adjust to minor stress lessens. And *anyone* can fall apart with too drastic a change in life pattern.

Whether a person is compulsive or not, an *erosion of life style* deprives him of many personal and social gratifications and defenses against loneliness, anxiety, and depression. Previously bound or sublimated impulses push for expression with greater urgency, and suicide as an egoistic or anomic event becomes progressively more thinkable. As one suicide note put it, "Why suicide? Why not?"[51] In Alice's life a definite erosion of stability rendered her more vulnerable to suicide.

Alice (cont'd.). When Don was 6 and his brother Joe was 4, Alice entered into a second marriage with Rolfe, an engineer who was very strict with her boys ("to keep them from turning out like their father"), but who babied the son born a year after their marriage. Their social life was stable; for many years Alice made friends and participated in the PTA, country club, and other social activities.

After Don's car accident, Alice silently blamed Rolfe's heavy-handed discipline for Don's behavior, became increasingly dissatisfied with the marriage, and listened to her friends' suggestions that she leave Rolfe. At the same time that Joe was being dishonorably discharged from the Army, Alice filed separation papers. She anticipated going into business with Joe and Don, who was within two months of discharge on parole. Shortly thereafter Don and Joe pulled an armed robbery together; both received five-year sentences.

This did it. Alice withdrew from her friends, started drinking, and met Bradley, who quickly left his wife and moved in with her. They drank and went through Alice's money, and she completely fell away from her old friends and activities. She and Bradley started traveling across the country. Bradley promised to set up a business and divorce his wife, but he succeeded only in passing a few bad checks and skipping from one town to the next.

For some, *risk-taking* is a way of life. One woman, in a showdown with her boyfriend and the other woman, took an overdose of sleeping pills. Later she said, "All my life I've been a gambler; I wanted to show them I was willing to gamble my own life." For a long time this woman had played the stock market and enjoyed the risk-taking involved. She transferred this psychology to the resolution of her romantic dilemma.

For many, risk-taking is part of the "good life." Perhaps the Kennedy family is the most noteworthy public example of the risk-taking style of high-achieving, flexible people. In examining the role of the victim in assassination attempts, Weisz and Taylor[52] suggest that the propensity of the victim to take risks increases his likelihood of being murdered.

Obviously, *chronic predisposing psychiatric conditions* play an enormous role in the choice of suicide. Among the more important are

1. *Drug or alcohol problems.* Fifty percent of the male suicides have measurable blood alcohol levels. Ruth Fox[53] says the suicide rate is fifty-five times higher for alcoholics. It is estimated that about 10 percent of addicts, alcoholics, and drug abusers will die by suicide, not counting their many accidental deaths.

2. *Manic-depressive disease.* The depressed phase is a highly dangerous time, and the patient should almost always be hospitalized.

3. *Depression.* People tend to commit suicide more often when depression is improving or after a period in which they have begun to feel better. Two reasons have been advanced to explain this pattern. First, patients who have been slowed by the intense psychomotor retardation of an exhausting psychotic depression do not have the energy to kill themselves or to formulate a plan. When they begin to improve, their energy returns, and suicidal behavior again becomes a possibility. Second, these patients dread a return to their formerly depressed states. A minor setback after a period of improvement may threaten the patient with another long bout of emotional paralysis. Recognizing that chronic depression is just around the corner, a patient may choose a time when he is feeling relatively well to kill himself. Experienced clinicians are very cautious during the improvement of severe depression and often resist pressure from the patient and family for premature discharge into an environment where suicide can be accomplished.

4. *Schizophrenia.* The schizophrenic patient most often commits suicide during the early phase of his illness, in contrast to the depressive patient, who commits suicide during the convalescent phase. Schizophrenic patients also commit suicide during times of change. Times such as when they enter the hospital, go into or come out of the psychotic phase, or when they are discharged are especially high risk.

5. *Personality disorder.* Most clinicians would describe Alice as having a personality disorder. Her distress became part of her character and led her to seek out partners who would hurt her. Menninger[54] uses the term *chronic suicide* to describe this process. From the time she made her first choice, choosing a husband, Alice seems to have been acting unconsciously

against herself. Suicide attempts were just one aspect of an overall pattern of self-destruction. Much of this pattern appeared as an adverse fate over which she had no control. But had she nothing to do with the choice of four alcoholic men and with two sons being sent to jail? When she did consider this, the insight seemed malignant and only made her hate herself more.

6. *Past suicidal history*. The *history of a previous suicide attempt* is the single most important prognosticator of suicidal potential. Alice had made two such attempts. In a man over the age of 50, a serious attempt within the past ninety days would almost certainly demonstrate a period of high risk.

Other forms of self-destructive activity should be regarded as part of the suicidal history. It is customary for therapists to regard these as *suicidal equivalents*. Alice, for instance, chose brutal, alcoholic men and a lifestyle (presumably motivated by shame and guilt) that amounted to social suicide in the group to which she had belonged. Other patients give even clearer histories of actions that although not directly suicidal are self-destructive. A formerly suicidal woman may turn to prostitution or heroin addiction. A suicidal air force officer may volunteer for an unnecessary mission. A young psychiatrist may begin treating his own anxiety with barbiturates. An adolescent girl may have many therapeutic abortions. At any point in his history the patient may exchange one of these suicidal equivalents for suicidal behavior. (An overzealous therapist may precipitate a suicidal crisis by forcing a patient to give up some "masochistic" behavior whose real motivations neither he nor the patient understand).

7. *Negative therapeutic history*. It is common to find in the histories of those who kill themselves a dismal story of *past failures in psychotherapy and unsuccessful medical treatment*.

Alice (cont'd.). After Don's first imprisonment, Alice saw a psychotherapist three times, did not find therapy helpful, and did not return. The therapist remembered her as "very skittish; underneath I had the feeling she was very confused, maybe crazy." For two years preceding her most recent suicide attempt she had been having heavy menstrual bleeding. Gynecologists had recommended a dilatation and curettage, but in her travels with Bradley she had never found the money for this minor surgery.

Recent Precipitating Factors

The chronic background of most suicidal crises can be summarized as the combination of negative life expectation with a character style which does not leave the environment much room to counter that expectation. The immediate background is a major current frustration. Suicidal patients act when the going gets tough. Certain acute life situations are especially apt to precipitate the suicidal act in susceptible individuals. These include loss, health problems, social disgrace, loss of the reason to live, and plastic surgery.

Loss. Loss stands out in almost every suicidal history. In an otherwise normal person the loss of a loved one can precipitate suicidal thinking. In the person with a chronic expectation of loss, starting with the loss of a parent in childhood, further loss can be catastrophic. Thus the emergency therapist finds himself taking an inventory of loss as he talks to his potentially suicidal patients. What may be difficult to remember is that the *threat of loss* can be as upsetting as actual loss. It may be likelier to precipitate suicide and is far more difficult to identify.

Alice (cont'd.). Alice's therapist was puzzled about why Alice attempted suicide at that particular time. Don's escape attempt had probably contributed, but some pieces of the puzzle were still missing. Alice insisted she was through with Bradley and seemed to believe that leaving him would be a gain, not a loss. The resident and ward staff supported her decision.

Therefore the resident was surprised to learn a day later that Bradley was visiting Alice and holding hands with her. In a joint interview he learned that Bradley was threatening to leave Alice and return to his wife, and that Alice's threats to leave Bradley were mostly a strategy to convince him to obtain his divorce and marry her. Since her sons' imprisonment, Bradley was the only person that mattered to her. Whatever society thought, she loved him, and she held the secret belief she could change him enough so that they could be happy together. She had been deeply threatened by his new talk of going back to his wife at a time when she wanted to make final arrangements for a permanent move across the country. At this point the resident perceived that he was dealing with a couple problem.

As Freud pointed out, loss hits harder when the thing lost is regarded ambivalently. But any loss is hard: death, divorce, military duty, urban renewal. Almost always the individual regrets not having done the best with what he had, and self-recrimination is usual.

A common issue in the lives of suicidal patients is the loss or threat of loss of a supportive professional. Frequently a therapist's vacation precipitates a suicidal crisis, a syndrome called the *caretaker crisis*. Often only the caretaker can resolve it by returning or promising to return. Although the issue is dependency, the caretaker crisis does not occur only in passive-dependent individuals. High-achieving, compulsive personalities, who usually have strong guilt feelings over dependency and stoically deny their needs feel the absence of nurturant others most. And they are the ones who find it most difficult to ask for substitute help. Quite frequently they signal their needs by serious suicide attempts. For this reason, discharge planning for patients with involutional depressions is extremely difficult. Patients may move compliantly through the planning stage of discharge and make serious attempts soon after they return home. In some cases they are not able to *say* that they still felt the need for support. As a matter of routine, many therapists tell their patients: "You probably won't agree, but in the first days at home you are going to miss this place a great deal, whatever you think now, and you should expect a return of the suicidal feelings. I expect you to call me when this happens, even though you may think it is unimportant."

Health Problems. Loss of another sort comes when a healthy person, proud of his body and used to activity, is forced into invalidism, and the patient may doubt that life is worth continuing. Two-thirds of the old people who commit suicide have painful or disabling diseases.

In checking up on the patient's health, *medications that have a depressing effect* should be identified. Rauwolfia alkaloids, prescribed for hypertension, have precipitated severe depressions that look primary. Diazepam (Valium®) and chlorpromazine have also been reported to have this effect. Surgical residents in particular are prone to overprescribe diazepam, which causes later appearance of depressive symptomatology in hospitalized patients.

Social Disgrace. Here too a kind of loss is involved—the loss of face. Suicide may follow sudden arrest or bankruptcy, disclosure of child molesting, and so on.

Some suicidal crises occurring after encounter groups are of this type, seemingly caused by too rapid a dissolution of the ego defenses that acted as supports.[55] Loss of face can occur in a group as small as two, and traditional one-to-one psychotherapy can also be a place where social disgrace occurs. Some patients seen in emergency rooms are in flight from therapeutic situations that have brought about confrontations with extremely unacceptable parts of themselves. *Homosexual panic* can also lead to suicide.

Loss of Reason to Live. To understand suicidal metapsychology, Freud started with the question, "Why should the normal instinct for self-preservation fail?" In evaluating suicidal patients, the emergency therapist must learn to reverse the question: "Why does this person live?" In searching for the factors that affect an individual's potential for suicide, it is easy to forget to ask this question. Yet when a suicide is actually completed, it is often because the one reason for staying alive no longer exists. The late actor George Sanders perhaps epitomized the *existential suicide* when he wrote, "I am committing suicide because I am bored."

Others stay alive because they harbor hopes of future interests. If a symbolic purpose keeps them alive, its disappearance may be unknown to anyone else. And they themselves may not always know what it was. Alice apparently found her reason to live in her dream of establishing a new life with Bradley. When this hope became threatened, the suicidal impulse, strengthened by her tragic background, broke through.

A paradigm for this type of suicide is the *vacation suicide.* For many, a vacation is anticipated as the solution to long-standing problems. When at last the vacation comes, but not the expected relief, a suicidal crisis may appear "out of the blue."

Plastic surgery too may precipitate a suicidal crisis. The issue again involves false hope. The surgery was expected to work magic by restoring long-absent self-esteem.

SPECIFICS OF INTERVIEW EVALUATION

Focus on Recent Changes

Despite its chronic background, the decision to commit suicide is always an acute event. In the emergency room the key question is "Is the patient moving in a suicidal direction now?" In the short range the prognosis is *worse* when the onset of self-destructive behavior is recent. (Of course,

the long-term prognosis is better for those whose pattern is not chronic.) Recent loss, recent appearance of depressive signs, and recent concern on the part of friends and relatives are all important signs. If suicide is an issue, evaluation should be prompt and follow-up frequent. The patient should not have to wait several days before the therapist can see him. Here, as with the evaluation of possible homicide, information about the development of the immediate crisis is essential. The resident decided to hospitalize Alice almost entirely on his evaluation of her present circumstances. Here, he reasoned, is a divorced, middle-aged woman in the acute period of a romantic breakup, with no job, no place to live, and a suicidal gesture, who says, "Next time I'll do it right." Whatever the long-range prognosis for her ending her life, another rejection now (in the form of accepting her denial and letting her go) could tip the balance in favor of suicide. Only later did the resident learn about the long lead-up to her attempt.

Inquire about Suicide Planning

Beginning therapists often find it difficult to ask detailed questions about the patient's fantasies of killing himself and about the steps he has taken to do so. Usually there are two reasons for this reluctance. One is the fear that detailed questioning will suggest suicide to a patient who has not thought of it. Actually, there is *no* evidence that it is detrimental to ask these questions. The therapist should be reassured that no suicide has been recorded in which the patient got the idea from a therapist.[56] There is probably more danger of intensifying suicidal intent if the patient feels he *cannot* talk about his ideas with anyone; the suicidal motivation thrives when it is closed off from communication.

The second reason the inexperienced emergency therapist is reluctant to delve into suicidal planning is a feeling of awkwardness. This is a specialized interviewing skill, but the principles are the same as for any other awkward interview topic. The therapist tries to lead into the subject naturally by following a stepwise line of questioning. A typical sequence of questions might be: "I gather things have been falling apart for you lately?" (Pause) "And that you're getting pretty depressed?" (A pause for the patient to reply, cry, or ventilate.) "Has it reached the point that you've thought of taking your life?" (The therapist deliberately implies that this is a normal part of the depressive process and that he recognizes the extremity of suffering necessary before such usually unacceptable thinking starts. This should enable the patient to answer honestly.) "Have you actually found yourself thinking of a way you might kill yourself?" Often the patient resists at this point with a vague answer such as, "All kinds of ways." But the therapist can insist, "I mean, have you thought of a specific way of ending your life?" *The answer to this question is the central one in any suicide evaluation.*

> *Alice (cont'd.).* The resident did not ask Alice what ways she had thought of for ending her life. After all, she had made a suicide attempt with pills. Moreover, her two previous attempts had been with pills. As we shall see, he should have asked what other ways she had thought of and what she meant by her ominous statement, "Next time I'll do it right."

Facts about the Suicide Plan. *Suicidal thoughts* must be distinguished from actual planning, and in evaluating the degree of intent the *lethal potential* of the plan, the *availability of means,* and the *sophistication of the patient* must be taken into account.

Probably more than half the population has had suicidal thoughts. The ratio of people who think about it to those who act on it is very large. Thus the fact that someone has thought about suicide is not sufficiently important to consider him a serious risk.

The plan provides the bridge between a passing thought and a definite action, and here the *lethal potential of the plan* is the most important issue. When the patient mentions shooting himself,

jumping off a bridge, or taking poison, his determination to die is obvious.

However, the interviewer should discover if the intended means are available. In New York, where jumping from high buildings is the method in 15 percent of all suicides,[57] a threat of suicide by this method is realistic. In a rural community, a plan to use this method would probably be a dramatic statement. The common threat, "I think I'll jump off the bridge," is more than a figure of speech in San Francisco, where 20 percent of the suicides occur when people jump off the Golden Gate Bridge. Guns and pills are available everywhere, and specific inquiry into whether the patient keeps a gun at home or has sleeping pills is a necessary part of evaluation. Alvarez, for instance, reports that he had been stockpiling barbiturates for months before his "impulsive" suicide attempt.

In deciding the degree of suicidal risk from the plan, *the degree of sophistication of the patient* must be taken into account. The university professor who thinks of shooting himself but who has no gun can use the same skills that earned him tenure to acquire one. The adolescent girl who swallows a bottle of aspirin in a slum may really think it will work. Lack of sophistication should be regarded as a high-, not a low-risk, factor because the chances for accidental death are greater. In their study of equivocal deaths Litman et al.[58] reported the following case:

> *Example 2-4.* When her husband threatened to divorce her, a woman ingested poison in front of him. He immediately took her to a hospital. After emergency treatment for arsenic poisoning she felt better and told the doctors she did not really want to die. However, she developed severe kidney damage and died after two weeks of uremia and cerebral hemorrhage. After some consideration, the recommendation was suicide.

The resident who treated Alice acted wisely by assuming she meant to kill herself, even though she used an over-the-counter medication. She had said, "I thought on top of the alcohol it would work."

Learn about Past Suicide Attempts. Incredibly, it is easy to forget to inquire if the patient has tried suicide in the past. The patient is often glad to leave an old attempt buried.

The full history has an important bearing on the prognosis. It should be taken carefully, with attention given to the method, timing, circumstances of the attempt, feelings about death, and the reasons why death was successfully prevented.

Notice How the Patient Communicates in the Interview

Eli Robins' group's[59] classic study on the communication of suicidal intent revealed that more than two-thirds of those who committed suicide had communicated suicidal ideas and 41 percent had specifically stated their intent. In the majority of instances the suicidal communications had been recently and repeatedly espressed in words, and to many persons. A neglected conclusion is that 31 percent of suicides do *not* communicate their intent clearly. Another 28 percent do not state directly that they plan to kill themselves. And some of the direct communications are made in such a joking or offhand way that they are not recognized as statements of intent. Thus *indirect* communication, as well as direct threats, must be picked up and heeded by the emergency therapist.

Affective Clues to Suicide. In the interview situation, three kinds of moods suggest the possibility of suicide: *hopeless resignation, euphoria,* and *psychomotor retardation.*

Resignation, a calm communication of hopelessness, is an extremely serious clinical finding. Rare but lethal, extreme calm is the mark of a paranoid person who may be planning homicide and suicide in a logical, methodical way. In the interview situation, the paranoid person with a well-organized delusional system may show studied calm. If paranoia is a defense against depression, the paranoid system may include a nonemotional plan for suicide as the last step in a well-worked-out strategy for revenge that also includes murder.

Depression followed by euphoria of recent onset is also a serious finding. Here the dynamic reason for improvement in mood may be that a decision has been reached. Suicidal people are notoriously ambivalent. Not knowing whether to live or die exhausts them, and there is great relief in finally knowing that they have decided to die. In Robins'[59] study, the husband of a 42-year-old woman said, "On the morning of the day of her suicide she was sweeter and more attentive than ever before, she kissed me better than she ever had before."

Psychomotor retardation, i.e., long reaction times to questions and a generally slowed, immobile appearance, is the hallmark of severe depression. At this stage many patients do not have the energy to commit suicide, but some might. This condition, possibly the end stage of long-standing ambivalence and confusion about living, is extremely painful for the patient. Suicides *do* occur in the retarded phase of this malignant process often enough.

Fantasy Clues to Suicide. There are several common fantasies, one or more of which may accompany the suicidal affect. The emergency therapist should ask the patient to imagine out loud his own death, its effect on others, and its long-range outcome. Often one of the fantasies will become apparent, and the therapist can use it in treatment. The most common fantasies are revenge against the hated self (as in the puer aeternus or incomplete Renaissance man), revenge against others, death as reversible sleep, and death as a reunion with loved ones.

As revenge against others, patients may express a version of "You'll all be sorry (and guilty) when I'm dead and gone." The others usually are members of the patient's immediate ecological group (lovers, spouses, parents, therapists). The patient's fantasy may be that after the suicide they will all feel intense guilt for the rest of their lives for their sins of omission and commission. After hearing out this fantasy, the therapist can point out two contradictory elements of reality. One is that although everyone would probably feel some grief and sadness if the patient died, each would, after a suitable period of mourning, return to the business of living, and the patient's death would recede to the background of his consciousness. The second is that however much anguish the patient's death causes others, the patient will not be around to see and enjoy it. For these two reasons the therapist can argue that although the patient's vengeful feelings toward others are understandable, there are more effective ways of expressing them than through suicide.

The concept of death as irreversible (except perhaps in religious persons with a strong belief in the afterlife) does not become fixed in the ego until the age of 5 or 6. Before that time children believe death is a variant of sleep from which they will always awaken. They play "Bang, bang; you're dead": the victim falls limp on the floor for a moment, and then comes back to life. Certain patients with primitive ego functioning have never fully assimilated the irreversibility of death, and this may come out in fantasy. When it does, the therapist can point out to the patient that dead is dead, that there will not be any physical reawakening to see the effect of the death on others. Surprisingly, the therapist's challenge to this fantasy may be sufficient to cause the patient to relinquish a fixed idea that suicide can be used in a temporary way.

Lonely patients may view death as a reunion with already departed loved ones; they will find the company and comfort in heaven that they cannot find on earth. To the extent that this fantasy is a remnant of magical childhood fantasies about afterlife (rather than a carefully developed adult philosophical view), the therapist can challenge the unrealistic hopes for reunion and at the same time offer a real relationship on earth.

Indirect Suicidal Communications. Many suicidal people communicate their despair indirectly, even seek to deny it, only to turn with vengeful anger on the therapist who has failed to appreciate the depth of their distress. Above all, suicidal people have difficulty locating their own feelings, and often they cannot communicate them clearly. The

wise therapist will not restrict himself to what the patient knows or admits about his feeling-life; he will look at other material.

Dreams provide valuable clues. Typical suicidal dreams involve the opening of a door onto a black, forbidding territory, escaping into a peaceful unknown territory, or jumping through a window. Dreams of enclosed spaces and of falling also may hold a suicidal meaning.

Self-deprecating remarks should not be taken lightly. In involutional depressions, statements such as, "I'm no good, you don't need me around, I'll only depress you," are extremely common. Frankly psychotic statements arguing, "I have sinned, I deserve to die," are often expressed by patients in severely depressed states. Cynicism in describing himself may identify the potential suicide to a sensitive listener who should be cued to inquire more deeply about those depressive ideas.

Behavioral clues are abundant. In Robins'[59] study, a patient phoned his ex-wife's mother and asked her to burn a candle for him. Another repeated a pantomime of shooting himself without a gun in his hand. A would-be suicide may begin to plan for his death by showing increased concern for others, visiting his friends for a series of intense chats, and giving away prized possessions. He may buy a gun, increase his life insurance, or change his will. Often the entire sequence can be reconstructed only when several people in the patient's social surroundings have been interviewed. Each will have seen only part, yet the patient may feel that everyone should have understood his intention clearly.

Direct Suicidal Communications. Robins' study positively contradicts the idea that those who threaten suicide never commit it. Among the direct statements his team collected were "I won't be here tomorrow," "Don't be surprised if you find I walked into the water," "You won't see me again except in a hearse," and, when a physician suggested an appointment with a psychiatrist, "By that time it will be too late." Such comments can be made so casually that others may not believe they are sincere. Suicidal patients are past masters at self-disqualification, and it is easy to be misled into believing they do not mean what they say. Also, the statements may be made in an altered ego state, in the heat of a quarrel or when drunk, for instance. When he returns to his "normal" state, it is easy for the patient to say that he did not mean it. If he has a drinking problem or is a frequent quarreler, he is likely to enter that "abnormal" state again and kill himself. It is good practice to *note down the patient's statements of intent* as made in the interview and as quoted by others. Often the meaning of these statements will become apparent later, although in the confusion of the initial interview they may seem trivial.

Alice (cont'd.). The initial notes of the resident who saw Alice read, "She took 'everything I had on hand'—seven Darvon, Sominex (some)—thinking, 'On top of the alcohol I'd had, it would work.' Then she called the police to 'Come get me, take me to jail. . .' She was brought to the emergency room and stated she would 'do it right' next time. She saw the situation as a 'mess' and refused to go into a mental hospital for fear 'of what it would do' to her youngest son."

Reading these notes much later, the resident was impressed by the amount of meaning lost in his later, inexact translations. He remembered her as saying to the police, "You'd better come and get me, I just took something." The distorted wording was deliberately left in the initial description to show how progressive clarification is part of the evaluation process. There is a definite threat and the hint of an "I have sinned" motif in the patient's curt "Come get me, take me to jail."

Suicidal patients often show *discrepancies between words and deeds.* Despite her overt rejection of help, Alice's actions were an invitation to someone to intervene. The resident was correct in insisting that her veiled communication suggested suicide if help were not offered. His insistence on

hospitalization was his way of communicating to a denying patient that he would not participate in her denial, that he had heard her. If he had let her go, Alice might easily have made a suicide attempt to revenge herself against his heedlessness, just as she had in part acted against the police and Bradley earlier in the evening. The treating person is often sorely tested by the patient's verbal denials.

Example 2-5. A 30-year-old nurse came to the emergency room from her doctor's office. She was staggering. Tests showed some barbiturate in her blood. "It's just a bad habit." she insisted. When she was offered hospitalization, she said she could not afford time off from her job; she'd been out sick too often already and her invalid mother was dependent on her for support. She insisted she had no suicidal intent. The emergency therapist instituted involuntary hospitalization for seventy-two hours until her situation could be clarified. He said that her unexplained actions spoke louder to him than her vociferous denials.

At the beginning it is extremely difficult to learn the art of listening to the patient's behavior rather than to what he says. Patients, however, are grateful when their behavioral cues are taken seriously. They often feel rejected when their words are accepted at face value.

Alice (cont'd.). Alice and Bradley formed a strong, positive attachment to the resident who had hospitalized Alice. Alice told him he was the best doctor she had ever met. When her situation remained uncertain, she asked if she could stay on the ward longer than seventy-two hours. She was surprised to learn she had been on voluntary status all along and was glad to continue on that basis.

Response of the Ecological Group

The context of suicide may involve a large and surprisingly varied network of people. Because people related by blood or law may not be the only important participants, this system is not best described in terms of the family. Indeed, the idea that only family members can be contacted may be restricting, as seen in the example of the young resident who felt he did not have a right to contact Bradley because he and Alice were not legally married.

Warren Miller[60] uses the term *ecological group* for the social network. He argues that suicide, like other crises, may be seen as an event registering strain in the entire system, *ecostrain*. Thus a suicide may appear in an ecological group that has recently suffered a move, cancer, a heart attack, or a graduation in one of its members. The suicidal crisis may be a ripple effect in a long wave of strain that has been triggered by a major shift in the structure of the group, as, for instance, from some important member's marriage, death, or divorce. (This view of crisis as "news of a difference" is developed in Chapter 1.)

Thus data from other members of the ecological group are important in understanding the dynamics of the crisis. They also contribute corroborative data that can give factual backup to an intuitive sense of high suicidal risk. Important data on suicidal potential can come from interviewing significant members of the ecological group. Finally, and very importantly, *interpersonal resources open to the patient* can be evaluated by interviewing the significant others in his life.

The Immobilization Response. The question of interpersonal resources is raised when the reaction of family members faced with a suicide warning is examined. Robins' series of cases points up a curious nonreaction in the face of clear suicidal messages. This nonreaction seems to occur when relationships regress to almost nonverbal, symbiotic states. Litman[61] has coined the term *immobilization response* to describe this nonreaction. Generally the immobilization comes from a stronger member who fails to react to a weaker member's plea for support in an interpersonal situation.

Alice (cont'd.). Bradley sounded angry when he called the resident who had hospitalized Alice. And he did not appear on the psychiatric ward until well into her second day. The nurses did not like him, and they felt his handholding with Alice was a kind of grandstanding. Moreover, he confided to the resident that he was "getting kind of tired" of her complaining. He wanted to know how sick she was. "Could she be depressing me is what I want to know? I don't want to be dragged down, if you understand what I mean."

Often the nonreaction comes from the therapist who himself is suffering a loss and does not hear his patient's complaint of neglect.

Alice (cont'd.). The emergency resident had not originally planned to take Alice as a patient. The ward was not his primary assignment, and his own caseload was already full. But both full-time residents were having marital problems, and they were tired and irritable. Neither wanted Alice in his caseload. Each was sure she would be too great a drain.

The Lifeline. An understanding of isolation and immobilization has led to the concept of *lifeline*. The single most important question for a therapist to ask himself when evaluating a patient is, "Is there a lifeline open to this person?" A lifeline is one or more interested persons who want the patient to stay alive. An immobilized other, no matter how significant, is not a lifeline. In fact, if he is immobilized enough, he may unconsciously drive the patient to suicide.

When a suicidal patient is referred, the experienced therapist takes a consultative set as he listens to the referring therapist. If the therapist on the other end of the phone is rejecting, moralistic, and stereotypes the patient in a pessimistic manner ("This is a masochistic gal. . . ."), the emergency therapist can assume that an immobilization response is present. If, on the other hand, the referral is made in a sympathetic and encouraging manner, he can assume that the patient has a lifeline. (The presence of a lifeline becomes especially important if the patient is ready for discharge.)

In all fairness, it must be recognized that the closed world of suicide can produce contagious exhaustion. Endless ambivalence, vengeful dependency, repetitive pressure for reassurance, and frustrating denial wear out those who want to help. Passive negativism is so exasperating that it regularly elicits lecturing and rejection.

Alice (cont'd.). Whenever the nurses talked to Alice about Bradley's limitations they met with denial. She insisted her love would change him, despite the fact that he divided his time between her and his wife and blatantly teased her about her jealousy. Gradually the nurses began to tease the resident, saying, "You sure know how to pick patients." The effect of this was to make him insist that Alice could be treated. Secretly he wondered *how.* Bradley used their joint sessions not to assist in planning for Alice, but to parade his own symptomatology before the resident in a scene-stealing fashion while he dropped hints about his ambivalence about Alice. Because Alice could not conceive of life without Bradley, the resident continued the couple's sessions on an outpatient basis. If their relationship could stabilize, possibly a way out of the impasse would emerge. In this way the resident quietly became the lifeline for Alice, and the couple's therapy her main avenue of hope.

In the next chapter we shall examine the treatment of suicidal patients in both the crisis intervention and the longer-term phases. The case of Alice will again be used to illustrate problems that occur frequently. The reader now may wish to ask himself: How would he proceed, confronted with the same patient? How would he formulate the situation, and what would his treatment plan be? He can check his approach with the suggestions offered in the next chapter.

REFERENCES

1. Alvarez, A.: *The Savage God,* Random House, New York, 1972, p. xiii. Copyright 1972, Random House.

2. Jung, C. G.: "Psychological Types," *Collected Works,* Princeton, Princeton, N.J., 1971, vol. 6, p. 433.

3. Hillman, James: *Suicide and the Soul,* Hodder, London, 1964.

4. Lester, David: *Why People Kill Themselves,* Charles C Thomas, Springfield, Ill., 1972. (Originally published as "Suicidal Behavior: A Summary of Research Findings," supplement to *Crisis Intervention,* vol. 2, no. 3, Suicide Preventation and Crisis Service, Buffalo, N.Y., 1970.)

5. Farberow, Normal L., and Edwin S. Shneidman (eds.): *The Cry for Help,* McGraw-Hill, New York, 1965.

6. Stengel, Erwin: *Suicide and Attempted Suicide,* Penguin, Baltimore, 1969.

7. Durkheim, Émile: *Suicide,* Free Press, Glencoe, Ill., 1951.

8. Freud, Sigmund: "Mourning and Melancholia," in *The Complete Psychological Works of Sigmund Freud,* Hogarth, London, 1957, vol. 14, pp. 243–258.

9. Adler, Alfred: "Suicide," *J. Individ. Psychol.,* 14:57–61, 1958.

10. Hillman: loc. cit.

11. Litman, Robert E.: "Sigmund Freud on Suicide," in Edwin S. Shneidman (ed.), *Essays in Self-Destruction,* Science House, New York, 1967, pp. 324–344.

12. Plath, Sylvia: "Daddy," in *Ariel,* Harper & Row, New York, 1966, p. 51.

13. Freud, Sigmund: *Beyond the Pleasure Principle,* J. Strachey (trans.), Liveright, New York, 1950.

14. Klein, Melanie, Paula Heimann, and R. E. Money-Kyrle: *New Directions in Psychoanalysis: The Significance of Infant Conflict in the Pattern of Adult Behavior,* Basic Books, New York, 1955.

15. Heimann, Paula: "A Contribution to the Re-Evaluation of the Oedipus Complex–The Early Stages," in ibid., p. 25.

16. Hendin, Herbert: *Suicide in Scandinavia*. Grune & Stratton, New York, 1964.

17. Menninger, Karl A.: *Man Against Himself*, Harcourt, Brace & World, New York, 1938.

18. Lester: op. cit., p. 132 (orig. pub.).

19. Ibid., p. 146 (orig. pub.).

20. Hillman: op. cit., p. 67.

21. Von Franz, Marie-Louise: *The Problem of the Puer Aeternus*, Spring Publications, The Analytical Psychology Club of New York, Inc., 1970.

22. Henderson, Joseph: *Thresholds of Initiation*, Wesleyan, Middletown, Conn., 1967, pp. 22–29.

23. Milford, Nancy: *Zelda*, Harper & Row, New York, 1970.

24. Alvarez: op. cit., pp. 279–283.

25. Hillman: op. cit., pp. 56–76.

26. Ibid., pp. 92–94.

27. Neuringer, C.: "Methodological Problems in Suicide Research," *J. Consult. Psychol.*, 26:273–278, 1962.

28. Shneidman, Edwin S.: "Sleep and Self-Destruction," in Shneidman (ed.), *Essays in Self-Destruction*, Science House, New York, 1967, pp. 510–539.

29. *Palo Alto Times*, Palo Alto, Calif., Feb. 23, 1972, p. 30.

30. Lester: op. cit., p. 5 (orig. pub.).

31. Farberow and Shneidman: op. cit., pp. 19–74.

32. Parkin, D., and Erwin Stengel: "Incidence of Suicidal Attempts in an Urban Community," *Brit. Med. J.*, 2:133, 1965.

33. Stengel: loc. cit.

34. Schmidt, E. H., Patricia O'Neil, and Eli Robins: "Evaluation of Suicide Attempts as a Guide to Therapy," *J. Am. Med. Ass.*, 155: 549–557, 1954.

35. Weisz, Alfred E., Donald C. Staight, Peter Houts, and Michael Volen: "Suicide Threats, Suicide Attempts, and the Emergency Psychiatrist," *Proceedings of 4th International Conference for Suicide Prevention*, Norman L. Farberow (ed.), Delmar Publishing Co., Los Angeles, 1968.

36. Beall, Lynette: "The Dynamics of Suicide: A Review of the Literature, 1897–1965," *Reflections*, 5(5):12–38, 1970.

37. Delong, W. B., and Eli Robins: "The Communication of Suicidal Intent Prior to Psychiatric Hospitalization," *Am. J. Psychiat.*, 117:695–705, 1961.

38. Dublin, Louis, in Erwin Stengel, op. cit., p. 33.

39. Robins, Eli, Seymour Gassner, Jack Kayes, Robert Wilkinson, Jr., and George Murphy: "The Communication of Suicidal Intent: A Study of 134 Consecutive Cases of Successful (Completed) Suicide," *Am. J. Psychiat.*, 115:724–733, 1959.

40. Dorpat, T. L., and H. S. Ripley: "The Relationship between Attempted Suicide and Completed Suicide," *Compr. Psychiat.*, 8:74–89, 1967.

41. Hendin, Herbert: *Black Suicide*, Basic Books, New York, 1969.

42. Retterstol, Nils: *Long-Term Prognosis After Attempted Suicide*, Charles C Thomas, Springfield, Ill., 1970.

43. Lester: op. cit., p. 194 (orig. pub.).

44. Douglas, Jack: *The Social Meanings of Suicide*, Princeton, Princeton, N.J., 1967.

45. Alvarez: op. cit., p. 81.

46. Choron, Jacques: *Suicide*, Scribner, New York, 1972.

47. Moss, Leonard M., and Donald Hamilton: "Psychotherapy of the Suicidal Patient," in Edwin S. Shneidman and Norman L. Farberow (eds.), *Clues to Suicide*, McGraw-Hill, New York, 1957, pp. 99–110.

48. Hilgard, Josephine, and Martha F. Newman: "Anniversaries in Mental Illness," *Psychiatry*, vol. 22, May 1959.

49. Weiss, E.: "The Clinical Significance of the Anniversary Reaction," *Gen. Pract.*, 17:117–119, 1958.

50. Alvarez: op. cit., pp. 268–269.

51. Ibid.: p. 128.

52. Weisz, Alfred E., and Robert Taylor: "The Assassination Matrix," *Stanford Today*, pp. 11–17, Winter 1969.

53. Fox, Ruth: *Alcoholism*, Charles C Thomas, Springfield, Ill., 1967, p. 245.

54. Menninger: loc. cit.

55. Yalom, Irvin D., and M. A. Lieberman: "A Study of Encounter Group Casualties," *Arch. Gen. Psychiat.*, 24:16–30, 1971.

56. Litman, Robert: "Management of Acutely Suicidal Patients in Medical Practice," *Calif. Med.*, 104:168–174, 1966.

57. Massey, J. T.: *Suicide in the United States*, PHS Publication 1000, ser. 20, no. 5, U.S. Department of Health, Education, and Welfare, 1967.

58. Litman, Robert, T. Murphey, Edwin S. Shneidman, Norman L. Farberow, and N. Tabachnick: "The Psychological Autopsy of Equivocal Deaths," in Edwin S. Shneidman, Norman L. Farberow, and Robert E. Litman (eds.), *The Psychology of Suicide*, Science House, New York, 1970, chap. 30.

59. Robins, et al: loc. cit.

60. Miller, Warren: "The Ecological Group," this book, chap. 32.

61. Litman: loc. cit.

Treatment of the Suicidal Patient

Some people turn to suicide to resolve interpersonal struggles; others want only to be done with struggle. For the first kind of patient, the seemingly introverted act of suicide has the extraverted meaning of influencing another person. The second type has given up on the extraverted world, and an introverted plunge into self-destruction seems the only way out of despair.[1] If the patient uses suicide to influence others, the therapist should aid at helping him find another way of getting himself heard. If suicide expresses loss of connection, the therapist must try to reconnect the individual with life. Both themes may be present in a given patient whose ambivalence reflects a tension between his extraverted and introverted feelings.[2,3] At different stages of treatment, one or the other theme may be dominant, and the therapist must be guided accordingly. Throughout the treatment the therapist must expect to be *active* and vitally involved with the patient in seeking alternatives to suicide as the solution to external and internal problems.

THE ACTION RESPONSE

The therapist counters the immobilization response (Chapter 2) of the patient's ecological group by a strong *action response*. By word and deed he indicates that he is vitally interested in keeping his patient alive and that if need be he is willing to be the lifeline. He counters the patient's ambivalence with firmness. For instance, the therapist may sit through a meal hour with an elderly patient who will not talk and insist that he eat all the food on his hospital tray.

The therapist must also open the patient's closed world to the feeling-responses of others and mobilize those in the ecological group who have been immobilized so they can share the extremity of the patient's predicament and stay involved with the treatment.

Finally, the action response dictates that the therapist be available to the patient in both the physical sense of being readily accessible by phone and willing to set up extra appointments as they are needed and in the emotional sense of being able to put his own feelings into clear, unambiguous verbal statements. In addition to talking, considerable caring behavior is required.

Example 3-1, Alice (cont'd). The resident working with Alice soon found that if he were slightly late for his appointment she would be sullen and uncommunicative. He made a point of being on the ward when he said he would, and the sessions became more productive. Throughout, Alice maintained that she could not understand why he should bother about her and said she did not need therapy:

The therapist soon will be tested to show that he has mastered nonverbal language, that he understands behavior signaling distress, and that he is able to convey concern by his own behavior. To pass the test, the therapist must express verbally what the patient's behavior leads him to feel and conjecture and must show by his own behavior what he wants the patient to understand.

Alice (cont'd). The night Alice was admitted the resident told her, "The fact that you want to leave this emergency room without any more plans than you had when you took the pills makes me think you still feel like killing yourself. Therefore I have to keep you in the hospital until I'm convinced you aren't going to take your life."

Alice immediately said, "If I tell you I won't take my life, will you let me go?"

The resident replied, "No, because your situation hasn't changed."

Alice then said, "I can get a lawyer to make you let me go."

The resident replied, "If I put a hold on you, you're entitled to a lawyer. But I'll say in court what I've said to you: your situation makes me think there's a great risk of suicide." He maintained his position through several minutes of cross-examination by Alice, who was keeping her eyes averted.

The resident used the style of communication he had learned to use with suicidal patients: (1) he told Alice in words what her behavior said to him, and (2) he backed up his verbal expression of concern with caring behavior, in this case a willingness to place a seventy-two-hour police hold on her if she did not accept voluntary hospitalization. This action response was in marked contrast to those made on her two previous discharges from emergency rooms after ingestions, when she was let go without recommendations for further treatment. A verbal statement of concern along with an offer of outpatient therapy would have seemed perfunctory to this hardened veteran of rejection.

THE ECOLOGICAL GROUP APPROACH

Rationale of the Approach

The members of the patient's ecological group should be included in the treatment process from the beginning. Too often, however, the therapist feels he has adequate information for treatment decisions from interviews with the patient alone. Failure to include others often results from binds the patient tries to place on communication.

Alice (cont'd). Although the resident did rather well in standing up to Alice's denials of the precariousness of her situation, he was considerably less effective in establishing his right to talk to several others who might have been included in her treatment planning. Because of Alice's assertions that she was "through with Bradley," the resident felt inhibited about including him in what seemed to be a confidential relationship. Her ex-husband Rolfe was now ill with cancer of the liver, and their 14-year-old son Billy lived with Rolfe and his new wife. Don and Joe were in jail. Alice's brother, a stable, married policeman, lived across the country, as did her mother, who had a heart condition.

Alice and Rolfe's new wife were concerned about Rolfe's terminal illness and the planning that should be done for Billy. Alice wanted to take Billy to live with her and Bradley after Rolfe's death, but the resident did not feel he had the right to contact Rolfe and his wife and make them participants in Alice's current treatment. Alice had said she did not want Billy, a shy, wilting adolescent, involved. She said, "That kid's been through enough already." Neither did she want her brother involved in her current difficulties with Bradley, even though he had offered Billy a home. The jailed sons seemed inaccessible. Alice did not want to worry her mother and possibly aggravate her heart condition.

The resident and the ward staff were trapped by Alice's denial and her insistent focus on her romantic vicissitudes with Bradley. They failed to deal with other areas of significance to Alice, especially with Billy's future. This major error in focus was reinforced by the patient's and staff's almost total avoidance of Rolfe's terminal illness. It was as if not talking about it would make it go away.

Unconcious collusion of the therapist and ward staff with a patient's denial is not uncommon. Careful supervision by someone outside the treatment process can be of great help in avoiding such collusion. The decision to exclude members of Alice's ecological group drastically limited the scope of the crisis intervention. Although the immediate threat of suicide was reduced by the strategy adopted (couple therapy), Alice's entire course of psychotherapy was affected by the failure to start with the widest possible evaluation.

When information is not obtained from members of the ecological group, the immediate results may be tragic.

Example 3-2. A previously active 45-year-old divorced mother of one married daughter and two teenagers had been paraplegic for two years following an auto accident. The week after losing a $150,000 lawsuit she visited her urologist, who noted a serious exacerbation of her chronic depression. Although she was adamant in refusing to see a psychiatrist, the urologist sought psychiatric consultation anyway. The emergency therapist called the patient at home.

Over the telephone she described her recent suffering, and when asked if she were unhappy enough to kill herself, she replied that she had often thought of it but did not plan to commit suicide for at least two or three years because she still had two teenagers to take care of.

The reassured resident discussed outpatient psychiatric treatment with her, but she continued to resist the idea. He left his name in case she decided to seek help.

Three weeks later the patient killed herself by hooking a newly purchased garden hose to the exhaust of her car and starting the motor.

The resident interviewed the patient's three daughters. The eldest, 22, told him, "Mother threatened every day to everyone that she was going to commit suicide. Sometimes she was sarcastic, sometimes she was bitter, and sometimes she was humorous about it." She said that all her mother's hopes had depended on the court case, and she had noticed the depression following its loss. She felt this was "only normal." This daughter had discovered the newly purchased garden hose sitting in the front seat of the car. She had asked her mother about it and was told in a characteristically dry way that this hose would be more effective than the old one.

The 18-year-old daughter had also noted the recent purchase of the hose. She lived in the house but took no action because "She was always threatening, I couldn't watch her day and night." She added that during the past week the mother had visited several wheelchair clubs and had commented with surprise on the happiness of the members.

The youngest daughter, 14, said that her mother had frequently confided her despair to her. She said she had repeatedly said to all of them, "If I try to kill myself, I don't want to fail."

This case illustrates the danger of an individual approach to the resistant suicidal patient. The emergency therapist blundered in relying on the patient's statement that she would stay alive to take care of her children. If he had insisted on interviewing them, he would have recognized their immobilization. The children could have been advised that the depression they accepted as usual in their mother was a treatable illness, and hospitalization could have been pursued. In later treatment their anger and immobilization would be important targets for intervention if the mother's hopeless feeling about herself were to be countered.

Crisis Resolution by Means of the Ecological Approach

After a suicide threat or attempt, the therapist gathers together the patient and key members of the group and states openly that the patient has been having suicidal feelings and is a definite risk. He tells them that the danger poses a problem for all of them and that he wants to help them as a group to find a solution to the crisis and any issues which have led to it.

In the drama that ensues, and with the supportive presence of the therapist, members of the ecological group are often able to resolve long-standing difficulties (see Chapter 1, "Principles of Crisis Intervention"). This way of working with the suicidal patient has particular advantages. First, it reinforces the effectiveness of verbal communication because the therapist's authority lends credence to the patient's stated threat to die. His own words translate the patient's ambiguous or nonverbal communication into intelligible statements. Second, sufficient drama and attention are given to meet whatever threatrical need-signaling is present in the patient. The drama of a group confrontation in the therapist's office accomplishes much that an actual attempt might. It gives others the message that the patient is suffering and allows them to present evidence of their concern.

Finally, the ecological approach enables the therapist to discover to what extent the group is providing a lethal context for the patient. Key members may wish the patient gone or dead. (Studies of voodoo deaths show dramatically that group wishes can be fulfilled.) When the group is bent on extruding the patient, the therapist may have to help the patient realize that membership in *this* group is no longer a viable option.

> *Example 3-3.* A 25-year-old man was brought into the emergency room by his parents-in-law. Their daughter had left him, and he had recently taken to hanging despondently around their kitchen. At first he insisted his wife would return and refused to accept their assertions to the contrary. Their patience and

sympathy for the son-in-law began to wear thin. When he began talking openly about suicide, they were relieved to have a legitimate reason to get him out of their house and into the hands of "someone who could talk some sense into him." They made it clear to the emergency therapist that their involvement with the patient was now at an end. They felt that they had discharged their responsibility by bringing him to treatment.

Thus the ecological approach can help to mobilize resources or identify the permanent extinction of old resources. Often this approach has two outcomes: (1) the patient is helped to achieve some long-desired interpersonal goal (e.g., a mother-in-law agrees to baby-sit or a husband to quit his second job) or (2) the group is helped to dispose of the patient. In either case the ecological group approach attempts to do in a life-preserving way what a suicide attempt might try to accomplish self-destructively.

This neat formulation of suicidal crisis resolution somewhat obscures the *ambivalence* that pervades the suicidal process in the ecological group as well as in the patient. Although group members often make superficial changes to please the patient and the therapist, it is usually more difficult to find out from them whether, at bottom, they really want relationships with the patient.

> *Alice (cont'd.).* In couple therapy and on the ward, Bradley acted eager to help and to make a new attempt at a relationship with Alice. But when the resident was leaving the ward, Bradley would often follow him, saying, "Do you think she's really schiz? I mean I don't want to get stuck with a psycho on my hands, if you know what I mean."
>
> The resident was troubled by Bradley's ambivalence, but he didn't know what to do about it. Following advice he had been given, he tried not to see Bradley or Alice individually once the couple sessions had begun. He did see Alice alone during the time she was on

the ward, but her suspiciousness made him wary of seeing Bradley without her.

Uncertainty in the ecological group about the patient's belonging is a major factor in the patient's ambivalence about living or dying. This uncertainty cannot be well resolved without a frank discussion of the possibility of separation. The significant others cannot work through their negative feelings about the patient in a setting where they are not able to air their views. The presence of a recently suicidal person is distinctly inhibiting to direct expressions of disaffection. The therapist, therefore, should also hold separate individual sessions with group members. He should not allow himself to be bound by pseudoconfidentiality; he must be judicious about sharing what he hears. He should make it possible for the various group members to state their feelings honestly, fully, privately, and without the fear that in doing so they will provoke the patient to suicide.

Example 3-4. A 28-year-old woman brought her 25-year-old husband to the emergency room. She tearfully admitted that he was suicidal because of her; she could not make up her mind whether or not to leave him. Couple therapy started, but no progress was made. The wife continued to vacillate, and the husband remained suicidal. The therapist decided to see them separately.

The wife revealed in her individual session that she was in love with another man and the only reason she stayed with her husband was her fear he would kill himself so that she could be free. This thought made her feel extremely guilty.

The therapist asked the husband what he would do if his wife actually left. (In the couple sessions the answer to this question had always been unequivocal: "I'd kill myself for sure.") The husband said, "I'll tell you *this*. If my wife really left for good, I don't think I'd kill myself. I'd ask you to put me in some quiet place, and I'd cry on somebody's shoulder until I was ready to get out and find somebody else."

Before the next joint interview, the therapist encouraged the wife to tell her husband the truth, and he prepared to support the husband. The husband first broke down, then accepted hospitalization. After a week of hospitalization and a week of day care he was able to enter productive outpatient psychotherapy without a return of serious suicidal feelings.

His wife did not continue in therapy. During her husband's hospitalization she filed for divorce. Eventually she married the other man.

When Not to Use the Ecological Approach

Obviously not every suicidal patient should be approached through his ecological group. Experienced therapists may well be dismayed by the recommendation for *routine* use of extensive contacts with significant others. They know of well-motivated patients who have sought individual therapy at a time of active suicidal thinking and have done well in it, without any outside contacts. Such patients are capable of recognizing when a formerly sustaining social ecology has dried up, and they are capable of initiating contact with new people to put their lives in order. For them therapist-initiated contacts with others might well be infantilizing or restricting and might possibly inhibit movement *out* of an undesirable life situation. Also, the therapeutic relationship is often more effective when it is kept entirely between two people.

Example 3-5. A 40-year-old single, professional woman contemplated suicide when a five-year homosexual relationship ended. She sought therapy a week after a mild overdose of pills. At the initial interview she seemed ready to begin depth therapy with an experienced, analytically oriented therapist. She soon formed a close bond with him.

During the first months of therapy the patient was able to enter into a sexual relationship with a man. A year and a half after treatment began the patient married. She continued therapy through the first year of her marriage and terminated when the marriage seemed assured of going well. Throughout the course of treatment, the analyst's only contact was with the patient.

Experiences similar to this one are common in private practice, where the fee and the referral process tend to select patients who are highly motivated to change and able to use an intense transference relationship positively. When the patient is met in the midst of crisis in an emergency room setting, his degree of motivation for change is still unknown, and the ecological group approach offers the best chance for adequate crisis intervention. The occasional disadvantages of overinvolving others in a patient's treatment are far outweighed by the advantages this approach holds for opening up a potential suicide's closed world.

THE INITIAL INTERVIEW

The initial interview is particularly critical for the suicidal patient: if it goes badly, it may be the *only* interview. Mintz[4] suggests a checklist of tasks the therapist ought to accomplish during the initial interview. The checklist, with slight modifications, is

1. Obtain the necessary personal data immediately. These include the patient's name, age, telephone number, place of occupation, residence, and the names of his closest friends and family members.

2. Bring the subject of suicide into the open. Also obtain information about suicidal thoughts, plans, preparations, and attempts.

3. Insist on the removal of all firearms and potentially lethal medications from the patient's home.

4. Notify and arrange to meet with one or more significant responsible others in the patient's life.

5. Discuss the natural history of depressive illnesses and their favorable responses to treatment.

6. Formulate and communicate a specific initial treatment plan.

7. Specifically schedule a next appointment for patients who are not hospitalized.

8. Be sure the patient is able to contact you.

There are a number of other points to be considered in utilizing Mintz's suggestions and conducting the first interview. First, even though the interview may be conducted by a nonmedical mental health worker, it should take place in a hospital, clinic, or other place where medical tradition and authority are in evidence. An atmosphere of medical authority can help to influence the ambivalent patient and ecological group to take seriously the life-protective measures that are recommended.

The therapist must consider how he presents psychiatric intervention to the patient. His primary concern is to preserve the patient's life, but if he tries to accomplish this in an overzealous, authoritarian manner he may drive the suicidal impulse underground, and it will surface again in a lethal form when he is unavailable. This is as true for involuntary as for voluntary patients. Consistently the therapist must regard the patient as someone who is, or soon can be, responsible enough to choose treatment when its goals are made clear to him. It follows that the patient is, or soon will be, free to withdraw from any treatment he finds unreasonable. For this reason a special challenge is to demonstrate sufficient courtesy, compassion, and tact to induce the involuntary patient to continue treatment.

Finding out the patient's name, address, and phone number *immediately* can be crucial because many suicidal people isolate themselves by using unlisted phone numbers, post office box addresses, and changed names. The anonymous patient is difficult or impossible to trace if he hurriedly leaves his office or becomes disconnected on the phone. Some patients even call the emergency room, give only meager identifying data, and announce they are going to kill themselves. The emergency therapist must make it clear from the beginning that he wants to establish and maintain contact. He should keep phone numbers and other information with him for later use in case of an emergency.

Example 3-6. A 30-year-old alcoholic man called his former therapist several months after he had broken off treatment. He asked the therapist to forgive him for what he was about to do and hung up. When the therapist called the telephone number the patient had given his answering service, he found the line busy. A check with the telephone company revealed that the phone was unlisted, and no address could be found. Fortunately the therapist still had the address and phone number the patient had given him at the time of their first contact. The phone number was the same, and the therapist called the police to investigate at that address. They found the patient nearly comatose from barbiturate ingestion. His life was saved in a nearby emergency room, and a crisis team took over his care. Two days later the patient called the therapist, thanked him, and announced his intention to enter an alcohol treatment program administered by the local hospital.

To bring suicidal thinking into the open, the therapist should permit the patient to talk about his thoughts, plans, preparations, and attempts. Suicidal emotion thrives if it is not disclosed. To share his frightening, "selfish," or "immoral" suicidal thinking with someone else is almost always a great relief to the patient, and his gratitude is the beginning of a firm bond with the therapist. The few patients who become angry at this questioning usually become less depressed and are determined to prove the therapist wrong.

Example 3-7. A gruff teamster in his mid-50s, widowed and alcoholic, became increasingly depressed following prostate surgery for a benign enlargement. When he refused food, the nurses became alarmed and notified the surgeon, who in turn called in a psychiatric resident consultant. The young man inquired gently about the teamster's state of mind and met with stiff, resistant denial that anything was wrong. Finally the resident asked if the teamster had ever thought of suicide. The older man became furious, delivered a dressing down to the resident, and loudly threatened to sue the hospital for "vile insinuations." It turned out that he was a good Catholic and suicide was against his religion. The nurses asked a priest to see him, and the priest arranged a reunion with a widowed sister who was glad to arrange care for him during his convalescence. Although he never ceased to berate the "headshrinker" who visited him, everyone noticed that from the morning of the psychiatrist's visit the patient began to eat heartily and show signs of his former vigor.

If weapons, poison, or pills are in the home, every attempt should be made to have them surrendered. It is wise to involve other members of the family in this effort. In some cases they are the suppliers of the weapons, and in others they have knowledge of the stockpiled drugs or weapons. Often it is easier at a first interview to insist upon "total disarmament" than it is later in treatment, when transference resistance may push the patient into an "arms race" of escalating suicidal riskiness with his therapist.

Example 3-8. A middle-aged man came to the Veterans Administration (VA) Hospital one afternoon. He was well-dressed and appeared healthy. He admitted to the resident that since the breakup of his marriage several weeks before, he had grown despondent. The resident asked if he felt the need to enter the hospital. The patient broke down in admitting that he did and confessed he had thought of killing his former wife and himself. The resident asked if he had a means to do it, and the patient revealed that he kept a loaded pistol in the glove compartment of his car. The resident arranged admission at once and walked with the patient to his car, where the gun was surrendered. The patient said, "I was going to use it on myself if I didn't get admitted today."

It is important to secure the permission of the patient before contacting others in his life. When the patient is present, the therapist can phone the other person and explain that there is a serious risk of suicide. This procedure provides an initial model for talking openly and directly about the situation. The therapist also establishes his right to communicate with others and to act as the patient's advocate in discussing a painful subject. With extremely rigid, compulsive personalities who feel guilty about burdening others, a stern insistence that frank communication is necessary usually works to secure the needed permission.

Depressive illnesses remit and respond to treatment. Without treatment, a depressive illness may last a few weeks or months. With treatment, improvement begins in days or weeks. The depressed patient and his ecological group should be told that his present suffering will not last indefinitely because depressive illnesses tend to remit with a full return of usual function.[5,6] Therefore, the emergency psychiatrist can counter stereotyped notions about the irreversibility of "mental illness" as far as depression is concerned. Firmness is necessary to deal with the pessimism characteristic of depression.

The therapist should formulate a specific initial treatment plan. The suicidal person lives in a vague, indecisive state, and the decision to die usually comes when there is nothing definite in his life. The therapist must give direct, unambiguous statements that leave no doubt about what he means. His initial plan should be simple, clear, and definite, and he should take pains to be sure that the patient understands exactly what is expected of him.

If the plan involves a trial period of outpatient treatment, the therapist may say to the patient,

> I would like you to start treatment immediately. I want us to meet twice a week for the next three weeks. Our sessions will be fifty minutes long, and we will try to understand together what is causing this depression and what can be done to help you find relief. Between sessions you may feel panicky or upset, and I expect you to call me. If I am going to be away, I will let you know, and someone who knows that you may be calling will be available.
>
> Under no circumstances are you to hesitate to call if you feel upset. If you feel pressed to act on your suicidal feelings, I expect you to call me before you act. During the next three weeks I will be in touch with people who are close to you, and we will schedule joint sessions when necessary. I will expect them to call me if they have any concerns. At the end of the three-week period we will all evaluate the situation again and make a decision on where to go from there.

If the therapist is not this definite, the patient may conclude that he does not care or appreciate the depth of his confusion. The patient may then signal his dilemma by a nonverbal "appeal" such as a suicide attempt.

It is important that the other members of the ecological group also understand the plan. Occasionally the treatment plan that seems reasonable to the patient and therapist will not meet with favor from important others. Their feelings are significant and should be taken into account. For example, an anxious wife may want to be present during her husband's interview or may not want to assume the burden of having him remain an outpatient. The wise therapist will not regard her as a nuisance, even if her presence complicates the therapy. He will recognize that he needs her active cooperation if treatment is to succeed, and he may have to make concessions to secure that cooperation. A good plan must be acceptable to the entire ecological group and must give all the members a sense that they are in competent hands and have a good chance of resolving their difficulties. Unspoken disapproval of the treatment plan may result in immobilization toward the patient and thus increase the risk of suicide.

The therapist should not end the first session until a next definite appointment has been made, even if the patient has not yet agreed to enter psychiatric treatment. For example, when the paraplegic woman in Example 3-2 declined treatment on the first contact, the psychiatrist left her his phone number in case she changed her mind. Instead, he could have said, "I want you to take a whole day to think about your decision to decline treatment, and I want to hear from you between four and five tomorrow. I will be in my office waiting for your call. This is my telephone number." If he had heard from her at that time, the resident could have continued negotiating about treatment and might possibly have secured an agreement to talk by telephone at regularly scheduled intervals during the period of acute crisis. If he had not heard from her, the resident could have telephoned her to express his continued concern. He could probably also have expressed his concern about her to her urologist, who might have helped him to persuade family members to attend an emergency strategy meeting.

In short, the definite appointment becomes a focus around which the degree of suicidal intent can be gauged and can also be used to demonstrate concern to an ambivalent patient. A patient's failure to keep the appointment can be interpreted as a presuicidal communication and should be responded to immediately. A failure on the therapist's part will be interpreted by the patient as a lack of concern. The therapist must take care in noting down and arranging to keep the appointment he makes. This is true whether the appointment is set up over the telephone or in the office.

The patient must be able to reach the therapist. Confused patients easily forget names, and they tire of fighting busy switchboards and indifferent answering services. Before the first interview ends, the therapist should write down his name, professional address, and phone number, preferably on an appointment card or prescription blank, and give it to the patient. The patient should be able to say the therapist's name, know his exact title, and know how to reach him in case this written information is mislaid. The first interview can be brought to an end with the lines of communication clearly established and with the explicit understanding that the patient and therapist expect to use the channels discussed.

It is the therapist's responsibility to make sure emergency room staff, clinic secretaries, hospital or answering service operators, and members of his own ecological group know how to reach him at all times. It is his responsibility to ascertain that the intermediaries between him and the patient have sufficient information to communicate for him during his temporary absences. It helps for the therapist to explain to the others that the patient is a suicide risk and that if he cannot be reached in a reasonable time, he wants a backup professional to be notified.

Sometimes an emergency therapist will conclude the first interview by referring the patient to another professional. As a consultant, he should ensure that the patient will be able to reach the professional and that a definite appointment has been made. Almost always he will need to speak personally to the other professional. He must also serve as a backup until the patient is solidly established in treatment with the other person. Thus the referring emergency therapist could say to the patient, "I expect you to call me back if any difficulties arise with this referral. I will be checking with your therapist to see that you have started." And he must do so. Again, if the therapist is not meticulous in following up on his referral, the patient may feel rejected and act out his ambivalence about treatment by attempting suicide. Even after he has referred a patient, the emergency therapist must assume that he is the lifeline until the patient is connected to another source of support.

THE DECISION TO HOSPITALIZE

The resident handled many of the tasks of the first interview by hospitalizing Alice. Although this decision relieved him of immediate anxiety concerning Alice's committing suicide, it also created problems in treatment. In this section we shall examine the criteria for hospitalization and the problems that occur after the decision to hospitalize has been made.

Initial Aspects of Hospitalization

The criterion for hospitalization is simple. If the therapist does not trust the patient to call him before making an attempt on his life, he should recommend hospitalization. This criterion does *not* mean that hospitalization, any more than outpatient treatment, guarantees the patient will not kill himself or that the therapist can assume final responsibility for the patient's decision about death. What it does mean is that the therapist stands against the *impulsive* decision to die. The strategy is similar to the use of Antabuse® with alcoholic patients. The drug cannot assume the responsibility for the patient's decision about abstaining from alcohol, but it does give him three days, the time it takes the medicine to leave his system, to think about returning to alcohol. Seventy-two-hour involuntary hospitalization is permissible in the state of California when a patient is unable to care for himself or is a danger to himself or to others.

The therapist can say, "I would like you to come into the hospital for at least three days. During that time we will all be able to take a closer look at this situation and come to a decision about how to proceed with treatment. It may be that a longer period of hospitalization will be necessary, or it may be that we can continue on an outpatient basis after that. I do think we need to make this decision inside, not outside, the hospital." The therapist neither presents hospitalization as a "cure for suicide" nor as a judgment of the patient's and the group's ultimate ability to resolve

the crisis. He presents the hospital as an environment more conducive to the therapeutic process that hopefully will reconnect the patient with his normal desire to live. The same need for his cooperation, the same need for outside support, and the same ultimate risk follow the patient into the hospital. After all, he is the same patient.

Certainly the therapist should not be afraid to use the hospital. Keeping the patient *out* of the hospital becomes an end in itself for some therapists, almost a proof of therapeutic macho. Others fear the anger patients sometimes show when hospitalization is suggested. Such considerations obscure the initial purpose of therapeutic work with suicidal people—the clear, unambivalent expression of concern. Neither the therapist's vanity nor the patient's anger is important when hospitalization becomes the appropriate expression of that concern.

Once the decision to hospitalize has been made, a new crisis occurs. Having just been told that a professional does not think he can control himself, the patient should not be sent home unguarded to pick up a toothbrush, razor, or any other personal belongings. Also, the therapist should recognize that the anxiety which attends entry into a new environment can lead to a suicide attempt the first night on the ward.

Ideally the therapist should take the patient to the ward himself, introduce him to the head nurse, explain in his presence that the patient has had impulsive thoughts of suicide, and request the ward staff's or family's help in bringing personal necessities from the patient's home to the ward. Such arrangements are usually easy to make. Occasionally the therapist may have to accompany the patient home to pick up the items.

Alice (cont'd.). After he had made it clear to Alice that he was determined to put her in the hospital, the resident met with stiff resistance over the issue of getting her belongings. She raised a number of objections to being accompanied by Bradley or by her son but finally acceded to the resident's suggestion that he go with her. Her small, ugly hotel room with clothing strewn around was a reminder to the resident of the squalor of her life. She gave the pills in the room to the resident and collected her possessions. They returned to the psychiatric ward.

The resident introduced Alice to the night nurse and explained that she had made a suicide attempt earlier in the evening, that they had gone together to get her belongings, and that she would have to remain on the ward until he could see her the following day. He told Alice that he would see her at 2 o'clock the following afternoon and left her in the care of the night nurse. He wrote a brief admission note, admitting orders (including ward restrictions and suicidal precautions), and his home phone number in the chart.

Medical Hospitalization

Patients who have attempted suicide with pills (especially aspirin, barbiturates, and tranquilizers), poisons (especially arsenic and carbon monoxide), or violence (knives or guns) *must* be medically treated and cleared before they are admitted to a psychiatric ward. Contrary to occasional belief, psychiatric wards usually are *not* equipped to evaluate either the acute symptoms or delayed complications of physical trauma. Patients whose medical status is in doubt should be treated on a medical or surgical ward by internists, neurologists, and surgeons, and they should stay on the medical ward until they are given medical clearance.

The psychiatrist should make himself available to the medical staff as a consultant and should use the principles described in Chapter 31. Internists may want to make a premature transfer of patients to the psychiatric ward because they are afraid that the patient will make another suicide attempt while he is under their care. Psychiatric consultation can help to assure and support the medical staff in their treatment of the patient as well as assist with proper referral for further psychiatric treatment on either an in- or an outpatient basis.

Psychiatric Hospitalization

The advantages and disadvantages of psychiatric hospitalization for suicidal patients are many and varied. Some of the themes to be discussed are developed further in Chapter 10 ("Acute Inpatient Intervention"), which treats hospitalization as a separate topic.

Psychiatric hospitalization per se performs no miracles. The patient may use the period of hospitalization to plan for death while he makes a token "recovery" to convince his therapist that he has "gotten over being silly." The ecological approach to establishing a lifeline can be used with a maximum degree of safety in the hospital.

The therapist should present a detailed history to the ward staff, and together they should work out a careful treatment plan with explicit goals. The patient should be told about these considerations so he can allow the staff to help him open up his closed world. As time goes on, the staff can offer the often lonely and discouraged therapist consultation and companionship through personal contact and nursing notes. He in turn can serve as a model to the staff by telling them what he is trying to accomplish. The staff that is listened to by the therapist is more likely to listen to the patient, and, as we have already seen, suicidal people require much support in making their feelings heard.

Alice (cont'd.). One positive feature of Alice's hospitalization was the degree of give-and-take between the resident and the ward staff. The resident made a point of talking with the nurses each time he visited Alice on the ward. The nurses in turn gave him a great deal of information about their contact with Alice, and they paid a good deal of attention to her. Alice's mood improved markedly as the hospital stay continued. From her initially guarded, suspicious style of communication, she moved toward an increasingly friendly openness and began to reach out to other patients. The ward staff regarded this change as progress, and they began to like her.

Structure and Expectations. The patient should be expected to participate in a structured program, i.e., attend group meetings, eat meals, observe ward rules, and so on. Patients often test the concern of others by failing to participate in any or all of these activities, disappearing without notice, and so forth. The therapist must carefully observe the patient and consult with the nursing staff during his daily visits so he will be able to detect such testing and bring it to the patient's notice. This is further proof to the patient of the therapist's unambivalent wish for him to live.

The therapist does not have to be a "nice guy" to set limits. Rather, his should be a clear and unemotional stance that insists on participation, that will believe the patient's stated interest in treatment when it is demonstrated by his behavior. The therapist may have to stand over an ambivalent, psychotically depressed patient and insist that he eat his food. He may say, "No, you have to stay here, you have to finish your plate; no, I expect you to eat," and so on.

If the patient makes a suicidal gesture in the ward (usually minor wrist cutting with a stray razor), the therapist should make it clear that he will not tolerate this behavior and should immediately offer an acceptable way for the patient to signal his distress to the ward staff in the event a similar situation arises. If a more serious attempt on life is made, the therapist should arrange a special conference between himself, the ward staff, and the patient. In addition to hearing the patient out, the therapist should make it clear that he expects the patient to communicate verbally to someone when he feels driven to hurt himself. A patient will almost always hear this message when it is given in the atmosphere of crisis following a serious attempt in the ward. The experience may be the turning point for a depressed patient in taking the ward and his treatment seriously.

Potential Dangers. Before a patient is hospitalized, it is important to be aware of the potential negative effects of the inpatient experience. Among these are the opportunities the hospital affords the chronically suicidal patient to establish *hostile dependency* on the unit, to *split the staff,* and to form *"sick" friendships.* These themes are illustrated by some of the events that took place during Alice's stay in the hospital.

Alice (cont'd.). Alice accepted hospitalization only grudgingly in the first place. After all, it had been the psychiatric resident's idea, not hers. Technically, however, hers was a voluntary admission. She lived in a state that offered medical insurance to indigent patients, and to avoid a large bill she had to establish her inability to pay.

Alice simultaneously passively thwarted efforts by the hospital business office to establish her eligibility for assistance and complained to the resident that she didn't see how she could pay her bill. He didn't want to be bothered with what seemed to him trivial paperwork and mistakenly assumed it would automatically be taken care of at some point. The matter came to haunt the later course of Alice's treatment.

While the resident was taking a short vacation, Alice made an issue with the ward chief about the impossibility of paying her bill, refused to accept his reassurance, and angrily signed out against medical advice. This action defined her as a financial delinquent on the hospital records and precluded readmission until she paid her bill.

Alice expressed her anger at being taken care of through passive-aggressive tactics. She would not clarify her financial position, complained that it prevented her from being helped, and thus turned a resource into a liability. Hostile response to dependency is typical of the suicidal person's ambivalence.

Frequently the patient's ambivalence can be discerned by the way a staff splits in its response to him. Part of the staff believes one treatment should be used, and the rest believes another.

Alice (cont'd.). Alice's insistence on returning

to Bradley infuriated the nurses, who had spent many hours trying to talk her out of it. The resident found the idea at least plausible if not ideal, and in heated staff discussions he pointed out that if Alice and Bradley did separate, they would only seek out similar new partners. The staff told the resident he was a hero for wanting to try with Alice and that if she improved he would have performed a therapeutic miracle. The first-year resident was still naïve and susceptible to seeing himself in a heroic role. After Alice left the hospital he started outpatient treatment without first seeking consultation. If he had, he could have taken the middle course of neither encouraging nor discouraging the relationship with Bradley.

Sometimes it seems that an inpatient staff is furnishing adequate consultation when it is not. The resident and the inpatient staff, including the ward chief, thought that a reasoned decision had been made. No one recognized how much Alice's ambivalent psychology influenced everyone to accept both the hopelessness of her relationship with Bradley and the impossibility of her survival without it.

Another potential hazard of hospitalization is the opportunity it furnishes patients to find other people with whom they can interact in a mutually self-defeating manner.

Alice (cont'd.). After Alice left the hospital she moved in with Frank, a depressed patient on day care. She took care of him and in return he gave her money and a place to stay. Bradley moved in almost immediately. He and Alice reported this arrangement to the resident at the first couple therapy session after his vacation. To Alice's mind, this arrangement met the therapist's demand that she have a place to live and a means of support.

For several weeks Alice and Bradley systematically took advantage of Frank, who even signed over his car to Bradley. Finally Frank's exasperated therapist called the resident during a session with Alice and Bradley and handed the phone to Frank. Frank told the startled resident, "Tell Bradley to stop using me."

Long-Range Aspects of Hospitalization. Patients recovering from a severe depression may become more suicidal as they recover from emotional paralysis and regain energy and initiative. *They must be carefully observed during this period.* Proposed shifts from total hospitalization to day care or discharge may seem desirable to the therapist but may feel like imminent abandonment to the patient. He must be allowed to express this feeling. The therapist may even take the initiative in exploring such feelings by saying:

> I know it feels fine now, and that's progress, but you are just past a period when you were at the brink of despair. Conflicts have a way of coming back, and I think you should expect some bad days in the near future. You should expect more depression, especially when you think there's no one around to contact, and you should be willing to try doubly hard to ask for help when that happens. If it occurs on a day when I'm away, I expect you to contact my partner, Dr. Smith.

The rationale of such a *negative prediction* is both to inform the patient with a program of action for further relapses and to employ the healing properties of a paradox. The prediction protects the patient in that, like the watched pot which never boils, the unconscious finds it hard to move in where consciousness is awaiting it. If depression does reappear, the patient will have the therapist's words in mind and will know this is expected behavior for him, not a sign that his treatment is a failure. His attitude can then be like the driver's who steers in the direction of the skid.

SPECIFIC THERAPEUTIC STRATEGIES

Drug Therapy

Therapists are concerned with two kinds of drugs: those the patient has been taking (frequently alcohol, barbiturates, narcotics, or stimulants) and those he is thinking of prescribing (usually antidepressants). He should take a careful history of self-medication and employ generally accepted principles in effecting withdrawal. Often depression, anxiety, and insomnia are caused by these drugs and diminish markedly or disappear when their use is discontinued. If the use of drugs has been heavy, or the patient's ability to withdraw is doubtful, he should be hospitalized for supervised withdrawal.

The therapist should evaluate the patient in the drug-free state so he has a base line against which to measure change. Some patients are drug-free on first contact or on admission; others need to be withdrawn. Many hospitalized patients will improve significantly within the first week of admission and will show considerable diminution of the target symptoms of depression, guilt, anxiety, insomnia, psychomotor retardation, agitation, and loss of appetite.

Patients undergoing a severe unipolar or involutional depression are often in such piteous condition that they should be hospitalized and placed immediately on antidepressant medications. Similarly, patients with documented manic-depressive illness in the depressed phase may benefit from lithium carbonate treatment.

Depressed, suicidal patients in milder or reactive depressions who do not respond to an initial drug-free period of treatment, whether or not in the hospital, should be started on tricyclic antidepressants (Chapter 28, "Treatment of Mania and Depression"). These drugs can be used in suicide attempts, and so long as suicide remains a substantial risk they should be prescribed in sublethal doses of at most a week's supply at a time. The "bother" of a patient's having to see a therapist frequently to refill a prescription is an advantage because it enforces regular contact and is a nonverbal statement of the doctor's concern.

Drugs, like hospitalization and legal restraint, should be employed unambivalently in both dosage and timing. Published dosage schedules for the tricyclic antidepressants often border on the

homeopathic; consult the schedules in Chapter 28. The dose should be brought into the therapeutic range in three to five days.

Insomnia is a private hell for otherwise only mildly depressed patients and can be peculiarly intractable to psychotherapeutic intervention. (If the patient is severely depressed, the insomnia usually responds to antidepressant medication along with the other symptoms.) Currently two agents surpass all others in safety for treatment of insomnia: flurazepam and chloral hydrate. Neither should be given in large quantities. Other available agents cannot be recommended for use with suicidal people; their "track record" for completed suicides is frightening. Barbiturate sleeping medications particularly have *no* place in the treatment of suicidal people; they are often stockpiled by patients who dissimulate en route to a serious, and often lethal, attempt (vide Alvarez).

It is also important to establish good consultative relationships with other professionals in the patient's life because they may become additional sources of drugs. These include internists, surgeons, dentists, and pharmacists. They need to know that the patient is suicidal and in psychiatric treatment. Their own use of psychotropic drugs in treatment of the patient should be curtailed as much as possible and coordinated with the psychiatrist's. Usually they will be glad to defer to his instructions. Courtesy and tact are essential in consultation, and communication between members of the treatment ecological group is more important than complete agreement.

Alice (cont'd.). From the beginning, drugs were a problem in the treatment of Alice and Bradley. Both were chronic drinkers (Alice's two husbands had been, too). Bradley had signs of cirrhosis; Alice did not. Both agreed to take disulfiram (Antabuse®). The resident prescribed it, hoping that if they could not drink to excess, they could not recreate the circumstances of her suicide attempt.

Alice still complained of insomnia. The resident, unaware of its potential depressant qualities, prescribed limited doses of chlor-promazine at bedtime (remembering her old therapist's conjecture, "Underneath . . . she is very confused, maybe crazy"). Initially she responded well to 100 mg at bedtime.

As Alice became quieter, Bradley grew more restive. He complained she was "like a zombie" on chlorpromazine; her immobile sleep on the drug upset him. He disliked disulfiram because it made him feel tired. Alice came to one session alone while Bradley was out on the road trying unsuccessfully once more to reactivate his promotional advertising business. She said, "I don't mind telling you this, Brad is a happy drunk. He hasn't used that pill you gave him since the first week, and I don't mind. I take mine, though. And the other one. I couldn't sleep without that one."

Psychotherapeutic drugs can quickly become a part of the patient's world, to be used in ways not originally intended by the therapist. Therefore any prescription of drugs must be clearly thought out in advance.

Electroconvulsive Therapy

Electroconvulsive therapy (ECT) is of proven worth in treating severe recurrent and involutional depressions. It should be considered seriously if psychotherapy and medication fail. Suicidal ideation per se is *not* an indication for the use of ECT, nor is the frustration of a therapist who has difficulty tolerating a patient's ambivalence and seeks a quick solution to long-standing conflict. Two possible risks of ECT are the social consequences of receiving a treatment linked to "the snake pit" in the public's mind (for instance, the response to the revelation of Democratic vice-presidential candidate Thomas Eagleton's ECT history during the summer of 1972), and the still-debated possibility of irreversible memory changes. ECT is sometimes withheld when its use would be life-saving.

Example 3-9. A 55-year-old lumberjack was brought by his wife to a minimally staffed hospital. She complained that she was tired of watching him, that he had been threatening suicide, and that he was "all slowed down." He was treated on a medical ward that had locked rooms for severely ill psychiatric patients and seen daily by a psychiatrically oriented general practitioner who was supervised by an overworked psychiatrist. He recommended joint sessions for the husband and wife and a trial period of amitryptyline. The joint sessions were used by the wife to complain of her husband's irritability and by the husband to deny the accusations. Outside the sessions the patient looked bleak and showed signs of psychomotor retardation.

After spending several days in the locked room, the patient thought he could manage on the ward. Although he still looked depressed, the physician let him out on the advice of the psychiatrist, who said, "You can't keep him locked up forever." On the next morning the patient became irritated at a nurse who was calling him to breakfast and jumped out of an upper story window. He was killed instantly.

In retrospect it is clear that he should be been referred for ECT after the failure of the antidepressants and psychotherapy.

Psychotherapeutic Strategies

Intensive psychotherapy with suicidal patients is a specialist's art, and there are certain techniques the therapist must master if he is to be effective. These include mediating catharsis, interpreting anger and hostility, separating the thought from the act, having the patient imagine his own death, encouraging activity, using the telephone, and involving the law.

Ambivalent suicidal patients often find it difficult to express negative feelings in words. When this impasse occurs, the therapist can *mediate catharsis* by expressing negative feelings for the patient.

For instance, after hearing a circumstantial account of a difficult marriage, the therapist may say, "Under the circumstances a person would be forced to feel quite angry at his wife." Or in family sessions the therapist might express what he thinks are the patient's feelings directly to the wife. This provides a model for the patient that tells him it is permissible to express such feelings.

Initially the therapist does not insist that the patient take responsibility for these feelings because he realizes they pose too much of a burden. Instead he acts as a kind of midwife to the process of catharsis and performs a certain amount of therapeutic work until the patient gains sufficient courage to acknowledge the feelings on his own.

But it can be brutal to both the patient and his family to focus on hate and ignore love. It is better, in fact, to have the patient acknowledge his love for the members of his family first; it is easier for them to accept criticism from someone they know loves them. Indeed, the suicidal patient is usually acutely aware of his own potential for destructiveness and feels a great need to protect his loved ones from it. (Suicide notes that say, "My darling wife, I don't want to hurt you anymore, I love you," express this poignantly.) Almost every depression causes grief and exasperation in others, and the suicidal person knows only too well that he can be a burden to his loved ones. Encouraging the patient to put his negative feelings into words directed to his loved ones may seem to him to be adding insult to injury.

Interpretations therefore must voice *both* halves of the patient's ambivalence, not just the aggressive component. Thus the therapist will say to a man in a bind of hostile dependency with a controlling wife, "It must be very hard, when your wife has been so good to you, to admit that there are times when, good as she is, you find yourself angry with her." This careful, even protective, wording gives the patient a chance to express the complexity of his feelings without guilt.

Without such respect for the patient's ambivalence, the therapist may lead him into expressing extreme anger and bring on another bout of depression when the patient guiltily reflects on what he has said. Worse yet, the patient may grow uncontrollably angry in a process of injudicious catharsis. Then the therapist has replaced a suicidal crisis with a homicidal one.

The therapist can encourage the open expression of feelings, but he should nevertheless refrain from joining in any attack on significant others. He can do this by making statements such as, "It is terribly important that you know you are angry and that you let the feeling live. We can't condemn her of course, since she does what she does out of her own character and for her own reasons." Indeed, the therapist may have to take a stiff line against absolute judgments so the patient will not feel he has succeeded in making the therapist an accomplice in his homicidal feelings or his therapy a place where the reputation of others is damaged. If the patient regards his therapy as a place where a symbolic murder is taking place, he will feel intensely guilty. Over and over the therapist will have to protect his patient from the backlash of guilt by making it clear that he is not judging the loved one and by pointing out the loved one's position: "She has to be angry at you sometimes; you aren't always right." As this process advances, the patient will feel increasingly safe about saying what he feels because he knows the therapist will not let it lead to actual or symbolic harm to others.

Part of the dilemma of suicide is the blurred distinction between fantasy and action—inner feelings must be acted upon to be acknowledged. Thus suicidal action is often the only way a patient can find of expressing himself. One of the most valuable acts a therapist can perform is to teach the patient that there is an *inner* world of fantasy and emotion with its own laws, and this world is not the same as the outer world of action.

The therapist must recognize that the suicidal patient is often quite concrete, i.e., has only a weak ability to distinguish fantasy from action, and may take the therapeutic dialogue literally after the session. The therapist must explain repeatedly that emotion is not to be naïvely acted upon. He should explain at the outset that he is going to encourage the patient to express his feelings, but if the patient feels compelled to act on them outside the therapeutic situation, he must call the therapist.

Example 3-10. An intelligent divorced woman in her middle 50s entered psychotherapy after a suicide attempt brought on by her rage at an indecisive boyfriend. She called her therapist after a session in which she had begun to ventilate her long-suppressed anger at the man, whom she had previously mothered and forgiven. She said that she felt like killing him. The therapist said those feelings were important but that they belonged to the psychotherapy, and if she felt like acting on them, she should come in immediately. At the next psychotherapy session the therapist inquired about her homicidal concern, and she said "I've got it under control now." She reported a dream she had the night after she spoke to the therapist. In it she was holding a knife. In front of her was a wall on which the word KILL was written. Gripping the knife tighter, she moved to the right and saw the word MURDER. She was so frightened she dropped the knife, and from this point impulsivity was not a problem.

Imagining the Effect of One's Death. It is instructive and often therapeutic to ask the suicidal person to imagine out loud how he thinks he will die. Such exploration may lead to a confrontation with the fact that the effect of death is often different from what the patient imagines. Some patients need to pursue suicidal fantasy to overcome it. As mentioned in Chapter 2, the fantasy may be one of killing a hated part of the self, of inducing enduring guilt and grief in others, of coming back to life and watching them suffer, or of being reunited with loved ones in heaven.

Example 3-11. A 35-year-old divorced mother of one had since childhood been entwined in a frustrating, symbiotic relationship with her clergyman father. She pathetically sought but rarely received his approval unless it was accompanied by extensive moral admonitions. During therapy she struggled, with occasional success, to free herself from this tyranny. Her therapist was struck by how primitive (although not psychotic) her defenses were and had thought of her as "a flamboyant, childlike, hysterical character."

Usually he presented her bill at the end of each month, and she paid it promptly. During a midmonth session she uncharacteristically asked him, "How much do I owe you for this month?" and took her checkbook from her purse. The therapist asked her why she wanted to pay her bill then. Was it because she was thinking of suicide and wanted to leave no hard feelings? She was indeed. She had received a depressing letter from her father and felt pessimistic. She believed that *nothing* would ever please him, was tired of trying, and wanted to take her son with her to heaven.

With the therapist's encouragement, she described how wretched her death would make her father feel and how he would finally come to see how he had failed to appreciate her. She looked forward almost gleefully to the retribution. The therapist asked the patient to estimate how long the father's grief would continue, given his long record of imperviousness to her feelings and tendency to moralize away the meaning of her existence. She soberly estimated that he would probably "get over it" in several weeks at most. The therapist asked her how she would be able to perceive and enjoy even those several weeks. She had never thought of this before. The patient realized that if she were dead, she would not be able to see her father suffer, and her effort would have been in vain. She put her checkbook back into her purse, and the two began to talk of more effective ways by which she could register her disappointment.

Other patients need to be confronted with the

uncertainty of death and the brutal reality of suicide. In a letter to an anonymous correspondent, Jung[7] said:

> Anon.   *19. Novb. 1955*
>
> I am glad that you do understand the difficulty of your request. How can anybody be expected to be competent enough to give such advice? I feel utterly incompetent—yet I cannot deny the justification of your wish and I have no heart to refuse it. If your case were my own, I don't know what could happen to me, but I am rather certain that I would not plan a suicide ahead. I should rather hang on until I can stand my fate or until sheer despair forces my hand. The reason for such an "unreasonable" attitude with me is that I am not at all sure what will happen to me after death. I have good reasons to assume that things are not finished with death. Life seems to be an interlude in a long story. It has been long before I was, and it will most probably continue after the conscious interval in a three-dimensional existence. I shall therefore hang on as long as it is humanly possible and I try to avoid all the foregone conclusions, considering seriously the hints I got as to the *post mortem* events.
>
> Therefore I cannot advise you to commit suicide for so-called reasonable considerations. It is murder and a corpse is left behind, no matter who has killed whom. Rightly the English Common Law punishes the perpetrator of the deed. Be sure first, whether it is really the will of God to kill yourself or merely your reason. The latter is positively not good enough. If it should be the act of sheer despair, it will not count against you, but a willfully planned act might weigh heavily against you.
>
> This is my incompetent opinion. I have learned caution with the "perverse." I do not underestimate your truly terrible ordeal.
>
> *In deepest sympathy,*
> *yours cordially,*
> *C. G. Jung*

"Stick to your last" is wise advice for anyone who is depressed. *Self-assertion* in relatively conflict-free areas provides one channel for the problematic aggressive drives. The patient should be encouraged to go to his job or, if he is on a ward, to structure his day. Activity outside therapy builds self-esteem and lessens the risk of severe conflicts over dependency.

The *telephone* is a nuclear element in suicide prevention. The patient should be encouraged to use it whenever he feels the need. This channel may be used in the early phase of therapy—as it was by the intelligent but overcontrolled woman in Example 3-10—to mention particularly unacceptable thoughts and feelings for the first time. Always its use extends and dramatizes the emotional lifeline with which the therapist is trying to provide the patient. It is particularly helpful in dealing with a suicidal crisis over a weekend or holiday because the therapist can schedule specific telephone appointments and force the patient to stay in touch. If the telephone appointment is not kept, the therapist is probably being tested for concern and should telephone the patient himself. If the patient does not answer, the therapist may take this as a presuicidal signal and call other members of the ecological group or the police.

The therapist should be willing to take *legal steps* to prevent suicide when the patient impulsively breaks contact or makes specific suicidal threats. Police officers are usually helpful to suicidal people, and their presence expresses concern. The best way to use the law is as a means of bringing the patient into custody long enough for an evaluation to be made. When the therapist does use the law (see Example 3-6), he is making an unambivalent statement that he wants the patient to live. Sometimes in the later stages of treatment the therapist may say to a patient who habitually threatens to kill himself, "When you tell me you plan to kill yourself, I will take you seriously, and I will have to inform everyone concerned, including the police, that this is what you plan to do." Alternatively, the therapist may state, "If you are absolutely set on killing yourself, I can't stop you, and I'm not going to chase you. I will make sure that everyone around you knows the risk."

COUNTERTRANSFERENCE PROBLEMS

Countertransference means reactions in the therapist, unwittingly called forth by the patient, that stand in the way of the therapist's attention to and understanding of the patient's dynamics. Suicidal patients can be draining in their demands and negativism. The therapist should recognize his limitations. Probably he should serve as a lifeline to no more than one actively suicidal person at a given time.

He also must come to terms with his own negative feelings. Sooner or later every therapist realizes that there is a patient in his caseload whose death would unburden him. The therapist must be on guard against his own tendency to immobilize. Probably his best protection is to share his burden with a colleague and to communicate fully and often his difficulties in working with the patient. When the colleague starts to immobilize, perhaps it is time to change colleagues or patients.

Usually it is bad to refer a patient in crisis. It is, however, acceptable when a therapist is unable to summon the energy to continue supporting a patient to be honest about his own limitations. Without impugning the patient, the therapist can explain that he feels as a professional he cannot offer the best treatment. The reason lies in the therapist's own limitations at this time, and he would like the patient to accept referral to another professional who can help him. This message is usually accepted by patients because it is an expression of continued concern and not a repudiation.

Many countertransference problems can be resolved successfully when the therapist perceives that he has become an agency through which the patient's ambivalence is being expressed. The therapist who wonders if the patient would not be better off dead should realize that he is taking over the patient's fantasy. Although the exact process may be obscure, therapists who work with suicidal people should recognize that it is possible to feel the patient's emotions. In fact, the patient may be working unconsciously to make the therapist give up hope and behave rejectingly so that the suicide will become justifiable.

When the bind is intense, skillful consultation may be required to free the therapist to recognize that his hostile feelings are being elicited by the patient. Then the therapist can confront the patient with what he is doing, often to good effect. Some therapists say, "Stop putting your anger into me." Others may say, "I find that you are communicating with me in a way that makes me feel hopeless too. You shouldn't try to bully me into agreeing with your depression. When you do, I will confront you with what you are doing. Because you feel hopeless now doesn't mean I have to agree with you that it will always be this way."

Finally, every therapist who works with suicidal people has to accept the possibility of failure. His own skills may not be equal to the demands of a particular suicidal process. The failure to help may be a force in furthering professional growth if the therapist accepts that his own process is one of continuous development in the face of difficult challenges.

Alice (cont'd.). Alice killed herself. She had left the hospital against medical advice, with an unpaid bill that prevented her readmission. The resident had started outpatient couple therapy with Alice and Bradley and hoped, if not to restore the relationship, at least to let it dissolve amicably. They enjoyed the sessions, but Bradley used them to talk about himself, and Alice used them to watch Bradley and obtain refills of her chlorpromazine prescription. She said virtually nothing about her emotional life.

After several months Alice and Bradley left again for the East Coast. While they were on the trip, both Alice's mother and ex-husband died, and she and Bradley had to take care of

Billy. They returned to the resident. Alice was much more depressed, but could not talk about it. She and Billy moved away from Bradley. She took a job selling dresses, became more depressed, and made another suicide attempt with alcohol and drugstore medications. She was sent to a state hospital for three days, then returned to the resident and was morose and taciturn. When Billy reported finding her in the kitchen one day with the gas turned on, the resident again sought to help. He found another therapist who agreed to treat her at another hospital with county financing. The resident and the other therapist discussed the possible use of ECT.

The resident's consultant heard the case and recommended that when Alice was released he wait for her to ask for help before trying to rescue her. Among other things, the consultant said, "This is a dead woman."

Alice stayed in the other hospital a week, felt better, and called the resident to make an appointment. On the day of this appointment she called to say she had car trouble but that she would be there the following week. Following his consultant's advice, the resident waited.

Three days before the appointment Alice drove to the railroad station, parked her car, and lay down across the tracks. She was cut in half by the morning express. When he was interviewed later with Alice's brother, who had come to get him, Billy expressed great relief that his mother was dead. "She was always threatening, and I was tired of coming home from school wondering if I was going to find her dead. Do you know what happened that day her car broke down? She was driving to the railroad station then, and her car broke down on the way. You did everything you could."

Privately the resident wondered. Had he immobilized at the end, or was his consultant right to make him wait until Alice asked for treatment? He wondered if he knew all along

that she would kill herself if he stopped reaching out actively. Turning to the record he kept of his dreams for his own analysis, he discovered the following one. It had been written down on the morning of Alice's suicide a few minutes before her death:

"Am in some kind of subway or train station. I have with me the briefcase in which I keep my patient's records, only instead of tan it is unaccountably black. There is a woman who is living in one state and tells me she wants to go to another. She has had troubles with her husband. We are talking on the lower platform, and I know I have plenty of time to catch the train. Suddenly I realize I've left my briefcase on the upper platform. I rush up to get it, and I pick it up just as the train is pulling in, just in time."

The resident's dream reflects the paradox of his experience with Alice. On the one hand, he did not succeed in rescuing her, and this failure blackened his feeling about himself as a clinical worker. On the other, he came to accept this disappointment as a corrective to his overconfidence and was able to function at a higher level of clinical understanding.

REFERENCES

1. Stengel, Erwin: *Suicide and Attempted Suicide,* Penguin, Baltimore, 1969.

2. Jung, C. G.: "Psychological Types," in *Collected Works,* Princeton, Princeton, N.J., 1971, vol. 6, pp. 354–356, 387–388.

3. Hillman, James: "The Feeling Function," *Lectures on Jung's Typology,* Spring Publications, New York, 1971, pp. 101–102.

4. Mintz, Ronald S.: "Basic Considerations in the Psychotherapy of the Depressed Suicidal Patient," *Am. J. Psychotherapy.,* vol. 35, January 1971.

5. Lesse, S. (ed.): *An Evaluation of the Results of the Psychotherapies,* Charles C Thomas, Springfield, Ill., 1968.

6. Kalinowski, Lothar M.: "Convulsive Shock Treatment", in S. Arieti (ed.), *American Handbook of Psychiatry*, Basic Books, New York, 1959, vol. 2, pp. 1510–1511.

7. Adler, Gerhard (ed.): *Selected Letters of C. G. Jung,* Princeton, Princeton, N.J., 1975. Reprinted by permission of Princeton University Press.

Evaluation and Treatment of the Homicidal Patient

We have presented suicide as a personal decision to end life, as an ego decision. Treatment is also largely directed to the patient's ego, his awareness and ability to take responsibility for his often overwhelming feelings and thoughts.

To understand homicide, we must go deeper. The motivation for most homicide does not lie within the ego, in its internal self-divisions or its external failures of integration into society. Rather, homicide arises in the more impersonal and instinctive area that Freud called the "id" and Jung called the "collective unconscious." Homicidal motivation belongs usually to the purposes of the id, not to the decisions of the ego; to collective prejudices, not personal values. The suicidal patient may tell the emergency therapist, "I wanted to die"; the potential homicide is likely to report, "Something in me wanted to kill."

Thus homicide, for the therapist, is a greater challenge than suicide. In addition to rational clinical skills, he needs to develop a feeling for the irrational, an intuitive sensitivity to the logic of emotion. Effective intervention in homicidal crises requires the ability to appraise areas of functioning of which the patient himself may be totally unconscious. Effective intervention also requires the ability to recognize the patient who is not equipped to exert his own controls so that appropriate external restraint can be provided. Finally, effective intervention requires the ability to face human destructiveness as a reality and see it without the sentimental or wishful thinking that avoids the human, and frequent, desire to harm others.

PEOPLE WHO KILL

With the important exceptions of those who kill on military assignment or for monetary gain, people who kill are enacting a primitive response to an impasse for which they perceive another person as being responsible. The choice of the primitive killing response seems to be conditioned by a long, maladaptive background that is present in nearly all homicide offenders. The actual killing is usually triggered by an immediate frustration.

Anger[1] often appears when

> ... the development of the situation is such that the possibility of any resolution to the situation, any reasonable prompt satisfaction of need or elevation of self is contradicted by elements of the situation.[2]

Anger, of course, relocates the blame for the impasse outside the suffering individual, avoiding the continued experience of pain, uncertainty, and anxiety. By engaging in violent, homicidal behavior, the aggressive person punishes someone in the outer world and completes the process of putting all his distress outside himself.

In actual practice, people who kill show *varying* degrees of being out of touch with their own pain and of relocating it in the outer world. Thus pain, denial of pain, anger, denial of anger, homicidal fantasy, denial of homicidal fantasy, homicidal action, and denial of having acted homicidally may all occur at different times in the life of a potentially violent individual. An important part of the treatment of a homicidal individual occurs through his learning to experience pain, anger, and hostile fantasy without turning to action.

Homicidal individuals differ in their relationship to fantasy. Of course many people experience homicidal fantasy as an accompaniment to anger. Some persons, frightened by this fantasy, repress it, and the hostile content appears only in dreams or other symbolic substitutes such as hostile jokes and teasing. Other people retain the fantasy but repress the anger that goes with it. They entertain extremely violent thoughts in a "split-off," unemotional way. When a mild-mannered person of this type kills, everyone is usually surprised because he has not shown even anger, let alone a potential for violence. Megargee[3] calls such people "chronically overcontrolled types." Indeed, the majority of those who kill never commit another violent act,[4] and the only clue to homicide is the pre-existence of homicidal fantasies.[5]

Other violent persons seem to have much anger but little fantasy. Habitually aggressive patients show an impoverished fantasy life and little recognition of internal states. Pain is repressed in favor of the direct expression of rage.[6] Often a depression exists, unrecognized because it is masked by the angry behavior.[7] For persons in this group—whom Megargee calls the "uncontrolled agressive types"—homicide seems but a side effect of a habitual pattern of rage response to frustration.[8]

The Homicide Offender

Most of what is known about homicidal behavior comes from studies of arrested persons. "Criminal" homicide includes murder and manslaughter (both voluntary and involuntary); it excludes killing in self-defense, excusable and "justifiable" homicide, and homicide performed "as a legal duty" by a peace officer or executioner. Generally speaking, the therapist will find himself taxed by the need to prevent the loss of control that leads to criminal homicide. Psychotic homicide is much less frequently a problem for him, as the indications for intervention are so clear-cut. (The treatment of psychotic states is discussed in Chapter 5.) Rational, premeditated homicide is rarely discussed with a therapist, nor is "justifiable" homicide. Therefore much of the data relevant to everyday preventive work are drawn from the records of those who have lost control and have been held legally culpable, from studies of prison populations of convicted slayers, and from records of persons arrested for murder.

Marvin Wolfgang[9] has summarized much of what is known sociologically about criminal homicide:

> The typical criminal slayer is a young man in his twenties who kills another man only slightly older. Both are of the same race; if Negro, the slaying is commonly with a knife; if white, it is a beating with fists and feet on a public street. Men kill and are killed between four and five times more frequently than women, but when a woman kills she most likely has a man as her victim and does it with a butcher knife in the kitchen. A woman killing a woman is extremely rare, for she is most commonly slain by her husband or other close friend by a beating in the bedroom.

A recent report[10] on the epidemiology of murder gives the following facts and statistics:

Of the urban murders in this country, 66% are between blacks; 24% between whites, and 4% whites killing blacks. The black murder rate is 16 to 17 times that of the white rate; black females murder three times as frequently as white males.

In 62% of all murders, men kill men; in 18% females kill males; in 16%, males kill females; and in 4% females kill females . . . .

According to the Federal Bureau of Investigation's statistics, the circumstances of U.S. murders break down this way: spouses killing spouses, 12.5%; parents killing children, 2.9%; other family killings, 8.9%; "romantic triangles and lovers' quarrels," 7.1%; other extramarital arguments, 41.2%; murders committed during lesser felonies, 22.1%; and murders committed during possible felonies, 5.3% . . . .

Firearms are the preferred weapons of murderers, who use them 66.2% of the time. Handguns account for 54% of the killings, followed by knives or other sharp instruments in 19% of cases, and bodily force in 8.2% . . . . Among murdering spouses, wives tend to use knives twice as often as husbands. Murdering husbands outnumber murdering wives, 52% to 48%.

. . . Of all crimes of violence, murder is the likeliest one to result in arrest. In fully 86% of homicides, the perpetrator is taken into custody.[11]

From these and other statistics, generalizations can be made about homicide. People tend to kill people who resemble them in age, sex, and race; they know each other and act under circumstances in which it might be difficult to predict who would be the killer and who the victim. [12-15] When the killer and victim are of different sexes, the killer is more often a male who kills his wife or girlfriend. Even though only one-half as many women as men are killed in the United States each year, women living with potentially homicidal men are at a considerably greater risk. [16-19]

Persons in the 20- to 24-year age group are most likely to kill; the median age of killers in one study was 31.9 years, of the victims 35.1 years.[19] In 1960 nonwhites comprised about 11 percent of the total population but suffered 53 percent of the homicides.[20] Mortality rates for homicides per 100,000 population by race for 1959 to 1961 were Japanese, 1.5; Chinese, 3.0; white males, 3.6; American Indians, 12.9; blacks, 22.6. [21, 22] Of the 18,000 homicides in 1972, 70 percent of the victims were black; "the typical murderer in the U.S. is a young urban black; a male who is either out of work, a student, or a laborer."[10]

Backgrounds of People Who Kill. In contrast to suicide, homicide is primarily a problem of the lowest socioeconomic classes. Detroit has the highest homicide rate of any city in the United States, but the highest rate in the country for nonurban areas is found in the rural South, twice as high as the rest of the United States. (This increased rate still holds when only Southern whites are compared to Northern whites. The simplest explanation is that Southern whites are more likely to carry handguns.)[10]

Areas with the highest homicide rates also have the largest proportion of persons who did not reach high school. Convicted murderers have lower IQ and school achievement scores than other inmates of prisons. The educational level of convicted murderers is lower than the average for males committed for all crimes. There is a high positive correlation between homicide and social maladjustment, as indicated by juvenile delinquency, child neglect and dependency, private agency child placing, and illegitimate birth rate. Gillin's[23] study found that, during the boyhoods of murderers, the subjects' mothers were almost twice as likely to work outside the home as the average American mother.

The subject had often had to assume early economic responsibility for family support; in seven out of ten cases he was 14 years of age when he began, and in over nine out of ten cases he contributed to family earnings before he was 21. Furthermore, there was one chance in three that his family had had a history of intemperance and at least one chance in five of insanity, epilepsy, or mental defect in his family.

... the murderers left school earlier, had full-time jobs before the age of 14 in significantly greater numbers, married women with more education than they themselves had had in significantly greater numbers, lived less harmoniously with their wives, and remained on their jobs for shorter periods of time than their brothers.[24]

Wolfgang and Ferracuti[25] have postulated that these sociological conditions have brought into existence a "subculture of violence" that puts a high premium on physical rather than verbal forms of mastery:

A male is usually expected to defend the name and honor of his mother, the virtue of womanhood ... and to accept no derogation about his race (even from a member of his own race), his age, or his masculinity. Quick resort to physical combat as a measure of daring, courage, or defense of status appears to be a cultural expression, especially for lower socioeconomic class males of both races. When such a culture norm response is elicited from an individual engaged in social interplay with others who harbor the same response mechanism, physical assaults, altercations, and violent domestic quarrels that result in homicide are likely to be common.

Early History. In addition to the predisposing subcultural background, the personal background of the eventual murderer suggests considerable disequilibration within the family and within himself. Menninger and Modlin[26] list five factors commonly present in the personal childhood histories of those who later commit murder:

1. *Severe emotional deprivation or overt rejection in childhood:* prolonged absence of one or both parents, a chaotic family life, or actual removal of the child from his family to live with friends or relatives.

2. *Parental seduction:* ranging from subtle forms such as offsprings' sharing their parents' bedroom through adolescence; through overt actions such as a mother's bathing the early adolescent boy, or parading nude before him, or a father's forbidding his four adolescent daughters ever to close the bathroom door under any circumstances, or inflicting painful corporal punishment; to frank incest.

3. *Exposure to brutality and extreme violence:* witnessing violent episodes involving parents, neighbors, or others in the community, and/or being subjected to violent attacks and punishments by parents or parent-surrogates. This witnessed and/or experienced violence is often associated with sexual behavior . . . .

4. *Childhood fire-setting:* "accidental" arson, building bonfires, homemade fire bombs, etc.

5. *Cruelty to animals or other children:* as evidenced by intentional destruction or injury of a sadistic sort; setting fire to animals, torturing them, etc.

Hellman and Blackman[27] discovered that a triad of bed-wetting, fire setting, and cruelty to animals in childhood could be demonstrated three times as often in the early history of those who had committed violent, antisocial crimes as in the histories of those whose crimes were not violent. They consider this triad highly predictive of a potential for violence. John M. Macdonald[28] studied convicted offenders and control groups and found that the homicide-threat group and the homicide-offender group both had a higher incidence of four factors (when considered together): parental brutality, parental seduction, childhood fire setting, and cruelty to animals. The homicide-threat group had the highest incidence of attempted suicide; the homicide-offender group had the lowest incidence of attempted suicide. If the homicide offenders had taken more than one life, been more sadistic, or killed strangers, one factor—cruelty to animals—was significantly higher in the childhood background. Other factors such as alcoholism, a police arrest record, and arrest for assault were distributed evenly among the three groups. He was unable to verify an initial impression that fire setting was a predictive factor taken by itself.

The literature gives an overwhelming impression that the childhood of the person who kills is one in which the child's feelings are not heard and his privacy not respected, in which he is used by adults as an outlet for their aggressive and sexual needs, and in which he turns increasingly to highly antisocial, nonverbal ways of expressing his resentment: soiling, burning, and torturing objects in his environment. Within the subculture of the deprived, those who later commit homicide are the particularly deprived; those most mistreated in youth become the most violent later.

Character Traits of Undercontrolled Patients.
Menninger and Modlin[29] have noted the following characteristics of habitually violent patients:

1. A marginal tolerance for anxiety and tension
2. A proneness to act rather than use thought, words, and symbols
3. Limited, superficial, or highly ambivalent relations with others
4. Intense self-centeredness, with a tendency to see others as very powerful and themselves as weak, inferior, and inadequate
5. A tendency to make suspicious assumptions about the hostile intent of the actions of others

The effect of these traits is to make a relatively minor stress a major crisis, for the sensitivity of these patients is great, and their repertoire of response explicitly physical.

Kinzel[30] has researched this hypersensitivity in an ingenious manner: by measuring the closest distances tolerated on approach from an experimenter by violent and nonviolent prisoners. This distance is called the "body buffer zone"[31] and is defined as the "area around a person within which anxiety is produced, if another enters." This distance is known to ethologists as "reaction distance," and violation of it produces sham or actual violence in an animal.[32] Anthropologists have shown that different cultures define different comfortable limits for intimate, personal, social, and public distances.[33]

Kinzel discovered that assaultive prisoners were hypersensitive to physical closeness to others: their body-buffer zones were almost four times larger than those measured for nonviolent prisoners. Furthermore, the violent prisoners had larger rear zones than front zones, whereas the nonviolent prisoners had larger front than rear zones. After twelve weekly determinations, the zones of both groups decreased to one-half their original size. This decrease indicated that some desensitization could occur as the experiment grew familiar, but the difference between groups remained significant. Kinzel concluded that the large zones for the violent group reflected what he called "a pathological body image state," which was supported by misperceptions of the experimenter as "looming" or "rushing" at the subjects: "Violent individuals tended to perceive nonthreatening intrusion as attack." Many also experienced tingling or goose pimples across their shoulders and backs when approached from the rear. The same subjects tended to be highly defensive about homosexuality, denying it despite histories of homosexual contact (standard for prison populations) and stating strong aversion to taking the "feminine" homosexual role. One subject appeared to experience homosexual panic during the experiment.

These data demonstrate what the personal consequences of a history of parental brutality and seduction may be. Outside prison, violence-threatening patients often complain of too-close approach by heterosexual partners. Paradoxically, the background of parental neglect may cause the same people to make great demands on partners for a maternal sort of support. The combination of an unusual need for mothering and an unusual need for physical distance creates tension in a partner who is trying to meet these contradictory expectations. The patient too is tense, for usually he cannot meet one of his emotional needs without sacrificing the other. Thus the partnership is likely to produce anxiety, resentment, and the potential for violence, each partner misreading the nonverbal cues as the other approaches or draws away physically. Because neither partner may be skilled in the use of words, the process is likely to proceed without either being able to define what is occurring. Instead, each is likely to behave with hostility to the other's presumed affronts, and an escalating pattern of violence is set in motion.

Megargee[34] has called the sort of person showing these habitually aggressive responses to minor stress "the undercontrolled aggressive type":

> The Undercontrolled Aggressive person corresponds to the typical conception of an aggressive personality found in the literature. He is a person whose inhibitions against aggressive behavior are quite low. Consequently, he usually responds with aggression whenever he is frustrated or provoked. Since inhibitions are specific to the situation, he will, occasionally, be inhibited from expressing his aggression. For instance, he might not attack his mother or a judge even though they frustrate him. In such cases, however, the Undercontrolled Aggressive person will readily use the mechanism of displacement and find a substitute target for his aggression, or he may resort to the mechanism of response generalization and make a less drastic response to the original frustrating agent.

Character Traits of Overcontrolled Homicide Offenders. Megargee[35] spells out the differences this group has from habitually aggressive persons:

> The Chronically Overcontrolled type behaves quite differently, however. His inhibitions against the expression of aggression are ex-

tremely rigid so he rarely, if ever, responds with aggression no matter how great the provocation. These inhibitions are not focused on a few specific targets, as was the case with the Undercontrolled Aggressive type, but instead are quite general. He is, therefore, unable to make use of the mechanisms of displacement or response generalization. The result is that . . . his instigation to aggression builds up over time. In some cases, the instigation to aggression summates to the point where it exceeds even his excessive defenses. If this occurs where there are sufficient cues to aggression in the environment, an aggressive act should result.

Megargee[36] describes some examples:

> In case after case the extremely assaultive offender proves to be a rather passive person with no previous history of aggression. In Phoenix an 11-year-old boy who stabbed his brother 34 times with a steak knife was described by all who knew him as being extremely polite and soft spoken with no history of assaultive behavior. In New York an 18-year-old youth who confessed he had assaulted and strangled a 7-year-old girl in a Queens church and later tried to burn her body in the furnace was described in the press as an unemotional person who planned to be a minister. A 21-year-old man from Colorado who was accused of the rape and murder of two little girls had never been a discipline problem and, in fact, his stepfather reported: "When he was in school the other kids would run all over him and he'd never fight back. There is just no violence in him."

After the aggressive act, the overcontrolled person reverts to his usual rigid (though brittle) controls. In a study of fifty-three Michigan murderers, Tanay[37] found that 68 percent had overly strong superegos and "a self-image of benevolence, cooperativeness, and self-sacrificing love," a view that was shared by most of their associates.[58] Such persons experienced anger "primarily in the form of sudden explosions" and had noted an altered state of consciousness prior to the murder.

This is the type of murderer who may carry a schizoid or schizophrenic diagnosis. Indeed, mass murderers such as Winnie Ruth Judd and Emil Kemper are extremely complicated problems for psychiatric management because they may appear well integrated both before and after a bizarre crime is committed.

Some persons of this type experience loss of control because they have been under the influence of alcohol or amphetamines. Others are experiencing psychotic episodes at the time of the murders. Indeed, Tanay found that 14 percent of his subjects were psychotic. In dealing with people with rigid, brittle defenses, it is well to imagine what might happen if the defenses were to be undermined by some means, not what the *usual* level of control is. When an altered ego state appears in this kind of person, and he presents himself for psychiatric help, he should be evaluated carefully.

THE PREASSAULTIVE CRISIS

In Chapter 1 we defined crisis as "news of a difference affecting the pattern of relationships found within an ecological group." For homicidal people, the pattern of relationships is already unstable, tending toward rupture, and the difference that precipitates violent action is one that a member of another ecological group might easily take in stride. The first sign of crisis is often an *affective state*.

Rarely does a patient in the preassaultive state present himself to an emergency room therapist saying, "I'm afraid I'm going to kill someone." Rather, the patient's complaint is likely to be a nonspecific tension state. He will be manifesting affective cues such as tremulousness, breathlessness, and rapid pulse and be experiencing a vague uneasiness. He may be alarmed by the tension building within and say, "I'm afraid I'm going to blow." The patient makes a paranoid projection of his distress onto the other person who then "becomes" the anxiety, as in Kinzel's experiments in which the disequilibration was pictured as the looming or rushing in of the experimenter, not as an internal process of the subject. How all this looks in an actual patient can be illustrated by the following case:

Example 4-1, Ronald and June. Ronald was a 35-year-old white man who had spent half his years in jails and prisons for car thefts, assaults, and forgery. He had met his wife, June, two years younger than he, when he was on parole at age 28. He liked her because she was "game for thieving"; after living together for several months they married.

For four months preceding their first psychiatric visit their marriage had become increasingly strained, and they had quarreled constantly. During an argument a week before their first visit, Ronald choked June until she lost consciousness. As she fell to the floor Ronald "felt all the feelings for her I had never let myself feel," meaning love, concern for her safety, and remorse for what he had done. He ran out of the house; when he returned she had recovered and was gone. He was terrified that she had left for good. He drove around looking for her and nearly gave in to the temptation to drive into a brick wall at ninety miles an hour. When he returned the next morning, she was back, after having spent the night at a male neighbor's. They agreed to try to talk things out; Ronald hinted at a definite suicide attempt if she left him.

They came to the clinic. After the initial interview, first together and then individually, Ronald's care was taken over by a male psychiatric resident and June's by a female social worker. It seemed at the time that each would be more comfortable with a therapist of the same sex.

Ronald's past was amply documented with instances of brutality, neglect, exploitation, delinquency, shallow interpersonal relationships, and academic failure. His father drank and had often beat him. One of Ronald's elder brothers constantly bullied him, and many years later Ronald still felt he would like to "pound my brother into the ground." He recalled his mother as a "beautiful person" who understood him but would not intervene in his or anyone else's problems and who was subjugated by her brutal husband. Curiously, Ronald told his therapist that he still liked his father and wished he could be closer to him.

Ronald did poorly in school, rejecting teachers' efforts to reach out to him. He was first arrested at age 11 for stealing $20 from his school. Later he was arrested on several charges of car theft (he claimed he did it only for joy riding) and spent considerable time in reform schools during his adolescence. Later he was sent to a state prison for similar offenses. He had always been fascinated by cars and had become an expert mechanic.

Ronald was on parole when he met and married June. She became pregnant, but before the birth he was returned to jail for a parole violation. June and the baby visited faithfully every weekend. A prison psychiatrist asked Ronald if he had ever thought of having sex with his mother, and Ronald knocked him out with one punch.

The baby died after a few months of what was diagnosed as crib death. Ronald was released five months later, and June quickly became pregnant again. The second baby's delivery was normal, but when it was nine weeks old, it too died suddenly. Ronald rushed the lifeless infant to the hospital where an autopsy was performed; the diagnosis again was crib death. Ronald worried that these deaths were the result of either "something bad in my blood" or of negligence on June's part.

Four years elapsed between the death of the second child and their first psychiatric visit. During those years Ronald had become increasingly dependent upon June. They had spent only three days apart during that time, and he insisted that she always be near him, an intense demand she found difficult to tolerate. Although she remained present physically, both sensed that she was becoming psychologically distant. Privately, she was thinking of leaving him. It was this impasse between Ronald's intense need for June and her growing restiveness that produced the brutal quarrel that brought them into treatment.

Ronald had been helpless in dealing with his father, his brother, his wife, his teachers, and his schoolmates. Repeatedly he had resorted to action: robbing the school, stealing cars, punching the prison psychiatrist, rushing his dead baby to an autopsy, choking his wife. Sadly, these actions had served only to complicate his life. For Ronald the problem always had been "out there" somewhere, and it is easy to imagine him thinking that the right course of impulsive action would finally resolve it. For Ronald, life had been chronically insecure; he needed to rely more and more on his wife to stabilize him. This chronic disequilibration gradually became a haunting fear that she would leave and it could at any time flame into an acute crisis were she to indicate that she actually planned to do so.

During the crisis with June, Ronald had been flooded with a violent impulse. Presumably choking her promised to relieve the immediate situation, however unfortunate the long-term consequences for him. In the language of dynamic formulation, an unconscious, archaic solution had appeared in response to an impasse Ronald did not know how to resolve at the ego level. It is important to look more closely at this solution, at its meaning for Ronald in terms of unconscious problem solving. We turn now to the common meanings of the homicidal solution.

Meanings of the Homicidal Solution

Homicide As Freedom. Studies on the body-buffer zone measure the degree of physical proximity people can tolerate before they lash out to free themselves from intrusion. The therapist measures the degree of psychological, emotional, or subjective proximity his patients can tolerate and the subtlety of means at their disposal to free themselves from a sense of crowding or oppression from another's closeness. Often the therapist finds that a partner triggers an unconscious introject of the devouring mother who cripples the infant's initiative while perpetuating his dependent ties upon her.[39] Murderous rage toward a wife may be a continuation of anger toward a mother, as would appear to be the case with Ronald. If suicide is frequently an attempt to achieve an extraverted end that wears an introverted mask, homicide is often the reverse: an attempt to achieve introverted freedom by acting upon an external situation which threatens to engulf the homicidal person.

Homicide As Power. There is an archaic belief that if a man kills another man or an animal, the life force (or mana) of the other creature belongs to him.[40] This primitive idea seems still to operate in many homicidal people and is well supported by their surrounding cultures. In our own country, Mafia dons have a charismatic appeal, as exemplified by the success of *The Godfather*. This same psychology may operate for some persons who find the homicidal solution appealing. In their daily lives they are weak and ineffective; through murder they at last demonstrate power.

Homicide As Mastery. In analytic treatment, there is a class of "killing dreams" in which the patient stabs or shoots a threatening figure or is witness to a killing. (Some examples are given in Chapter 22.) The dreamer often feels profound satisfaction (an emotion that may alarm him when he wakes). After such a dream the patient often takes active steps toward mastery of a long-standing intrapsychic conflict. A phrase such as "getting to the heart of the matter" suggests the positive meaning of the homicidal idea.

There are some persons who turn to homicide to experience mastery of long-term interpersonal conflicts. Indeed, some murderers have reported that immediately following the killing they felt profound emotional relief, often for the first time in a long time.[41]

Homicide As Connection. Often homicide is a way of establishing a connection with a person who is felt to be so powerful or remote that no other form of communication suffices: physical force becomes the only way of being heard.

An example of this theme can be found in Shakespeare's *Julius Caesar*, in the scene in which the conspirators are pressing their arguments to Caesar, who imperiously brushes them away. Casca, the least articulate of the group, finally shouts, "Speak, hands for me!" and plunges the first dagger into Caesar's breast. The rest of the conspirators join him in stabbing the Emperor. Clearly Caesar was a man who could be reached only by attack.

Similar dynamics operate in everyday life. Every therapist knows some patients who dislike words, fear the verbal prowess of the therapist, and must be approached in nonverbal ways such as through painting or gestalt techniques. Outside therapy, less inarticulate patients frequently resort to physical means to settle disputes or to relate to others.

> *Example 4-2.* A 24-year-old woman who had excelled in sports was experiencing great distress in her relationship with her husband, a highly articulate and argumentative young professor of English. She subtly provoked him to assault until he pushed her down to the floor and began to choke her. She said later that she felt considerable satisfaction because she thought that it was a fairer fight than their usual verbal battles.

Her husband, it developed, had harbored conscious homicidal feelings toward his mother for some years, and she was taking a great risk by provoking him in the area of this strong residual hatred. Confronted by her therapist with the potential danger, she could for a long time reply only, "I know that, but I can't fight back when he uses words, and I can fight back when he attacks me physically."

Homicide may also represent a sexual connection, as shown in the frequent association of stabbing with sexual molestation. Homicidal fantasy directed toward wives often erupts in men who have become impotent. Presumably the aggressive impulse compensates for the fear that emotional connection has become impossible. Severely depressed men, humiliated by associated impotence, may resort to homicide to establish the desired connection with the powerful wife.

THE DECISION TO ACT

Many overcontrolled people enjoy Walter Mittylike fantasies of homicide; many undercontrolled people engage in at least verbal altercations. Few of either group actually commit homicide. Four factors illuminate the conditions under which the danger of turning fantasy or quarrels into violent acts becomes great: a history of past violent behavior, sanction of the ecological group, sanction of the victim, and impairment of individual ego functioning.

Patients who have a history of *past violent behavior* used as a mode of conflict resolution are more likely to employ it in the future than those who do not. Wherever the violence has been "successful," i.e., winning fights or receiving plaudits rather than punishment, the tendency will have been reinforced, as Berkowitz[42] has shown in a study of nursery school children.

It is true that the way people responded to stress and conflict in the past is the best single predictor of how they will respond in the future. In evaluating potential for violence, the emergency therapist should learn about a patient's history of fights, arrests and convictions for violent crimes, reputation for toughness among his peers, and having caused previous deaths in civilian or military life. He should gauge the patient's general regard for the value of the lives of others: are people subjectively real, or objects to be disposed of if they get in the way?

Homicide occurs more frequently when it has the *sanction of the ecological group,* as in the subculture of violence Wolfgang has described. Macdonald[43] describes the following case:

> *Example 4-3.* A wife who had been threatened sent for her father-in-law, who told her in her husband's presence, "If my son had killed you tonight, I wouldn't have blamed him."

Macdonald shows that often the family will provide the murderer with the weapons he uses to kill.

Murder often takes place with the *sanction of the victim.* In many cases, the victim was the first to show and use a deadly weapon, to strike a blow, or to start the interplay involving physical violence. In some cases the victim (usually a wife) virtually challenged the partner to kill her.

> *Example 4-4.* One case involved a wife who suffered repeated beatings and homicidal threats. In her living room she displayed a gift from a neighbor man with whom she had lived during a period of separation from her husband. Macdonald insisted that she get rid of this gift, and she did so, but only as far as her mother's mantelpiece, where her husband discovered it on the couple's next visit. Following a threat with a loaded shotgun, the wife said, "Go ahead, you might just as well kill me." Whenever the husband announced his intention of selling the shotgun, the wife would insist he keep it.[44]

Whenever homicide is threatened, the emergency therapist must ascertain whether the victim is actively provoking the homicidal attacks. Often considerable therapeutic pressure must be applied to counter ecological group pressure to a homicidal solution.

Homicidal behavior is id behavior. A healthy ego usually inhibits criminal homicide for the obvious reason that criminal homicide is not in the ego's best interests. Under circumstances of *impaired individual ego function,* homicidal impulses can break through more easily to concrete expression. These circumstances include the influence of drugs and alcohol, organic brain disease, psychotic conditions, and unusually strong emotion.

Saturday night is the time of the highest incidence of homicide,[45] and usually both the victims and offenders have been drinking. [45, 46] Homicide rates, like suicide rates, are highest where alcoholism rates (as measured from deaths from cirrhosis of the liver) are highest.

Drugs that may reduce ego control include LSD, cocaine, and barbiturates, but the most dangerous are amphetamines, which produce in the withdrawal phase symptoms nearly identical with paranoid schizophrenia. In a recent study of homicide offenders,[47] amphetamines were the most commonly used drug at the time violent crimes were committed (16 percent) by both habitual and nonhabitual violent offenders. Cocaine, incidentally, works like a very short-acting amphetamine and may lead to outbursts of suppressed rage in susceptible individuals.

Organic brain disease is a potential cause of violence.[48] Menninger's[49] concept of *dyscontrol* is important. He describes it as "varying degrees of disturbance in organization, failure in coping, escape of disruptive impulses, disruption of orderly thought processes, and confusion." If organic brain disease is present, dyscontrol occurs with minimal stimulation and greatly increases the potential for violence. Organic conditions associated with dyscontrol include psychomotor-variant dysrhythmia, temporal lobe dysrhythmia, occipital dysrhythmia, and brainstem glioma. Alcohol may unmask temporal lobe epileptoid states and associated violence in susceptible individuals. The possible relation of the chromosomal XYY karyotype to violence is still under investigation. [50, 51]

Any patient who complains of sudden outbursts of unexplained rage or struggles with uncontrollable homicidal thoughts should see a neurologist for a full evaluation, including a sleeping electroencephalogram (EEG). In many instances, an abnormal EEG will be the only finding. The therapist will be charged with helping the patient to cope with occasional outbursts of disruptive affect under minimal stimulation, just as he must help the patient deal with affects produced by emotional interaction.

Certain *psychotic conditions* predispose individuals to homicide, especially involutional paranoid psychosis and paranoid schizophrenia. The risk is much greater for schizophrenic patients who drink than for those who do not. The male involutional psychotic murderer often kills himself after killing his spouse, whom he unconsciously sees as possessing the soul he must regain. This kind of murder is illustrated in the film *The Blue Angel*, in which a rigid, 50-ish professor falls under the power of a young woman cabaret singer (Marlene Dietrich) and is progressively degraded by her. Eventually he is driven to make an attempt on her life, trying to regain himself, even at the cost of ruin. In evaluating depressed patients in middle life, it is important to explore ideation concerning the spouse; this may be the area where paranoid ideation lies hidden.

THE EVALUATION OF HOMICIDE RISK

Dealing with Homicidal Threats

The emergency therapist will see patients who impress him as high-risk for homicide as well as those who seek him out because of their own fears about violence. Macdonald[52] studied 100 patients who threatened to kill; at five-year follow-up 3 had killed, and 4 had committed suicide. His study suggests that when someone threatens to kill, it is impossible to predict what the outcome will be, except that the probability of a lethal outcome is very low. Nevertheless, the threat to kill indicates a troubled emotional state and must be taken seriously.

Often young mothers present fantasies of killing their new babies. Such fantasies are common and rarely acted upon. The mother should be evaluated for the ideational, affective, and behavioral strength of these fantasies. Although she is plagued by the idea, has she felt herself giving in to strong emotion to strangle, strike, or drown the baby? Has she felt herself to be on the verge of acting on any such urges? Has she struck the child or left it in a potentially dangerous situation and walked off? How much does she fear loss of control over her fantasies?

If the fantasies are almost entirely ideational, i.e., if she has not felt surges of anger and if she has not impulsively struck the child, then she can be reassured that such fantasies are common, and outpatient psychotherapy should be arranged. The goal of therapy is to allow her to understand better the disequilibrium in her life brought about by the birth. If others can help take care of the baby for a few hours a day, she may appreciate both the relief from being a full-time mother and the implied approval that it is natural to want to do something else.

If the fantasy has strong affective and behavioral components, or if the patient seems to be on the verge of a postpartum psychosis, the baby is at risk. The husband, family, friends, and social agencies must be prevailed upon to protect the child until the mother is once again able to care for it.

Many patients who think about killing are not made anxious by the presence of homicidal fantasy. Other patients are made so anxious that they deny the presence of the fantasy and experience only a nonspecific tension. Neither position is realistic. The therapist should explore any homicidal ideation patiently and in detail to enable both the content and the anxiety about the consequences of action to emerge. This is one situation in psychiatric work in which it is helpful to stimulate anxiety. Once the patient is made anxious by his own potential for violence, he is likely to be more careful. If the therapist believes a significant danger is present, it is mandatory that he communicate the risk to the patient and to significant others.

Essentials of Interview Evaluation

Few patients say outright, "I think I'm going to kill someone." Instead, they will expect the emergency therapist to recognize that people come because they fear they may be losing control. Indeed, the question, "Why did you come here?" may be met with a quiet, evasive answer, slow to come and blunted in effect.

The therapist will need to encourage his patient to talk about this area. He should indicate by his questions that he is interested in and capable of receiving information about the patient's capacity for violence. He does not from the outset lovingly assume good faith or virtue in the patient by a show of "unconditional positive regard" which is in fact deeply conditional and indicates to the patient that he would be disappointed to hear selfish, angry, or negative data. In short, the psychiatrist's stance should indicate that he is accustomed to the bad as well as the good in people, and that he wants to get down to specifics for the practical purpose of assisting the patient. As in other aspects of crisis intervention, the therapist seeks to understand the origins of the crisis, its current status, and its possible future outcome.

Past behavior is the single best predictor of how the patient is likely to behave in the future. Psychiatric history repeats itself. Has there been an association with anyone's violent death, accidental or otherwise? Has the patient been the cause of anyone's death, for whatever reason? Has the patient ever tied anyone up with a rope? Has he used knives or guns? Was he ever arrested or jailed? Has he been known to engage in fights? What has his behavior been like when he drinks? Have there been homicidal thoughts, plans, preparations, or attempts in the past? What was his childhood like?

Did he experience parental brutality or seduction, wet his bed, set fires, or torture animals?

What is the current status of his homicidal thoughts, plans, preparations, and attempts? Does the patient have a weapon at hand? Does he have ready access to a weapon? What is his current drinking pattern? Has he been anxious or depressed without apparent cause? Is he actively quarreling with anyone, or jealous of someone? Has anyone provoked him to attack? In many cases the therapist must obtain permission to talk to the family or friends to hear the full story of the patient's recent destructiveness. Quite often they have brought the patient in and are sitting in the waiting room assuming naïvely that he will tell the therapist everything that has concerned them. They should be interviewed privately and assured that the information they give will not be used in an impulsive way which could harm them. They should be encouraged to air *fully* any uneasiness they have about the patient. They should also be evaluated as potential accomplices and as willing victims: do they add to the homicidal risk?

Are there any future conditions under which the patient would resort to a homicidal solution? (A mild-mannered man may answer, "If my wife ever left me for someone else, I'd get the gun out of my top drawer and shoot them both.") What are the patient's attitudes toward punishment? (Some patients welcome punishment as a final, suicidal curtain to a homicidal drama.) Has the patient considered killing himself?

In the evaluation interview, it is helpful to consider those psychiatric patients who are especially likely to commit homicide:

1. Anyone who has made homicidal preparations
2. Involutional paranoid psychotic patients
3. Paranoid schizophrenic patients who drink
4. Antisocial personalities who are starting to settle down (Ronald falls into this category)
5. Either member of a sadomasochistic marital couple
6. Schizophrenic mothers

ESSENTIALS OF PREVENTION

The Psychological Approach

The key to controlling homicide is control of impulsivity. The psychiatrist should take the necessary steps to help the patient separate the thought of homicide from the act. The therapist "lends" his own ego to the patient's weakened ego-control by standing squarely against impulsive emotional discharge. The therapist should proceed slowly and systematically with such patients and avoid excessive emotionality of his own. He stands for thinking things out, coming to decisions only after time, and for order. Therefore, from the outset he should make it clear that he will not be rushed into impulsive decisions, especially these which involve therapy. For instance, if the patient suddenly decides he wants to switch from individual to couple therapy, the therapist should find out why before he hurries to the waiting room to invite the wife in. Abrupt cancellations of appointments should be questioned, and the patient should be confronted with his impulsivity if it manifests itself in treatment.

The therapist must explore all homicidal thinking thoroughly, but he should not side with these ideas. He guards particularly against a therapeutic process of injudicious catharsis in which the patient is allowed to rant at a family member without contradiction from the therapist. If the therapist does not actively point out the "other side" and the dangers of premature action, often such sessions are perceived as license to act on the feeling that has been expressed. A basic condition of psychiatric treatment is that the patient is free to feel, but not necessarily to act, and it is especially important that the therapist stress this distinction when homicidal emotion is discussed.

Another basic principle is that the ultimate responsibility for homicidal behavior rests with the patient. The therapist should make it clear that therapy is no guarantee that a murder will not be committed and cannot be used as a justification for committing this crime. He reminds the patient that if he is firmly launched in the direction of committing murder, there is no way a therapist can stop him or protect him from the consequences of his act. In the emergency setting, he makes it clear he will communicate with peace officers and those in danger to avert loss of life but that in the end the patient must learn to control himself.

Environmental Manipulation. In the early phase of intervention, the therapist is often called upon to *separate the warring parties.* He may have to advise a wife or husband to move out of a house or even a city to avoid harm. He may effect hospitalization to separate people who are likely to kill each other.

The therapist also needs to *undercut potential accomplices.* He does this by exposing them in the act of condoning homicidal behavior and by making them anxious about their responsibility for a possible lethal outcome.

He must also *identify the willing victim* and encourage that person to enter treatment. She is often the wife of a man with a drinking problem or severe personality disorder who feels responsible for his failings. She may want to leave him, but she may be so filled with guilt (partly as a result of his guilt-provoking tactics) that as soon as she expresses her desire she wants to be punished for it. Clearly this situation can provoke homicide because the man is not only aroused to anger but also encouraged to attack, and decisive therapeutic intervention is required for the woman to understand her role. Often a basically healthy woman gets caught up in this bind. Once she learns to stand up to the man she is leaving without provoking him, her later therapeutic progress can be highly gratifying. Early treatment, however, is a relentless pointing out to the potential victim what she is doing to invite attack.

Generally, it is effective to make the patient, his "accomplices," and his "victim" conscious of every prehomicidal communication. As with other impulsive behavior, homicide appears when it is not expected. Therefore, in dangerous situations it seems wise to teach everyone to expect trouble. (The watched pot is less likely to boil.)

Appealing to Narcissism. Homicidal people often have severe personality disorders, including major deficits in conscience. Because ethical imperatives or moral considerations are not generally inhibiting to antisocial people, therapeutic pessimism about their treatability has prevailed. A current useful tactic that makes use of one of their characteristics is a direct appeal to their narcissism. Antisocial people are often good-looking, enjoy life, and pride themselves on getting what they need without being "hung up" by the needs of others. These defenses against feeling can be mobilized against aggression.

Example 4-5. A Mexican-American man in his late 20s was referred for treatment by a facial surgeon who was concerned about the patient's violent anger at his ex-wife, an Anglo. She had stood by and laughed while her current boyfriend broke the patient's nose when he had dropped by, drunk, to harrass her. Now he was in the hospital to have the nose reset and could think of nothing but revenge against the wife. Even his dreams were full of it.

His therapist suggested that the wife was trying to degrade him further by stimulating him to revenge. "She just wants to see you in jail. Why should you let her drag you down to that level and wind up serving time yourself just to satisfy her?" Gradually the patient began to take pride in not letting his ex-wife "drag him down." He was able to find another woman who respected him, and he congratulated himself no end for being "too smart" to let his ex-wife "fix him for good."

Avoiding Complacency. No matter how stable a patient looks in the office, the therapist who treats homicidal patients must always fear the worst. At the beginning, a firm stand on alcohol and illicit drugs should be taken, and the therapist should insist that all weapons be removed from the home. As treatment proceeds, the therapist must listen carefully for communications that tell him the destructive situation is still raging outside the office—information about drinking bouts, quarrels, gun collections. He should continue to reflect the lethal possibilities to the patient whenever he hears such information.

Particularly, the therapist should recognize and not be fooled by the "mask of adequacy" in improving borderline people. At the first blush of improvement, they will try to leave treatment: it is almost as if they are testing to see if the therapist perceives their continuing potential for violence. If he has honest doubts about their ability to sustain a nonviolent adaptation, the therapist is thoroughly justified in being quite firm with them about their need for continued treatment.

Ronald and June (cont'd.). Ronald and June saw their therapist almost every day during the acute crisis. Ronald quickly formed an attachment to his therapist and thought of him as a benign older brother who was sympathetic to his concerns, who could offer sensible reflection and advice, and who could help him find more successful ways to deal with June. The therapist worked consistently with Ronald to help him convert his feelings into words instead of inarticulate rages and to help him anticipate situations instead of responding with impulsive violence.

At the beginning of his therapy, Ronald described episodes of "blindness" while driving. These episodes occurred only when someone was with him and forced the other person to tell him how to manipulate the car to the side of the road. Fifteen minutes later Ronald's sight would come back. A neurological examination was negative, and Ronald agreed with the therapist that these episodes were an expression of some unknown and overwhelming feelings and that he should let

June discussed with her therapist her ambivalence about living with Ronald and also mentioned it to Ronald. During the third week of treatment, Ronald toyed with a large hunting knife while he talked with June at home. The next morning it appeared at her bedside. She was terrified and called her therapist. They discussed the options of June's leaving the house and calling the police. Her therapist did not minimize the danger, and informed Ronald's therapist of the incident. June decided to stay with Ronald for the time being. Ronald's therapist discussed the knife with him and pointed out how terrified June had been. Ronald denied any sinister motive and elected to lock up the knife in a trunk for June's peace of mind.

Following this step, June decided to stay with Ronald permanently. Both gained considerably in their ability to talk about difficulties, first with their therapists and then with each other, and the risk of a violent confrontation diminished steadily. Ronald's trust of his therapist grew, and he was able to reveal things that he had never been able to tell anyone. In fact, Ronald had never even articulated many of these matters in his own mind. His therapist could, from his position of trust, transmit some of his own social and personal wisdom, lending Ronald some of his ego. Together they came to see how damaging and self-defeating Ronald's unthinking, impulsive actions could be.

The frequency of the visits diminished. For six months Ronald and June had been living together in greater harmony and were able to talk about and resolve their differences. The homicidal crisis had long since passed, and therapy ended by mutual agreement.

The turning point of the case was the handling of the hunting knife. Its appearance symbolized the dramatic potential for violence. June's prompt reporting of the knife to her therapist testified to lished) to play the role of a victim. The therapists' emphatic demand that the issue of the knife be dealt with and Ronald's decision to lock it up marked the moment when the violence model was abandoned, the verbal model was accepted, and the preassaultive crisis was resolved.

Learning to Relate to the Inner World. John R. Lion[53] has said of the explosive and antisocial personalities he treats at the outpatient violence clinic of the University of Maryland School of Medicine:

> . . . It is common to hear this type of patient tell what he would *do* about an unpleasant situation, but not how he would *feel*.
>
> Therapeutically, therefore, I have regarded one of the main tasks of therapy as promoting in these violent patients an ability to feel and appreciate the depression that accompanies any kind of frustration. It is my experience that if the patient can merely recognize some of his feelings and briefly reflect on them, less impulsive, aggressive action is apt to occur. . . .
>
> Second, it is extremely useful to deal with the fantasies and imaginations of this group of patients. Many patients with impulsive personality disorders seem to have an impoverished ability to fantasize, to think about the possible consequences of behavior, or even to indulge in any kind of daydreams connected with their feelings. To counter this, I spend time with the patient in getting him to elaborate upon the possible consequences of actions he plans, in talking about the possible solutions to his problems, and generally in getting him to talk about his feelings and fantasies concerning a particular act. This is a vital step for a violence-prone patient.
>
> The patient who tells me he wants to kill his wife, for example, must be made to dwell upon the fantasies surrounding the actual murder and the end result of his homicide— incarceration. Likewise, the patient who drives recklessly under the influence of alcohol must

be made to fantasize about the possible occurrence of an accident, revocation of his license, and jail, down to the last detail, for with the detail comes the affect. The fantasies surrounding incarceration are particularly important to elaborate on so as to bring home fully to the patient the consequences of his actions. These usually stir up many depressing feelings and make the patient squarely face his own vulnerabilities and limitations. These are what the violent patient must come to grips with. A violent patient is violent only insofar as he is unable to come to grips with his own weakness and helplessness and to tolerate the depression associated with realizing these feelings.

This excellent description of a difficult task in the treatment of homicidal people—opening up the inner world without eroding controls—shows how fantasy and affect can be used to strengthen the ego. Dream material, too, can be used in this way, especially when the dream content shows the undesired outcome of some particularly charged aggressive release.

> *Example 4-5 (cont'd)*. The Mexican-American man who wanted to kill his wife had a dream in which he kept shooting at her until she was filled with holes. Still she continued to stand in front of him with a mocking expression on her face. Filled with rage, he walked around her only to find he had been shooting at a cardboard image. It was easy for his therapist to point out that the flesh-and-blood woman had been gone for a long time and that he was locked into a fruitless, exhausting struggle with a memory. This dream and its interpretation were the point at which he was able to grieve for the loss of his wife and to engage seriously with another woman.

Lion's way of working with fantasy is to *relate* it to real-life issues. This method has much to offer the overcontrolled person, too. Potentially homicidal people who are overcontrolled need to discover their hurt and anger, not hide it behind rigid defenses. Their capacity for *unrelated* fantasy must be counted as one of the rigid defenses. Although violent fantasy may be present, even pleasurable, it is not integrated. The overcontrolled person does not relate it to his feelings or to the possibility that this fantasy is one he could enact. He needs to be taught to relate his violent fantasy to his life, not to discount it, and to assume that his usual controls will continue to serve him. He should accept the possibility that he may be rehearsing[54] for a big, one-time violent action, and he should be taught to look for the feelings which lie hidden behind the violent images. As these emerge, the patient will become more anxious, less in control, and more in need of therapeutic support. For the first time, he may need limit setting and reminding of the real-life consequences of violent behavior.

Pharmacologic and Physical Approaches

Psychological means alone are often not sufficient to bring homicidal patients under control. Sometimes drugs are helpful in reducing powerful affective states. A discussion of the use of drugs in combination with psychotherapy is found in later chapters.

Diazepam (Valium®) has rapidly become a popular psychotropic drug because it provides quick relief in a way most patients find pleasant. However, dissociative reactions, including rage reactions, have been reported with its use. The combination of diazepam and alcohol may lead to a classic "blackout" in which the patient behaves aggressively and later cannot remember doing so. Clearly diazepam is an inappropriate drug for control of homicidal behavior.

Phenothiazines and related compounds are preferable. Both trifluoperazine (2 to 5 mg one to three times a day) and haloperidol seem useful in controlling chronic anger and haloperidol seems especially useful in treating psychotic patients with a hypomanic component. Both drugs often cause Parkinsonian side effects.

All these drugs have atypical reactions. In general, close contact with the doctor is required if these agents are used. They should also be regarded as adjuncts to therapy, not as substitutes for psychotherapeutic intervention with the patient and his ecological group.

Some violent patients must be restrained. Many emergency rooms provide locked rooms for obstreperous patients who are dangerous or "high" on drugs or alcohol. Judicious restraints should be used with such patients. It is wise not to underestimate an acutely intoxicated or psychotic patient's potential for violence.

Most schizophrenic patients need not be restrained, and schizophrenia alone is not a indication of potential violence. Schizophrenic patients who are violent may require the same restraints as intoxicated patients. There is no contraindication to the use of physical restraint when a significant doubt exists concerning the patient's immediate potential for violence. The therapist should, however, have some positive sign or recent history of destructiveness before he applies restraints.

The most agitated patients require, in addition to restraints or a locked room, an injection of 75 mg of chlorpromazine followed four hours later by another injection or oral administration. Dosages depend on the size of the patient, the degree of agitation, and the degree of intoxication. Phenothiazines react synergistically with alcohol, barbiturates, and sedatives; lesser doses should be administered to patients already intoxicated on these drugs. The immediate goal, in any case, is to quiet or "snow" the patient safely when he cannot be controlled in any other way.

Assuming physical control of a situation is an art in itself. When he takes control, the therapist must accept that he has assumed total responsibility for the patient's behavior. It is up to him to see that the controls are instituted firmly, unambivalently, and smoothly.

It is best to make a concrete display of power that gives the patient no opportunity (in even his foggiest, most concrete state) to misperceive the situation. This is effectively accomplished if four or five men enter a room together. If restraint is to be applied, it should be administered without hurting the patient or allowing him to hurt himself. If an injection is to be administered, the nurse may give it as the male staff members hold the patient. Whenever possible the patient should be given a choice of drinking his medication or receiving it by injection. The male staff should stand by to ensure that no one gets hurt.

External controls administered this way offer security to the patient who is unable to control his violent impulses. When inadequate staff is used, chase sequences upsetting to both the patient and the staff are likely to ensue. There is every chance that someone will get hurt.

The treatment of homicidal patients involves a special sensitivity to their emotional needs, a willingness to be active, direct, and decisive in intervention, and the ability to avoid one's own impulsivity in dealing with them. A common and gratifying result of therapy is the patient's discovery of the use, rather than the misuse, of aggressive energy.

REFERENCES

1. Stearns, Frederic R.: *Anger: Psychology, Physiology, Pathology*, Charles C Thomas, Springfield, Ill., 1972.

2. Sullivan, Harry Stack: in Stearns, ibid., p. 3.

3. Megargee, Edwin I.: "Undercontrolled and Overcontrolled Personality Types in Extreme Antisocial Aggression," *The Dynamics of Aggression*, Harper & Row, New York, 1972, pp. 108–120.

4. *Medical World News*: "The Mind of a Murderer," **14** (43):40, Nov. 23, 1973.

5. Menninger, Roy W., and Herbert C. Modlin: "Individual Violence: Prevention in the Violence-Threatening Patient," in Jan Fawcett (ed.), *Dynamics of Violence*, American Medical Association, Chicago, 1971, pp. 71–73.

6. Gallup, Palmer: "Pain and Rage in Personality Disorders," unpublished paper.

7. Spiegel, Rose: "Anger and Acting Out: Masks of Depression," *Am. J. Psychotherapy* **21**: 597–606, 1967.

8. Tupin, Joe P., Dennis Mahar, and David Smith: "Two Types of Violent Offenders with Psychosocial Descriptors," *Diseases of the Nervous System*, **34**:356–363, October/ November 1973.

9. Wolfgang, Marvin E.: "A Sociological Analysis of Criminal Homicide," in Marvin E. Wolfgang (ed.), *Studies in Homicide*, Harper & Row, New York, 1967, p. 15.

10. *Medical World News:* op. cit., pp. 42–43.

11. Ibid.

12. Menninger and Modlin: op. cit., pp. 71–78.

13. Garfinkel, Harold: "Inter- and Intra-racial Homicides," in Marvin E. Wolfgang (ed.), *Studies in Homicide*, Harper & Row, New York, 1967, pp. 45–65.

14. Iskrant, Albert P., and Paul V. Joliet: *Accidents and Homicide*, Harvard, Cambridge, Mass., 1968.

15. Federal Bureau of Investigation: *Crime in the United States: Uniform Crime Reports*, U.S. Government Printing Office, Washington, 1963.

16. Macdonald, John M.: *The Murderer and His Victim*, Charles C Thomas, Springfield, Ill., 1963.

17. Cole, K. E., Gary Fisher, and Shirley S. Cole: "Women Who Kill: a Socio-psychological Study," *Arch. Gen. Psychiat.*, **19**:1–8, 1968.

18. Langberg, Robert: *Homicide in the United States, 1950–1964*, National Center for Health Statistics, ser. 20, no. 6, U.S. Government Printing Office, Washington, D.C., 1967.

19. Wolfgang: loc. cit.

20. Langberg: loc. cit.

21. Macdonald: loc. cit.

22. Wolfgang: loc. cit.

23. Gillin, John: "Murder as a Sociological Phenomenon," *Ann. Am. Acad. Polit. Soc. Sci.* **284**:20–25, 1952.

24. Iskrant and Joliet: op. cit., pp. 119–120.

25. Wolfgang, Marvin E., and Franco Ferracuti: "Subculture of Violence—a Socio-psychological Theory," in Marvin E. Wolfgang (ed.), *Studies in Homicide,* Harper & Row, New York, 1967, p. 275.

26. Menninger and Modlin: op. cit., pp. 74–75.

27. Hellman, Daniel S., and Nathan Blackman: "Enuresis, Firesetting, and Cruelty to Animals: A Triad Predictive of Adult Crime," *Am. J. Psychiat.,* 122:1431–1435, 1966.

28. Macdonald, John M.: "Homicidal Threats," *Am. J. Psychiat.,* 124:475–482, 1967. Copyright 1967, the American Psychiatric Association.

29. Menninger and Modlin: op. cit., pp. 76–77.

30. Kinzel, Augustus F.: "Body Buffer Zone in Violent Prisoners," *Am. J. Psychiat.,* 127:99–104, 1970.

31. Horowitz, Mardi J., Donald F. Duff, and Lois O. Stratton: "The Body Buffer Zone: An Exploration of Personal Space," *Arch. Gen. Psychiat.,* 11:651–656, 1964.

32. Hediger, Heini: *Studies of Psychology and Behavior of Captive Animals in Zoos and Circuses,* Geoffrey Sircom (trans.), Criterion Books, New York, 1955.

33. Hall, Edward T.: *The Hidden Dimension,* Doubleday, Garden City, N.Y., 1966.

34. Megargee: op. cit., p. 111.

35. Ibid.

36. Ibid., p. 110.

37. Tanay, Emanuel: "Psychiatric Study of Homicides," *Am. J. Psychiat.,* 125:1252–1258, March 1969.

38. Tanay, Emanuel: *Medical World News,* op. cit., p. 41.

39. Hillman, James: "C. G. Jung's Contributions to 'Feelings and Emotions': Synopsis and Implications," in Magda B. Arnold (ed.), *Loyola Symposium on Feelings and Emotions, 1968,* Academic, New York, 1970, pp. 125–134.

40. Jung, C. G.: "The Mana Personality," *Two Essays on Analytical Psychology,* Meridian Books, The World Publishing Company, Cleveland, 1956, p. 240.

41. Wertham, Frederick: *The Show of Violence,* Doubleday, Garden City, N.Y., 1949.

42. Berkowitz, Leonard: "Experimental Investigation of Hostility Catharsis," in Jan Fawcett (ed.), *Dynamics of Violence,* American Medical Association, Chicago, 1971, pp. 139–144.

43. Macdonald: "Homicidal Threats," op. cit., p. 480.

44. Ibid., p. 481.

45. Wolfgang, op. cit., p. 22.

46. Ibid., p. 83.

47. Tupin, et al.: op. cit., p. 360.

48. Gross, Mortimer: "Violence Associated with Organic Brain Disease," in Jan Fawcett, (ed.), *Dynamics of Violence,* American Medical Association, Chicago, 1971, pp. 85–91.

49. Menninger, Karl A.: *The Vital Balance,* Viking, New York, 1963.

50. Jacobs, Patricia A., Muriel Brunton, and Marie M. Melville: "Aggressive Behaviour, Mental-Subnormality and the XYY Male," *Nature,* 208:1351–1352, 1965.

51. Kessler, Seymour, and Rudolph Moos: letter to *Science,* vol. 165, Aug. 1, 1969.

52. Macdonald: "Homicidal Threats," loc. cit.

53. Lion, John R.: "The Role of Depression in the Treatment of Aggressive Personality Disorders," *Am. J. Psychiat.,* 129:347–349, 1972. Copyright 1972, the American Psychiatric Association.

54. Bandura, Albert: *Aggression: A Social Learning Analysis,* Prentice-Hall, Englewood Cliffs, N.J., 1973.

Evaluation and Treatment of the Psychotic Patient

WHAT IS PSYCHOSIS?

The initial contact with a psychotic patient can be a confusing, upsetting experience. One does not want to relate to the patient in this state; one wants to bring him or her out of it so a normal interaction can occur. The first suggestion of the diagnosis of psychosis, then, often comes with the interviewer's discomfort with a patient's way of being-in-the-world, a sense that the patient is somehow too extreme or dreadfully lacking. Thus the patient's behavior is too bizarre, too happy, too sad, too confused, too confusing, too aggressive, or too withdrawn; or it is not usual enough, not well-enough modulated, not clear enough, not logical enough, not "under control," not "in contact." In short, the patient's failure to meet others as they expect to be met is *drastic*. The professional judgment that someone is psychotic simply registers the fact of his drastic departure from the basic expectations of others.

> *Example 5-1.* Late at night, the police brought a woman in her 20s to the emergency room. She had been trying to hitch a ride on a dangerous stretch of freeway when they picked her up.
>
> She wore a torn, faded granny dress, was barefoot, and her curly mop of blonde hair was flung out in all directions. Unlike many similarly dressed young adults, she had a look of pitiful terror on her face.
>
> When the therapist asked her what was wrong, her eyes widened in terror, her whole body shook, and her head moved back and forth furiously. She could have been saying, "I'm not allowed to talk." To any question she repeated this violent gesture of refusal. Otherwise she would stare, peacefully enough, straight ahead, with a half-smile on her face, and seemed not to care about the impression she made.
>
> She had said nothing to the police and had not resisted arrest. On her the police had found an envelope with the name of a mental hospital in a distant state, with the name Bob and a telephone number written on it.
>
> The therapist asked her if he could call this number. She did not respond. He dialed the number, received a recorded message that the number was not in service, and let the patient hear the recording. She started to weep. Almost immediately the tears stopped, and she again stared ahead with the half-smile on her face.

"Do you miss Bob?" the therapist asked. She responded with a burst of high-pitched laughter. After this, no question brought any response other than a shrug, a shudder, or a half-smile. After half an hour, the therapist had not even learned his patient's first name.

A formal definition of psychosis is given in Freedman, Kaplan, and Sadock [1]:

> *Psychosis.* Mental disorder in which a person's mental capacity, affective response, and capacity to recognize reality, communicate, and relate to others are impaired enough to interfere with his capacity to deal with the ordinary demands of life. The psychoses are subdivided into two major classifications according to their origin: psychoses associated with organic brain syndromes and functional psychoses.

The traditional dichotomy between organic brain syndromes and functional psychosis is oversimplified and can be misleading. What appears to be typical paranoid schizophrenia (functional) can arise as the result of impaired cerebral circulation in an austere hospital setting or as a result of amphetamine use. The patient in Example 5-1 may have been schizophrenic, but she may also have had a brain tumor or have been reacting to drugs.

Thus two uncertainties must be taken into account in working with psychotic patients: the patient's uncertainty about reality (or in the case of some paranoid schizophrenic patients, an overcertainty about a reality others cannot perceive) and the therapist's uncertainty about the nature and causes of the psychotic phenomena in the patient he is trying to evaluate and treat. Throughout this chapter we shall give guidelines on (1) how the therapist can refine his abilities to make an accurate diagnosis without prematurely stereotyping the patient with an incorrect label, and (2) how best to initiate treatment.

Example 5-1 (cont'd). When the patient remained mute, the therapist handed her a pencil and pad and asked her to write her name. She took the pencil and drew four interlocking ellipses that looked like a highway cloverleaf. With a look of great urgency she handed the paper to him.

The therapist accepted the drawing but he could not understand it. He then ordered 200 mg clorpromazine for her. She sniffed it, then swallowed it all. He told her he was arranging for her admission to a hospital. She did not respond. He placed her on a seventy-two-hour hold and arranged for transportation to the nearby state hospital, the only facility that would take her and had a bed open.

The transfer diagnosis was "acute schizophrenia, suspected," and the admitting physician at the state hospital promised follow-up information that never came. The therapist heard no more about the patient.

Such episodes are common. Contact with the psychotic patient is limited and confusing. A tentative diagnosis is made on the basis of limited information, and drug and hospital treatment is offered (often with only implied consent, sometimes with no consent) based on the tentative diagnosis. It is not suprising that strong criticisms have been leveled at the current practice of psychiatry with psychotic patients.[2,3] On the other hand, studies indicate that these same practices lead to a later, voluntary entry into treatment by two-thirds of the patients who are so treated.[4] Indeed, it is probable that this woman would start to talk within a day or two and that a more precise understanding of the nature and origin of her peculiar communicative state would become possible.

Nevertheless, several chances for error in the brief interventions that make up most first contacts with psychotic patients exist. Foremost is the chance for *diagnostic error.* The therapist decided to give the young woman chlorpromazine because he suspected "acute schizophrenia." Such a precise diagnosis was impossible to make from the data at hand. In addition to chlorpromazine, he gave his patient a label that will now accompany her as others treat her. Such labels are like old bandages clinging to an inadequately cleaned wound, infecting it further; often they must be removed and changed before adequate healing can occur.

On the other hand, not making a diagnosis is a dangerous practice. Without diagnosis the patient cannot be given the best care. The proper use of ECT (shock therapy), lithium, antipsychotics, and psychotherapy proceed from diagnosis. It is especially important to know if the psychosis is of organic origin, for unrecognized it often means irreversible brain damage or death. Changes in the central nervous system, first detectable by psychological interview, are the earliest signs of many serious somatic illnesses.

Organizing the Interview Data into Syndromes

Making an exact diagnosis of a psychotic patient is seldom easy. The diagnostic interview may reveal many symptoms that could belong to several diagnoses. Lorr, Klett, and McNair[5,6] have sought to arrange such data with the methods of factor analysis. They have shown that psychotic symptoms detectable through interviewing techniques fall into ten basic psychotic syndromes. These syndromes,

which may be present in varying combinations in different psychotic illnesses, and the patient symptom variables that make up each of them, are shown in Table 5-1. Lorr has shown that eight of these syndromes can be organized around a circle (Fig. 5-1) showing their frequency of association. The distance of the syndromes from each other in the circle represents the likelihood of their appearing together in a given psychotic state. Adjacent syndromes appear together frequently, opposite syndromes infrequently.

A patient showing motor disturbance is likely to show conceptual disorganization or disorientation but less likely to exhibit paranoid projection. A patient showing paranoid projection is as likely to show grandiose expansiveness as anxious intropunitiveness. Such associations become important when, as often happens, a patient shows one syndrome prominently. Then the circle guides the interviewer in what to look for next.

Organizing the Syndromes into Diagnoses

In the case of the psychotic hitchhiker in Example 5-1, the syndromes of motor disturbances and retardation and apathy were present.

The Psychotic Syndrome Circle

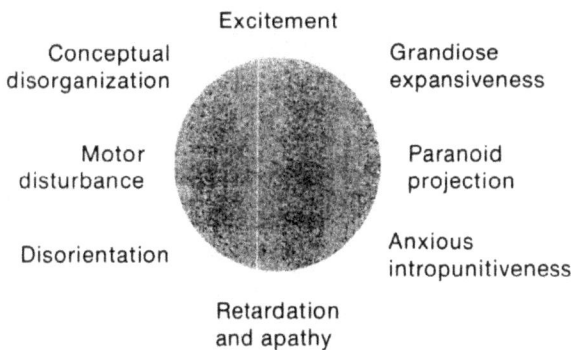

Figure 5–1 The psychotic syndrome circle.
[Adapted from [5], p. 116.]

Table 5-1   Psychotic Syndromes and Patient Variables Associated
with Them*

Psychotic Syndrome Name	Patient Variables Included
Excitement	Expresses feelings without restraint Manifests speech that is hurried Exhibits an elevation in mood Exhibits an attitude of superiority Dramatizes self or symptoms Manifests loud and boisterous speech Exhibits overactivity, restlessness Exhibits an excess of speech Tries to dominate the interview
Paranoid projection	Preoccupied with delusional beliefs Believes people talk about him Believes he is being persecuted Believes people conspire against him Believes people control his actions Believes external forces influence him
Hostile belligerence	Verbally expresses feelings of hostility Expresses an attitude of disdain Manifests a hostile, sullen attitude Manifests irritability and grouchiness Tends to blame others for problems Expresses feelings of resentment Complains and finds fault Expresses suspicion of people
Perceptual distortion	Distressed by hallucinatory voices Hears voices that accuse or blame Hears voices that threaten punishment Hears hortatory voices Sees visions Reports tactual, gustatory, or olfactory hallucinations Familiar things and people seem changed
Anxious intropunitiveness	Tends to blame or condemn self Anxious about specific matters Apprehension re vague future events Exhibits an attitude of self-depreciation Manifests a depressed mood Expresses feelings of guilt and remorse Does not show a lack of insight Preoccupied by suicidal thoughts Preoccupied by unwanted ideas Preoccupied by specific fears Believes he is unworthy, sinful

Retardation and apathy	Manifests slowed speech
	Indifferent to own future
	Exhibits a fixed facial expression
	Manifests slowed movements
	Deficient in recent memory
	Manifests blocking in speech
	Apathetic to self or problems
	Exhibits a slovenly appearance
	Manifests low or whispered speech
	Fails to answer questions
Motor disturbances	Exhibits peculiar, rigid postures
	Manifests overt signs of tension
	Grins or giggles inappropriately
	Exhibits peculiar grimaces
	Exhibits peculiar repetitive gestures
	Talks, mutters, or mumbles to self
	Glances around as if hearing voices
Conceptual disorganization	Gives answers that are irrelevant
	Gives incoherent answers
	Tends to drift off the subject
	Uses neologisms
	Repeats certain words or phrases
Disorientation	Does not know he is in a hospital
	Does not know where hospital is located
	Does not know name of one other person
	Does not know season of year
	Does not know calendar year
	Does not know own age
Grandiose expansiveness	Exhibits an attitude of superiority
	Hears voices that praise and extol
	Believes he has unusual powers
	Believes he is a well-known personality
	Believes he has a divine mission

*Drawn from material found in Lorr et al.[5], pp. 35–38, based on a factor analysis of ratings using the Inpatient Multidimensional Psychiatric Scale (IMPS).

The interviewer should have checked more carefully for signs of disorientation. It was not clear from the information whether the young woman's tears and laughter had any relation to the name Bob, or whether she intended the cloverleaf diagram to be an answer to the command to write her name. If the disorientation syndrome were present, it is likely that this young woman had an organic brain syndrome manifested by motor disturbances, disorientation, retardation, and apathy.

On the other hand, if the police description had stressed symptoms resembling those of an excitement syndrome on the freeway, the apathy she exhibited in the office could have been discounted and signs of conceptual disorganization should have been sought. If the cloverleaf diagram were an answer to the command to write her name, this impression would be confirmed. Acute catatonic schizophrenia manifested by motor disturbances, conceptual disorganization, and a history of recent excitement would be likely.

Treatment in the first instance would be an intensive search for the organic cause of the underlying disturbance; in the second, it might be a referral to a setting specializing in the treatment of acutely psychotic young adults.[7,8]

Three Approaches to Taxonomy

The American Psychiatric Association. In 1952 The American Psychiatric Association published its first *Diagnostic and Statistical Manual of Mental Disorders (DSM-I).*[9] The current edition, *DSM-II*[10] was published in 1968 and contains the preferred nomenclature. By and large, *DSM-II* preserves the traditional dichtomy between organic and functional psychoses and presents concise and useful descriptions of the various diagnostic entities, e.g., that *schizophrenia* can be broken down into subtypes of *simple type, hebephrenic type, catatonic type,* and so forth. The entities described in *DSM-II* are amplified upon by Freedman, Kaplan, and Sadock.[11]

Menninger. Karl Menninger and colleagues[12] took a different approach. They organized their basic patterns of psychosis around five major configurations of emotional, perceptual, and cognitive dysfunction: (1) pervasive sadness and guilt; (2) erratic disorganized excitement; (3) autistic regression; (4) delusional preoccupation; and (5) confused delirium. Any of these patterns encompasses a variety of the more traditional states. Menninger thinks that all of them represent a similar level of "dyscontrol" or ego failure.

A useful aspect of the Menninger approach is that it is phenomenological; i.e., it describes phenomena that the interviewer sees in his work with patients. Thus, if the interviewer notes pervasive sadness and guilt, or erratic disorganized excitement, he can then see what other symptoms

and signs described in those configurations are present. This approach may guide him to a more accurate diagnosis (which may be a traditional one) to aid him in treatment planning.

The five basic patterns of psychosis described by Menninger et al.[13] are

1. Pervasive feelings of sadness, guilt, despondency, and hopelessness, with convictions of inadequacy, incompetence, unworthiness, or wickedness—or several of these. Psychomotor retardation is usually present, sometimes stupor or restless activity, even agitation. Delusions or delusional trends appropriate to feelings of guilt, defection, unworthiness, and self-disparagement are common—such as fantasied offenses or fantasied punishment to come. (This picture has been called *melancholia, depression, thymergasia, affective disorder,* and other names.)

2. More or less continuous erratic, disorganized excitement, accompanied by a corresponding excess of verbal and motor production and emotional heightening, elation, excitement, irascibility, and so on. In this syndrome overactivity, volubility, and impulsivity may be at times self-injuring, at times bizarre, meddlesome, exhibitionistic, and socially annoying. The characteristic feature is the great and continuing overflow of poorly controlled energy. (This picture may be found in conditions variously called *mania, hypomania, delirium, furor, frenzy, recurrent mania, hyperthymergasia, moria, dysergasia, catatonic schizophrenia (excited stage), status epilepticus,* and many others.)

3. Autistic regression and self-absorption, silliness, mannerisms of speech and behavior, bizarre delusional ideation, irrelevancy and incoherence of speech, posturing and gross (apparent) indifference to social expectations. Inertness or automatonlike behav-

ior, often mutism or hallucinations, apparent indifference to the external world, but occasional sudden "impulsive" outbursts of speech or action are also typical. (This picture may be found in such conditions as *hebephrenia, parergasia, amentia, autism, chronic delirium, dementia simplex, catatonic schizophrenia (stuporous stage), chronic deterioration, regressed states, nuclear schizophrenia,* and many others.)

4. Delusional preoccupation with one or several themes, usually persecutory in trend, and usually accompanied by defensiveness, resentment, suspiciousness, grandiosity, condescension, irascibility, and so forth. A facade of dignity and sensibleness may partially or occasionally obscure the underlying picture. (This picture has classically gone under many compound names containing the noun *paranoia* or the adjective *paranoid.*)

5. Confused, delirious states with disorientation, bewilderment, amnesia, confabulation, and sometimes hallucinations and hyperactivity. These are commonly seen with severe injury, intoxication, or inflammation of the brain, hence with encephalitis, arteriosclerosis, alcoholic and other poisonings, Huntington's disease, Alzheimer's disease, and so forth. (These pictures have also been called *dementia* and *delirium.*)

Lorr, Klett, and McNair. Lorr et al.[14] used an empirical approach to taxonomy based on their earlier, phenomenologically defined psychotic syndromes. They tested several populations of acutely and chronically psychotic patients to see which syndromes were present or absent and how those syndromes that were present clustered together. They were able to establish nine regular types of psychosis for men and nine for women, representing different combinations of the basic syndromes.

All these psychotic types fell under four major categories: (1) paranoid, (2) disorganized, (3) excited, and (4) intropunitive. We shall use these four categories in the section on differential diagnosis.

From the work of Lorr et al. it is apparent that "disorientation," long considered the hallmark of organic psychosis, is in fact but one aspect of *psychotic disorganization,* which manifests itself along several dimensions: conceptual, affective, and orientative. In actual clinical situations, the sharp textbook distinctions between "functional" and "organic" illness do not hold up well: catatonia and hebephrenia are not always easy to distinguish from dementia and delirium.

THE DIFFERENTIAL DIAGNOSIS OF PSYCHOTIC STATES

The emergency therapist should accept the uncertainty of the initial contact with psychotic patients and explore the range of diagnostic possibilities. This chapter will attempt to help the therapist think intelligently about the range of diagnostic possibilities for any clinical situation. The material is organized under the four basic categories stemming from the work of Lorr et al.

Differential Diagnosis of Paranoid Conditions

Paranoid thinking may appear by itself (classical paranoia, rare) as a reaction to stress (common), or as part of another psychosis. It always involves a delusional interpretation of the motives, behavior, or intentions of others. The basic forms of paranoid thinking are *paranoid jealousy* (a profound, relentless suspicion that a partner is unfaithful, based on scant evidence and excessively argued), *paranoid eroticism* (the assumption that someone else, often a famous person, is infatuated with the patient and that even his avoidant actions are motivated by love), *paranoid grandiosity* (the patient's grossly inflated estimate of his own power), and the *persecutory paranoid state* (which may be the patient's nonspecific fear of retaliation for some hostile act or an active program of self-defense against a delusional "pseudocommunity"). The pseudocommunity, a typical part of the chronically paranoid patient's delusions, is "a group of real and imagined persons" assumed by him to be "bent on destroying his reputation or his life."[15]

The most common conditions under which paranoid thinking occurs are the paranoid stress reaction, the involutional paranoid state, schizophrenia, psychoses associated with drug use, organic brain syndromes associated with physical illnesses, and the manic phase of manic-depressive psychosis.

Paranoid Stress Reaction. This state is, as its name implies, an acute response to a crisis. Bellak says that the acute paranoid condition

> ... consists of an episode of delusions brought on by exhaustion or by a psychologically determined precipitating cause and is characterized by illusions which gradually develop into hallucinations and delusions. After the episode is over the personality is well-preserved and integrated.[16]

In *DSM-II*, this condition is classified under "other paranoid state." It is seen frequently in military settings and is part of the identity turmoil of young men. It can, however, occur at any age.

Involutional Paranoid State. This is a paranoid psychosis characterized by delusion formation that begins in the involutional period. Many feel that this condition is an alternate form of involutional depression. Divorced or separated women are at especially high risk. Twice as many women as men are hospitalized for involutional paranoid states. [17,18] Often, the wish fulfilling component of the dynamics is transparent, as in the following case:

> *Example 5-2.* A 47-year-old woman was admitted to the hospital from the emergency room, where she had been brought by her daughter. The woman had been living alone for the past ten years since her divorce. She had become extremely agitated that day after listening to the radio. During the interview, she said she believed herself to be engaged to a famous entertainer and had expected him to sing "their song" that day. When the song was not included in the broadcast, she became distraught and called her daughter.

Paranoid Schizophrenia. A question that should be asked early in the evaluation of anyone showing evidence of paranoid thinking is, "Is this schizophrenia?" Usually thought is more disorganized and delusional notions are more bizarre when schizophrenia is present than when paranoia occurs by itself. Kurt Schneider [19,20] has listed symptoms of first-rank importance for the diagnosis of schizophrenia:

1. Audible thoughts
2. Voices heard arguing
3. Voices heard commenting on one's actions
4. The experience of influences playing on the body (somatic passivity)
5. Thought withdrawal—the experience of having one's thoughts taken from one's mind
6. Thought insertion—the experience of having someone else's thoughts put into one's mind
7. Thought diffusion (thought broadcasting)—the experience of having other people directly privy to one's inner thoughts
8. Delusional perception—the crystallization of a set of delusional inferences on the basis of an everyday perception
9. "Made" feelings—the experience of having feelings which are felt to be the work of others

10. "Made" impulses–the experience of impulses to act which are felt to be implanted from outside

11. "Made" motor acts–the experience of being completely under the control of an external influence as one acts

This list of symptoms can be used to distinguish between paranoia and schizophrenia. Both paranoid and schizophrenic people are disturbed in relationship to an ecological group. The paranoid person has a suspicious, isolated relationship to his ecological group, fears its actions, mistrusts its motives, and misperceives its intentions. His ecological group is, in addition, a pseudocommunity: some of its members do not exist, although he behaves as if they do.

By contrast, the schizophrenic individual has an overly concrete relationship to his ecological group. Emotional participation, usually unconscious, with other persons is experienced by the schizophrenic person as a direct involvement in his conscious thinking. Moreover, the ecological group to which he relates is largely anonymous, such as arguing *voices* or *influences* playing on his body.

Finally, both paranoid and schizophrenic individuals are overly concerned with ordinary events and public experiences, for instance, with events they read about in newspapers or see on television, or with experiences with strangers on public transportation. The paranoid person personalizes public contacts; the schizophrenic person concretizes them. A paranoid schizophrenic patient may do both.

Some authors[21] doubt the existence of "pure paranoia," a state in which a single, fixed, false assumption underlies an intricate and internally consistent logical system, and mental functioning is normal in all other areas. These authors feel that schizophrenic thought disorder is always present in such cases, although it may be difficult to detect. In any event, some people who organize experience in a highly paranoid fashion exhibit few of the symptoms of the schizophrenias described by Schneider,[22] Bleuler,[23] and others.

Paranoid Psychoses Associated with Drug Use. Both schizophrenic and nonschizophrenic paranoid states may be associated with many organic conditions. Withdrawal syndromes from alcohol, amphetamines, bromides, barbiturates, and appetite-supressing drugs such as phenmetrazine may closely resemble paranoid schizophrenia. Amphetamine, LSD, marihuana, and cocaine may produce frightened or hostile paranoid thinking in the "high" state, with associated destructive or self-destructive behaviors (see Chapters 6, 8, and 9). Obtaining a single urine sample during an emergency can lead to identification of many of these substances if the patient is unable or unwilling to admit their use. In paranoid states of unknown etiology, it is always wise to suspect drug use and to be on the lookout for other signs of withdrawal or intoxication.

Paranoid Psychoses Associated with Other Organic Conditions. Sometimes a seemingly isolated paranoia in a clear sensorium is the first sign that a major organic illness is present. Patients over 45 who develop paranoid schizophrenic symptoms should receive careful neurological examinations for brain tumors. Cancers in other organs may also occasion paranoia; it is as if the patient senses a threat and projects it outside his body. When the patient confronts the reality of his physical illness, he can share the stress of preparing for an operation or for death with a physician, and the paranoia often disappears. As usual in psychosis, uncertainty appears to do more emotional harm than painful reality.

Paranoid reactions are common in physically ill patients who are confined to hospitals under conditions resembling sensory-deprivation experiments. In addition to environmental isolation, many chronically ill patients have organic brain syndromes that subtly or grossly impair their abilities to process information. Often these patients make paranoid explanations to themselves for poorly understood hospital procedures, personnel changes, or illness. In the treatment of such states, simple explanations, a lighted room at night, and frequent human contact often work wonders. These easily reversed paranoid reactions suggest that paranoia is a response to physical and emotional isolation and that it tends to disappear when the isolation can be interrupted through authentic contact with reality.

Manic-depressive Psychosis. An acute manic episode involves psychotic symptoms that progress through a sequence of stages. After the illness reaches its height, it remits by retracing the stages.[24] In the initial stage, the patient is *euphoric*; he talks too fast and demands too much. Kraepelin[25] called this picture "acute mania." In the intermediate stage, *anger and irritability* prevail, and the patient becomes angry and explosive. It is in this stage that paranoid delusions, both persecutory and grandiose, may appear, along with the classical flight of ideas. Kraepelin called this picture "delusional mania." In a final stage, the patient is *panicked*. He looks helpless. His thought processes, which are incoherent, are marred by loose associations, by bizarre and idiosyncratic paranoid delusions, and by ideas of reference. His movements are frenzied and pathetic. He may be disoriented or hallucinating. The picture is similar to that of a disorganized paranoid schizophrenia or to a delirium. Kraepelin called it "delirious mania."

The way to distinguish the intermediate delusional state of a manic episode from other paranoid states is to note the associated affective tone. The manic patient is irritable, and paranoid thinking emerges naturally from his anger. He can be talked out of it, distracted, mollified. As one therapist expressed it, "The way I could tell he was manic was that I still liked him when I was talking back to him." By contrast, the patient in a paranoid state is likely to present his delusions with reserved, controlled hostility and to remain unlikeably cool as he insists on preserving them.

One way to distinguish the final delirious stage of mania from deteriorated paranoid schizophrenia is to use Schneider's first-rank symptoms of schizophrenia. These first-rank symptoms were devised to distinguish schizophrenia from affective psychotic illness. None of these first-rank symptoms appeared in twenty manic patients studied by Carlson and Goodwin,[26] who established the three-stage sequence of mood changes in the manic episode. Another way to distinguish is to focus on the evidence for affective illness.[27] It should be noted that the progression from one mood stage to another can occur in a few hours or might take several days, but the sequence of stages seems to occur uniformly. Therefore, rapid progression of a seemingly paranoid psychosis through a series of moods in the stages described indicates a manic-depressive illness, and the therapist needs to consider lithium treatment (see Chapter 28).

Differential Diagnosis of Disorganized Psychotic States

Under these conditions, the ego fails to operate as a consistent center of consciousness and control. This failure may be represented in frank conceptual disorganization, disorientation, or the fragmentation of emotional responses so that thinking, sensory input from the outer world, and affective reactions are not properly integrated. When integration fails, the patient is in a vulnerable condition, at the mercy of his own uncontrollable reactions and of stronger people's wills.

When evaluating psychotically disorganized patients, the therapist must remember this *impressionability* and guard against premature feeling-reactions, diagnostic "labels," and treatment plans that encourage the patient to assume a *facade of pseudoorganization*. This facade conforms to the therapist's ideas, but the patient has not actually integrated his own experience. Indeed, many psychotic diagnoses are not made because the patient perceives that the therapist cannot tolerate "craziness," or the therapist structures the interview so that "crazy" material does not emerge.

In the differential diagnosis of disorganization, the most important distinction is between the *schizophrenias* (defined as "functional" psychoses having no clear basis in brain pathology) and the many *organic brain syndromes* (a change in the tissue structure or metabolism of the brain is the cause of the psychosis). A less frequent cause of the disorganized psychotic picture is the *third-stage mania* that has already been described.

The Schizophrenias. These disorders are a group of different behavioral responses to a similar kind of psychological deficit, involving the patient's inability to organize and maintain a consistent attitude toward his experience. There are many ways to understand this deficit,[28, 29] but Kurt Goldstein[30] offered a particularly clear formulation:

> ... an impairment of attitudes toward the abstract in the schizophrenic resulting therefore in concrete behavior similar to that in patients with brain disease. The abstract attitude of which Goldstein writes consists of: abilities to assume a mental set voluntarily, to shift voluntarily from one aspect of the situation to another, to keep in mind several aspects, to grasp the essentials of a whole, to break these up into parts and isolate them, to abstract common properties, to plan ahead, to assume an attitude of the possible, to think and act symbolically, to detach the ego from the outer world.[31]

The fact that often he does not utilize symbols in an abstract way does not mean the schizophrenic patient is impoverished in their use. Unlike the brain-injured patient whose language is frequently banal, the schizophrenic patient may show an arresting talent for metaphor. And although schizophrenic language is often difficult to comprehend, it is frequently interesting and intriguing. The major drawback is that the patient does not label the fact that he is using metaphors.[32] The effect is a little like a poet starting to speak modern poetry in the midst of an ordinary transaction.

Example 5-3. The senior editor of this book was doing therapy with a young schizophrenic woman. One day she greeted him with, "Hello, Mr. Rosenbaum, do you have any roses in your garden?" He responded that he didn't have a garden. Later he thought this answer missed the point. Translated (and taken in context), the question was: "Leaving your medical credentials aside, can you tell me if you are my therapist in name only, or do you really know how to make me bloom?"

A *symbolic mode* has come to replace the *cognitive mode* of ordinary communication. Moreover, the shift to the symbolic mode is not a conscious choice. Instead, the symbolic mode is substituted in situations that call for the cognitive mode. The patient may make these inappropriate substitutions most of the time or only some of the time. Almost all schizophrenic patients retain some healthy ego and can use the cognitive mode in well-structured situations. It is in ambiguous or unstructured situations that they turn most often to the symbolic mode.

Use of the symbolic mode is not in itself abnormal, of course; as Deikman[33] has recently pointed out, we all shift from the cognitive mode to a much more loosely structured mode of consciousness when we meditate or make love. The ability to daydream is part of mental health. What is abnormal is the *interference* with usual thinking by symbolic mode activity, the *archaic nature* of the symbolic intrusions, and the very substantial *loss of the normal ability to coordinate* cognitive mode with symbolic mode activity. As both Jung and Sullivan have noted, schizophrenia is like being unable to awake from dreaming as one tries to pursue everyday activities. The result is a disastrous fragmentation of personality. As Buss and Lang[34] note:

> ... when a schizophrenic is faced with a task, he cannot attend properly or in a sustained fashion, maintain a set, or change the set quickly when necessary. His ongoing response tendencies suffer interference from irrelevant, external cues and from "internal" stimuli which consist of deviant thoughts and associations. These irrelevant, distracting, mediating stimuli prevent him from maintaining a clear

focus on the task at hand, and the result is psychological deficit.[35]

Enoch Callaway[36] has compared schizophrenic thought processes to programs run in a computer constructed with unreliable components: the ability to make some reliable operations remains, but the risk of interference and interruption in the running of normal programs is ever-present.

The archaic nature of the symbolic mode in schizophrenia has been stressed by Freud and Jung, who saw striking comparisons to the preconceptual thinking of infants and to prescientific myths. Often the most archaic symbolic communications conceal the strongest affects. If this affect is discovered and released, the need to use symbolic communication is markedly reduced, as will be shown in Example 5-10.

Appropriate affective response is needed for the normal mediation between the symbolic and cognitive modes. When affect is lost, either mode can extinguish the other, with resultant disastrous restriction of personality. In the florid schizophrenic states, the symbolic mode tends to overrun the cognitive mode. In latent and residual schizophrenia, the cognitive mode gains a brittle, uneasy ascendancy, creating personality imbalance. Many observers have noted that such "borderline" patients are overly logical, poor in fantasy, and unable to relax. Instead of having a comfortable ability to loosen up, they use rigid defenses to wall off the symbolic mode, which is portrayed in dreams as a tidal wave threatening to break through. If affective response returns, some of the normal ability to shift into the symbolic mode may return, and the tidal wave subsides in the unconscious. If affective response does not return, the risk of a psychotic break is ever-present.

Bowers[37] has described the pathogenesis of an acute schizophrenic episode. First there is the *impasse*. The prepsychotic individual may be in considerable panic, unable to decide how to act or to communicate with others at a crucial point in his development. He may feel betrayed or rejected by a loved one, and he may be harboring intense

hatred and destructive fantasies toward the loved person. He cannot or dare not express these fantasies. This inability to communicate may stem in part from the patient's negative self-image. As Arieti[38] points out, recent failures in living may have confirmed a negative self-concept acquired much earlier in life. The patient really is a "bad me"; the world (like some earlier Terrible Parent), a "Malevolent Thou." Then, writes Arieti,

> In the totality of his human existence, and through the depth of all his feelings, the individual feels himself as totally defeated, without any worth or possibility of redemption.
>
> In most cases, only one solution, one defense, is still available to the psyche: to dissolve or alter his cognitive functions, the thought processes that have brought about conceptual disaster and that have acquired an ominous resonance with the original and preconceptual understanding of the self.[39]

At this point there is *destructuring of perception and affect*. The prepsychotic panic gives over to frank psychosis as the symbolic mode is allowed to overrun the cognitive mode. For many patients the experience is at first beatific, transcendent, and mystical. The patient may be elated by what he perceives as a "peak experience" of heightened awareness, and he will often want to share this "high" with others. The symbolic mode brings with it *symbolic perception*:[40] ordinary things take on a special meaning. Magical coincidences occur and are hailed. (Such perception is not quite delusional, but more like that of the Tarot reader who makes some accurate inferences by occult symbolic means but also may allow untoward associations to creep in.) *Projective identification* also occurs more easily in the symbolic mode: unacceptable parts of the self are rediscovered as a lurking presence of evil in the outer world, and "ideas of reference and influence" begin. (At this point the therapist may be viewed suspiciously or with scorn, even if he makes an effort to understand the patient's vision of the world. Any mention of the patient's former negative feelings is especially unwelcome, a sign of the therapist's "bad faith.")

Next, a *destructuring of the sense of self* occurs. The cognitive mode now gives way altogether to the symbolic mode. Identity dissolution begins and may be characterized by changes in the patient's mental image of himself, including major and bizarre changes in his body image. (For example, his left side may no longer seem to belong to him or his face may look unreal.)

Finally, *delusions are formed* as the symbolic mode supplies explanations for these changes to the shattered cognitive processes. The pressure to make sense of the experience aids in overcoming the realistic uncertainty that the delusional ideas are true, and crude delusional explanations may be welcomed with relief by ordinarily sophisticated patients. (A doctor with much experience in electronic technology may be satisfied that his room is bugged.[41]) Often the newly psychotic person naïvely shares his delusional explanations in an elated way.

A particularly common delusion is for the patient to believe that he is a messianic hero,[42] often Christ. In this case, the symbolic mode appears to be exerting its *reparative function*. Correcting the patient's helpless, evil, bad me, this delusional self-image not only improves the patient's self-esteem but gives him the energy to rechannel his life energies, especially his aggressive drives.[43] In this state the patient is often able to enter treatment, as Example 5-11 will show.

The *time course* of these stages is highly variable. The cognitive mode can disappear suddenly in response to overwhelming stress (such as the exhaustion of combat). The patient is likely to react to this sudden loss of ego with panic, excitement, and confusion (often expressed as the fear of being dead or of dying). These responses characterize "reactive schizophrenia," for which the prognosis is good.

Or the cognitive mode may be eroded insidiously (as in a family that subtly prevents vulnerable members from attaining a consistent point of view). The patient is able to make compensations for chronic interference with ego function, and panic does not appear. Instead, we see a major inability to think or to form coherent feeling-responses behind a facade that may be sad, silly, quizzical, apathetic, or paranoid—in any case, *resigned* to the presence of a deficit. This facade tends to put others off and to hide the schizophrenic person from himself[44]; it helps him do what his ego can not do, but at the cost of a permanent acceptance of dysfunction. This is the picture of "process schizophrenia," which has a poor prognosis. Prognostic features in schizophrenia are shown in Table 5-2.

Table 5-2 Prognostic Features in Schizophrenia [Herjanic [45]]

Associated with a Poor Prognosis
Insidious onset (more than six months)
Hebephrenic clinical picture
"Massive" delusions of persecution
Clear sensorium
Schizoid personality
Family history of schizophrenia
Striking emotional blunting
Associated with a Good Prognosis
Prominent depressive symptoms
Family history of affective disorders
No family history of schizophrenia
Good premorbid adjustment
Confusion
Acute onset (less than six months)
Precipitating factors
Concern with dying and guilt

The diagnosis of schizophrenia often implies a treatment fate. Certain typical courses for reactive and process schizophrenia have been described, each with a characteristic treatment. Involvement in aftercare becomes a major part of many schizophrenic patients' lives and strongly affects their ecological groups. According to Herjanic[46] and Rosenbaum,[47] typical courses are:

1. Acute onset with complete recovery. A later stress may precipitate another psychotic episode, which also responds to treatment. Response to psychotherapy is gratifying. A short hospitalization with or without antipsychotic medication may suffice; when high-dose phenothiazine treatment is used, the patient may be able to return to his usual activities in one or several weeks.[48]

2. Acute onset followed by recurrent episodes, with increasing residual impairment between episodes. Here antipsychotic drugs are needed intermittently, and long-term psychotherapy is indicated.

3. Insidious onset and chronic course broken by acute exacerbations and slight improvements. Both long-term phenothiazine treatment and long-term supportive psychotherapy are commonly used.

4. Insidious onset and slow progressive deterioration without acute exacerbation. Here long-term phenothiazine treatment and long-term social supervision are needed. Often such patients live in halfway houses, boarding homes, or state hospitals.

Despite many advances in society's understanding, tolerance, and treatments for the schizophrenias, they are not benign conditions. According to Herjanic, long-term follow-ups reveal that about one-sixth of untreated patients are eventually considered "cured with mild defect" (meaning a somewhat eccentric lifestyle and a blunted emotional life), another one-sixth show a moderate defect, and the remaining two-thirds become severely disabled. (Such statistics exclude the schizophrenias with the best prognosis as variants of affective illness.) A key point is that the patient be encouraged to seek treatment when schizophrenia is suspected.

In the emergency room, the therapist will see many forms of schizophrenia and many kinds of crisis situations. The patient may appear because he is distressed by the changes in his personality, or some peculiar feature of his behavior may distress a significant other. If his ecological group is in crisis, the schizophrenic person is more likely to appear in the emergency room. Affects belonging to the group in crisis are often perceived symbolically as direct interference with the patient's own thoughts. Yet if he communicates this distress, it may be the last straw for an already strained ecological group. His presenting picture will often be only part of a larger crisis situation. (This includes times of national crisis, which can be extremely trying for schizophrenic individuals.)

The schizophrenic patient's need for specific intervention and the ecological group's need for crisis intervention must be kept separate. It is true that the patient will settle down when the emotion in his group becomes less intense, but failure of the cognitive mode requires special individual support that an ecological group approach alone cannot provide. The balancing of these two needs is described in Chapter 10, which presents the treatment of an acutely schizophrenic young man and his ecological group.

The diagnosis of schizophrenia is not easy because of the wide variability in presenting pictures. In many instances acute schizophrenia is difficult to distinguish from delirium. If confusion and disorientation predominate, organic causes, including intoxication, must be ruled out before the diagnosis of schizophrenia is made. Chronic schizophrenia may resemble organic dementia or mental retardation.[49]

In describing the signs and symptoms of the schizophrenias, and from these a typology of schizophrenia, Bleuler[50] drew heavily from the work of Kraepelin. A primary symptom is *autism*, which reflects the shift from the cognitive to the symbolic mode. Some cognitive mode function always remains to the ego, but it is often grossly impaired by the continual intrusions of the symbolic mode. As a consequence, *attention* is no longer focused for tasks but scans the perceptual field; it ignores usual boundaries and becomes overinclusive. We have already stressed the loss of appropriate *affective response*, which may trigger the turn to the symbolic mode. *Ambivalence* characterizes emotions that are communicated by the symbolic mode; entire response tendencies organize into pairs of opposites and paralyze decision making. Finally, will, behavior, and activity undergo changes. A concise review of Bleuler's original descriptions may be found in Rosenbaum.[51]

Recently, Schneider's first-rank symptoms of schizophrenia (already described) have gained considerable importance in diagnosis. Some therapists insist on their presence before the diagnosis can be made; others remain faithful to Bleuler. A useful table of the symptoms that have been related to schizophrenia has been prepared by Herjanic (Table 5-3).

The last step in diagnosis is the classification of the kind of schizophrenia. Usually it is not difficult to distinguish acute from chronic schizophrenia, paranoid from hebephrenic (silly) or catatonic (excited or stuporous) schizophrenia. Subtleties emerge when the schizophrenic picture grades into one resembling affective disorder (schizoaffective schizophrenia, excited or depressed), neurosis (pseudoneurotic schizophrenia), or sociopathy (pseudosociopathic schizophrenia). In *DSM-II*, the latter two schizophrenias are called "latent schizophrenia." Additional labels include simple, residual, childhood, and chronic undifferentiated schizophrenia. Since Bleuler and Kraepelin there have been few changes in this unsatisfactory classification. Further discussion of the differential diagnosis of the schizophrenias is beyond the scope of this book, but the reader is referred to others [52, 53] who also provide a key to the current taxonomy.

Organic Brain Syndromes. Frequently disorganization is found in organic brain syndromes.[54] Because they may occur in an entirely clear sensorium, organic brain syndromes are difficult to distinguish from schizophrenia. Usually there is a reduction in the *level* of awareness and a reduction in the *efficiency* of cognitive functions that suggests organic difficulty. Spheres of mental

Table 5-3 Symptoms Related to Schizophrenia [Herjanic [45], p.76]

A. Almost Pathognomonic Symptoms
Audible thoughts
Voices conversing with one another
Voices commenting on one's own actions
Somatic passivity experiences
Thought withdrawal
Diffusion of thought
Delusional perception
Feelings of being controlled by others
Flat affect

B. Highly Suggestive Symptoms
Neologisms
Tangential speech
Blocking
Catatonic symptoms
rigidity
waxy flexibility
posturing
Autism

C. Symptoms Commonly Seen
Incongruous affect
Delusions
persecution
reference
body change
Hallucinations
auditory
somatic
Apathy
Inappropriate or bizarre behavior
Social isolation
Poor occupational or academic performance
Poverty of thought

functioning in which impairments are most likely to appear can be remembered from the acronym EMOJIAC;

> Emotion
> Memory
> Orientation
> Judgment
> Intellect
> Attention
> Concentration

Emotion becomes labile and shallow; recent memory is more impaired than past; orientation to time and place is more impaired than to persons; judgment of social realities may be poor; intellectual functioning (such as the ability to compute) is compromised; attention to environmental events is reduced; concentration on work and the general level of mental functioning is reduced.[55] All these issues are treated more fully in Chapters 14 and 30 and the appendixes.

Delirium derives from a Latin word meaning "derailed." It implies a sudden insult to consciousness that is based on a failure of brain metabolism or depression by toxins. The effects of this sudden "cerebral insufficiency"[56] are a reduction in the level of consciousness, a lessening of the ability to attend, and a marked disturbance in cognitive function. Diffuse slowing in the EEG "is a regular finding in delirium regardless of the cause" and provides "an accurate reflection of the metabolic adequacy of cortical neurons."[57] The EEG is slowest when the level of awareness is lowest; it tends to recover as treatment produces a return of a clear sensorium and is the most reliable indicator of the continued presence of the delirium. These EEG findings are not present in schizophrenia.[58]

The delirious patient may not look ill to cursory examination, or he may be obviously "out of his head." Profiles of patients include the (1) quiet and torpid, (2) blandly confused, (3) anxious and panicky, (4) hallucinating, and (5) muttering and incoherent patients. Types 1 to 3 are easily confused with depressed, habitually stupid, or neurotic patients; only a careful mental status examination can reveal the underlying cognitive defect.[59]

Dementia, which denotes a permanent loss of function in higher cortical neurons, produces an irreversible intellectual deficit. The deficit is stable, marked by a *loss* of function rather than by a distortion of function, as is delirium. Disturbances in memory stand out, and the personality deteriorates as the patient becomes progressively more unkempt, lacking in initiative, and emotionally unstable. In addition to diffuse loss of higher intellectual functioning, *judgment* fails in the demented patient. Occasionally a patient will be admitted to a psychiatric unit with the diagnosis of acute schizophrenia or affective psychosis, and only later will the diagnosis of dementia of recent onset become apparent. Among the causes of dementia (which will not be considered further in this book) are (1) senility; (2) degenerative brain diseases (such as Alzheimer's and Pick's diseases, and Huntington's chorea); (3) arteriosclerosis; (4) syphilis; (5) encephalitis of other cause; (6) brain injuries; (7) brain tumors; and (8) end-stage alcoholism.[60]

Psychoses Associated with Drug Use.* The most common drugs are amphetamines, alcohol, LSD, marihuana, and cocaine. *Amphetamine withdrawal psychosis* may closely resemble acute paranoid schizophrenia. In the early withdrawal phase there may be frightening visual and auditory hallucinations, disorientation and confusion, irritability, muscle cramps, headaches, sensations of heat and cold, sweating, and alternations of weakness with aggressive and sometimes violent behavior. Amphetamine and its metabolites, which can be demonstrated in the urine, lead to the diagnosis. Both during intoxication and after withdrawal, other symptoms may be very similar to those of chronic paranoid schizophrenia.[61]

Alcoholic psychosis include acute and pathological intoxication, delirium tremens, alcoholic auditory hallucinosis, and the Wernicke-Korsakoff syndrome. All these conditions are described in detail in Chapter 6.

LSD psychosis is discussed in Chapter 8. In contrast to schizophrenia, a "bad trip" on LSD is characterized by predominantly visual hallucinations and a heavy dose of what Sullivan called the "uncanny" emotions: awe, dread, horror, and

---

*Psychoses associated with drug use, toxic conditions, and diseases of the body and the brain are other kinds of organic brain syndromes. Because it is important to consider their individual characteristics, we shall consider them separately from the organic brain syndromes just described.

loathing. The average LSD trip lasts eight hours and can be managed successfully by "talking the patient down" with occasional support from diazepam (see Chapter 8). However, LSD use has precipitated a full-blown paranoid psychosis in susceptible individuals, so the emergency therapist should not be complacent when someone comes in on a bad trip. Unknown agents mixed in street drugs—the most common being strychnine and arsenic—also produce organic psychoses if they are taken in quantity.

Marihuana psychosis[62] has been reported in patients who required admission to a hospital after they smoked marihuana. Initially they exhibit aggressive behavior, gross motor disturbances, bizarre grandiose delusions, passivity, and amnesia. Later there may be an indefinite period of amnesia, flattening of affect, and mild-to-moderate thought fragmentation. When cannabis and alcohol are combined, visual hallucinations can also occur.

The effects of *cocaine* are similar to those of a short-acting amphetamine. When the user is high, or during the early withdrawal phase, he may become belligerent and grandiose. In four to six hours the trip ends. Damage to the mucous membranes of the nose (nosebleeds) are a sign this drug has been used.

Carbon Monoxide Psychosis. Cases of carbon monoxide poisoning are becoming more frequent. The clinical picture combines confusion with the expression of anger that would ordinarily be suppressed. Headaches and a characteristic cherry-red color to the skin suggest this diagnosis. Although leaking home refrigerators are the commonest cause, this syndrome has been reported after freeway driving. It also may result from a suicide attempt.

Metabolic and Endogenous Psychoses. Tumors of the brain and endocrine system can produce schizophrenic pictures. Other endocrine abnormalities can also produce significant behavioral alterations.

Brain tumors are the bane of the emergency therapist's existence because he usually forgets to consider them as a possible cause of psychological illness. Patients who develop paranoid schizophrenia after the age of 40 should always be evaluated for brain tumors. A good neurologic evaluation is part of the routine treatment for the first appearance of any psychotic state in a person of any age. Psychosis and confusion may be a compensation for compromise or loss of brain tissue.

Hypoglycemia may produce a range of symptoms from passive-aggressive behavior to psychosis. Many prediabetics show hypoglycemic symptoms, although the most florid symptoms are found in diabetics who use too much insulin and in patients with insulin-secreting tumors of the pancreas. The symptoms usually include a sense of "jitteriness inside," hunger pangs, sweating, muscle weakness, apprehension, disorientation, and delusions. Hyperactivity of reflexes and seizures have been reported.

The patient may be brought raving into the emergency room. If hypoglycemia is suspected, a blood glucose determination should clarify the diagnosis, and, if confirmed, an intravenous injection of 50 cc of 5% glucose should produce a dramatic clearing of the symptoms. Such glucose infusions should be made only after it has been ascertained that the patient has not been drinking heavily. A comatose alcoholic patient may be unable to metabolize glucose because of an excess of pyruvic acid secondary to thiamine deficiency. Unless thiamine is administered first and given time (usually thirty minutes) to take effect, a serious or fatal reaction to glucose may ensue.

Other endocrine conditions that may produce behavioral alterations are hyperthyroidism, pheochromocytomas, and high doses of steroids. Often the organic nature of these conditions is betrayed by the *lability* of the patient's affect. In the most severe forms the symptoms mimic delirious and manic states.

Infections and Inflammations of the Brain. Psychosis characterized mainly by confusion and a clouding of consciousness is one of the first signs of *meningitis* and *encephalitis*. Additionally, *temporal arteritis* may manifest itself in this way. Often the patient is well until a few hours before the appearance of the symptoms; the family is anxious but otherwise normal, and there is no history of stress. Often the psychosis is present before other signs of organic disease such as fever or underlying pneumonia can be demonstrated. There will be pressure from a medical service to accept this patient as a "schizophrenic." Generally, nonspecific psychosis characterized mainly by confusion without other signs indicating schizophrenia should be evaluated medically for several days before the patient is transferred to a psychiatric unit.

Epilepsy.[63] It is well known that the "psychic seizures" of *temporal lobe epilepsy* can produce a schizophrenialike picture. These episodes may last for days or weeks and may not be accompanied by EEG changes that clearly diagnose epilepsy. On the other hand, temporal lobe EEG changes are present in many patients diagnosed as schizophrenic. All of Schneider's first-rank symptoms of schizophrenia may be present. Other psychotic reactions belong to the "twilight state" following a *grand mal seizure.* Periods of excitement may occur and in rare instances last several days. These periods are characterized by extreme agitation, paranoid ideation, hallucinations, and delusions that cause aggressive outbursts.

Differential Diagnosis of Excited Psychotic Conditions

Alcoholic psychoses, hypoglycemia, epilepsy, and LSD are common organic causes of psychotic excitement. Among the functional psychoses, the *manic phase of manic-depressive psychosis, acute catatonic schizophrenia, acute homosexual panic,* and the *sociopathic personality in a state of rage* are the most frequent excited conditions. And certain *side effects of phenothiazine drugs* and *chronic schizophrenia in exacerbation* can lead to excitement.

The Manic Phase of Manic-depressive Psychosis. This phase was partially described before to distinguish it from paranoid schizophrenia. To make the diagnosis of primary affective disorder, manic type, Feighner and his associates[64] seek

A. Euphoria or irritability

B. At least two of the following:
   1. Hyperactivity
   2. Push of speech
   3. Flight of ideas
   4. Grandiosity
   5. Decreased sleep
   6. Distractibility

C. At least a two-week course before reaching the hospital

It must be emphasized, however, that in a single, brief contact the patient may look quite good—quiet, reasonable, and charming—not at all as described by his ecological group. The therapist may emerge from the initial interview feeling that he alone understands the patient and that those who insisted he come to the emergency room are scapegoating him. Splitting the therapist and the ecological group is characteristic of the acutely manic patient: he has an unparalleled ability to manipulate.

Indeed, on initial contact the therapist's only clue to the presence of mania may be the "interpersonal havoc"[65] that the acutely manic patient can create. Janowsky et al. observed in a recent article, "Playing the Manic Game":

> Possibly, no other psychiatric syndrome is characterized by as many disquieting and irritating qualities as that of the manic phase of manic-depressive psychosis. These characteristics seem specific to the acute attack. . . .

> The acutely manic patient is often able to alienate himself from family, friends, and therapist alike. This knack is based on the facile use of maneuvers which place individuals relating to the manic in positions of embarrassment, decreased self-esteem, and anxious self-doubt.[66]

These authors found that the manic patient uses five types of activity to induce discomfort in those around him:

1. Manipulation of the self-esteem of others: praising or deflating others as a way of exerting interpersonal leverage

2. Perceptive exploitation of areas of vulnerability and conflict

3. Projection of responsibility

4. Progressive limit testing

5. Alienating family members

Thus, one way to recognize the manic patient is from the size and exasperation of his ecological group. Many people will call the emergency room, angry with the patient and with each other, each with a different idea of what must be done. The appearance of a *manipulated ecological group* at war with the patient and with each other is strong evidence of mania.

Acute Catatonic Schizophrenia (Excited Phase). This syndrome differs from mania in the *fragmentation* of the patient's personality. The patient is wildly excited by vivid hallucinations and delusions that he may or may not offer freely to the therapist. This form of schizophrenia often has a good prognosis. The patient often shows considerable insight into psychotic material and is intensely interested in sharing it with a therapist: thus he is a good candidate for psychotherapy.

The patient's willingness to share his psychotic attempts at regaining his sanity poses problems for the emergency therapist. A real liability of many paranoid and manipulative psychotic patients is their need to impose their idiosyncratic solutions upon others. The therapist can help such patients only if he stands up to this psychotic attempt at problem solving and insists that the patient come to terms with his deficit in realistic thinking.

On the other hand, many schizophrenic patients are seriously engaged in rebuilding their own egos, and they use their fantasies to help them, not to exert power over others. They behave as if the symbolic mode is helping them. The therapist who cannot accept the archaic solutions presented by the symbolic mode may pressure his patients to substitute cognitive mode thinking. He will get it, but only by forcing his patients to assume a facade. The symbolic thinking will continue beneath this facade but will not develop into cognitive thinking because the patient has been taught to distrust it.

The acutely catatonic patient may be either wildly excited or stuporous and may require several days of tranquilizing medication before he is able to open up.

Acute Homosexual Panic. The picture of this syndrome is described by

> . . . intense agitation and panic, confusion, delusions and hallucinations of persecution, occasional assaultiveness, and considerable preoccupations with homosexuality and fears of homosexual attack per anum. [67]

There is often a precipitating event, such as

> . . . seductive closeness or actual attempt at seduction by a member of the same sex, loss of a close friend of the same sex, failure in heterosexual performance, separation from home and friends, etc. [68]

Recently Ovesey[69] has demonstrated that apparently homosexual concerns are often really *pseudohomosexual* in many men, who symbolize their conflicts over power and dependency in terms of sexual submission to a feared or envied rival. Whenever their power is threatened, such pseudohomosexual men often turn to violence, as in the following case reported by Woods: [70]

> *Example 5-4.* A businessman entered treatment because of severe depression precipitated by competitive defeat at the hands of an old business rival. The patient's fantasy of wealth and status was shattered by his rival's completely legal but unethical manipulations which won a coveted contract. In treatment

the patient alternated between fits of depression and fits of rage with plots of vengeance and violent destruction. He finally hired someone with instructions to beat and cripple the offender on the anniversary of the incident. The patient clung to his plan until one day he appeared panic-stricken following a dream. In the dream he encountered a cripple on the street whose attempts to walk appeared ludicrous and caused the patient to laugh loudly. However, he jumped into the cripple's immensely powerful arms and was promptly stipped naked and impaled upon a huge erection. A crowd gathered and hooted at his humiliation.

Clearly, such men live close to panic, and psychotherapy may precipitate a frank psychosis. As Woods points out:

Patients may experience psychotherapy as having their nose rubbed in their passivity and dependency, and the therapist's interventions as the equivalent of rape. They view the unfolding of their inner life as a submissive humiliating surrender of masculinity. Such patients often have strong paranoid dynamics, and when there is significant or psychotic ego disorganization the therapist may indeed be in danger.[71]

It is important to remember that the patient in a homosexual or pseudohomosexual panic is likely to turn to violence. Often the treatment resembles the treatment of the homicidal patient described in Chapter 4, but with the frequent additional need for brief hospitalization.

The Sociopathic Personality in a State of Rage. This kind of patient is excited, hostile, and manipulative. The usual explanation is that he has begun to fail in his attempts to manipulate others or in his attempts to control himself. Usually his psychosis reflects the ambivalence between his need for help and his desire to dominate. The following case is adapted from Lorr's illustration of his excited-hostile type:

Example 5-5. A 38-year-old white male, unemployed, married, and the father of two children, was admitted to the hospital when he complained of feeling as if he were "losing his mind." His long drinking history had begun in the military service.

Six weeks before his admission to the hospital he had come to the city to look for work. He started drinking before he was on the bus, played card games, and passed checks on a closed account. He thought of jumping out of his hotel room window, but the idea struck him as so ridiculous he became hysterical. One day he awoke in "somebody's boathouse." He felt ill, vomited frequently, and was so frightened by the ideas flying through his head that he came to the hospital for help.

After his admission, the patient acted anxious to please and promised never to get into trouble again. He worked well at hospital jobs and had a good memory and good orientation. He was continuously boisterous and jocular on the ward and in groups because, he said, he would rather be that way than cry. In spite of his promises to do better and his anxiousness to please, he refused group and individual therapies because he felt he had only two problems: financial difficulties and the fear of his wife's leaving him. A week before he was to be discharged he became upset when he received legal papers for his wife's divorce. He became destructive and disturbing to other patients on his ward and was discharged. He was diagnosed as a sociopathic personality with alcoholism.[72]

Often in retrospect such admissions appear to be the sociopathic patient's attempts to obtain sympathy, an excuse for misbehavior, and an appeal for a second chance. He may try to fulfill these needs by simulating any of the psychotic syndromes just described, especially mania and panic.

Often the manipulative patient is alienated and needs a treatment setting to satisfy his wish to complain with the theater's aging salesman, Willy Loman, that "Attention must be paid!" Like Willy, the manipulative patient may need to hide his dependent need behind a belligerent, help-rejecting facade. It may be adequate therapy to pay attention briefly, even if the hospitalization ends when the patient, no longer feeling the need for help, angrily departs against medical advice.

Side Effects of Phenothiazine Medications. Certain side effects of phenothiazine medications resemble excited psychotic conditions. The most important are *akathisia* and *tardive dyskinesia*.

Akathisia appears *early* in treatment with phenothiazines. Akathisia

> . . . is the inability to sit still. The patient experiences symptoms of restlessness and tends to move about. Inactivity produces a feeling of extreme discomfort, resulting in shifts of the legs, tapping of the feet, or rocking the body. The patient who is unable to remain seated and must get up and walk about is said to have tasikinesia.[73]

A clue to this untoward reaction to phenothiazines (usually trifluoperazine and fluphenazine) is the patient's complaint that he finds the medication unpleasant. However, he may complain of being unable to sleep and to lie down, and the emergency therapist, noting his restlessness, pacing, and anxiety, may assume that the patient's hyperactivity represents an exacerbation of his psychosis. Tardive dyskinesia occurs *late* in treatment with phenothiazines (see Chapter 26).

Of course, excitement is often the reason for long-term phenothiazine treatment, not the result of it. Recently Kline[74] reported the case of a schizophrenic woman whose tendency to hostile, belligerent excitement has required high-dose treatment with phenothiazines for eighteen years. She has shown no physical ill effects from these drugs and has maintained an adequate social recovery.

Chronic Schizophrenia in Exacerbation. This produces dramatic, excited picture, often when the patient stops his medication in defiance of someone who has displeased or expected too much of him. Such patients are often dragged by police into emergency rooms in astonishing states of excited disorganization that require several men to contain. Occasionally a patient will come himself for a "booster dose" of a phenothiazine drug that helped him in the past.

Example 5-6. The wife of a middle-aged man called to say that her husband was coming into the emergency room. His previous therapist also called and said that this man would probably come in as he had seven years before, screaming loudly that he was going to lose control. After a single dose of chlorpromazine, his former therapist predicted, "He will most likely calm down and be able to go home." The therapist offered to see him in his office the following day.

The patient came in screaming, "I'm going to blow, I'm going to blow!" and had a pale, "possessed" look that was distinctly frightening. The emergency therapist immediately gave him 200 mg of liquid chlorpromazine to drink; the patient quieted down almost immediately, and his wife said there would be no problem at all taking care of him until he could see his therapist.

The entire transaction took less than an hour and was an exact repeat of the patient's behavior seven years before.

Differential Diagnosis of Intropunitive Conditions

Intropunitive means the continuous self-torture of the psychotically depressed individual. The neurotically depressed patient's jury is still out, but the psychotically depressed patient has already been found guilty and has begun to serve his sentence. When he accepts this internal judgment, the patient may become anxious or resigned, and his preoccupations leave no doubt that he feels he has sinned and must pay through incessant self-questioning, a period of inactive silence, or death. Thus agitation, psychomotor retardation, or dread may be the predominant affective symptoms, and the depressive thought content may involve obsessive concerns with bodily decay, the conviction that life is over, or accusation by voices that insist on self-mutilation or execution. Where neurotic ambivalence centers on the degree of guilt, psychotic ambivalence concentrates on how the sentence may be carried out: suicide (a risk in all depressions) is most likely here.

The important diagnostic considerations for intropunitive psychotic states are *psychotic depressive reactions, primary affective disorders, schizoaffective schizophrenia, depressions related to drug use,* and *depressions caused by organic illness.* Many examples of patients with psychotic depressions are found in Chapters 2 and 3, together with material concerning the dynamics of depression. Here we shall concentrate upon the diagnosing of such states. Depressions belong to the class of psychiatric illnesses that have been called "the affective or mood disorders." The current classification of these disorders by George Winokur[75] is depicted in Figure 5-2.

Psychotic Depressive Reactions. Most people react to loss or precipitating stress with a certain degree of depression. Some, especially so-called depressive characters, may react with a depression so severe and incapacitating that it assumes psychotic proportions. The depression may occur in response to a loss or threatened loss, such as the death of a loved one, the onset of old age, a major life-threatening illness, or major surgery. Or depression may occur with pre-existing psychiatric illness, such as hysterical personality, anxiety neurosis, antisocial personality, alcoholism, or drug addiction.[77] Winokur[78] found such depressions frequently among patients admitted to a psychiatric hospital for a variety of primary diagnoses, such as neuroses, acute and chronic brain syndromes, schizophrenia, and alcoholism. He suggests we call such depressions "secondary depression," noting that it is entirely possible they are reactive "to a chronic life of psychiatric disabilities" caused by the primary disorder. Our chapters on suicide and alcoholism (Chapters 2, 3, and 6) give much information concerning the lives of persons chronically susceptible to such "secondary depression," which can in fact be more

The Affective Disorders

Primary depression

Secondary depression (associated with psychiatric illness)

Depression related to physical illness

Reactive depression (bereavement)

Manic-depressive disease (bipolar)

Depressive disease (unipolar)

Pure depressive disease

Depression spectrum disease

Figure 5-2 The affective disorders. [76] [Adapted from [76], p. 2.]

incapacitating than the primary disorder, requiring intensive acute intervention without prejudice based on the prognosis for the underlying chronic condition.

Primary Affective Disorders. In the primary affective disorders the symptoms are thought to arise primarily from biological and physiological causes and only secondarily as a response to life stress. Often there is a family pattern of mood disturbance, indicating a hereditary aspect.

Some psychotic depressions are part of a manic-depressive cycle. The patient has had clearly documented episodes of mania and depression,

usually with a normal period separating them, although sometimes one phase proceeds directly from the other. This is called *bipolar* affective disorder, and it seems to run in families.

Patients who become psychotically depressed one or more times and who have never had a manic period are said to have a *unipolar* affective disorder.[79] Usually their families are also free of a history of mania. A special kind of unipolar disorder is involutional melancholia, which is profound depression arising in the middle age of persons who had been previously extraordinarily conscientious, virtuous, and responsible.

Some patients with *unipolar* depressions are the

Primary Depression

Manic-depressive disease (bipolar)

Characteristics

Periods of mania and depression

Strong family history of affective disease

Five or more episodes in lifetime

Patients in their 20s or 30s

X-linked transmission

Depressive disease (unipolar)

Characteristics

No periods of mania

Fewer than five episodes of illness in lifetime

Onset in late 30s or 40s

Pure depressive disease

Characteristics

Typical patient is male in his 40s

Equal number of male and female relatives with depressive illness

Depression spectrum disease

Characteristics

Typical patient is female under 40

Male relatives have tendency toward alcoholism and sociopathy

Female relatives have tendency toward depressive illness

Figure 5-3 Primary depression. [76] [Adapted from [76], p. 3.]

only members of their families to become depressed. Others have relatives who show depressive equivalents such as drinking and sociopathy. On this basis Winokur[80] distinguishes pure depressive disease from "depression spectrum disease." His summary of the kinds of primary depression is given in Figure 5-3.

Even though all these kinds of psychotic depressions may seem quite similar clinically, making such distinctions is important for treatment: lithium carbonate seems to offer prophylaxis against the depressive as well as the manic phase of bipolar illness; ECT may work wonders in unipolar depression; and tricyclic antidepressants should not be used in bipolar depressions. (Drug treatment of depressions is discussed in detail in Chapter 28.)

Three stages in the development of a psychotic depression have been described, akin to the three stages of a manic attack. The *first stage* of a depressive attack is marked by fatigue, inertia, and dissatisfaction. The patient may cease to take care of himself, report bodily discomfort with bizarre tinges ("his chest is heavy as a stone . . . he feels no sensations but his weight"[81]), start to berate himself, or make suicide attempts. Typically, the patient will have difficulty falling asleep, wake early in the morning, feel worst just after getting up, and feel most like himself in late afternoon.

The *second stage* is sometimes called the acute stage. It brings major focus on the body and its sensations, but the explanations for the physical distress are weird. We hear from the patient that "his brain is melting, his bowels are stopped up, his heart fails to beat, his stomach is rotting away."[82] One patient said, "I had a bowel movement several months ago that took the life out of me." In addition to such *somatic delusions*, the fixed belief that a major illness is present may appear. Furthermore, a kind of negative grandiosity appears: the patient has become the worst person in the world, the source of its evils and problems; he thinks he has engendered wars and catastrophes. He feels unreal, and hallucinations and paranoid ideas appear. Although he expects death, he fears poisoning and stops eating. (At this

point food has lost its flavor and looks peculiar.)

The *third stage* is stupor. The patient refuses to get up, talk, or respond visually to stimulation. He will not eat, go to the bathroom, or control his urination or defecation. Such patients often develop major fecal impactions or bladder infections. He is preoccupied with fantasies of sin and death, delusions, and hallucinations.

Anxiety comes early in the depressive process; weight loss is late. Early in depression the patient may try suicide; later he may starve to death.

Abstracting from these and other descriptions of psychotic depression, Feighner and colleagues[83] propose these criteria to make the diagnosis:

A. Dysphoric mood (depressed, sad, blue, and so on.)

B. At least four of the following:
   1. Anorexia or weight loss
   2. Sleep difficulty
   3. Loss of energy
   4. Agitation or retardation
   5. Loss of interest in usual activities (includes decreased libido)
   6. Self-reproach or guilt
   7. Diminished ability to think or concentrate
   8. Recurrent thoughts of death or suicide

C. At least a one-month course prior to admission to the hospital

Schizoaffective schizophrenia is distinguished by the evidence of conceptual disorganization favoring the symbolic mode, which is characteristic of schizophrenia. Many clinicians feel that this disorder is a variant of primary affective illness, from which it is sometimes indistinguishable.

Depressions Related to Drug Use and Organic Illness. Serious depressions are seen after alcohol and amphetamine withdrawal, during active marihuana and barbiturate use, and as a side effect of reserpine and diazepam (Valium®) medication. The psychotic manifestations tend to clear when the patient has been free of all drugs for several weeks, although the amphetamine and alcohol user may show sleep disturbances for months after withdrawal. These issues are discussed in greater detail in Chapters 6 to 9.

Organic illnesses, such as anemia, cancer, and heart disease, may show the dispiritedness, anxiety, retardation, sleep disturbances, and weight loss of a primary depression yet be entirely secondary to the hidden physical condition. They are a reminder to the therapist to wonder always if a true organic condition lies behind the psychotic somatic delusion. Endocrine abnormalities—such as hypothyroidism, diabetes mellitus, and estrogen insufficiency—provide a realistic basis for weird-sounding complaints of bodily decay and depletion of vital force.

One of the aftereffects of an attack of viral influenza may be serious depression in depression-prone individuals. Suicides have been known to occur two to four weeks after apparent recovery from such an infection.

INITIAL TREATMENT OF PSYCHOTIC PATIENTS

The therapist's job is to protect a personality that is disintegrating. He must be conservative (to avoid further disintegration) and constructive (to set the stage for reintegration). It is helpful to think of the therapist's responsibilities in the initial contact in terms of *mistakes to be avoided* and *steps to be taken*. We start with a discussion of mistakes because the management of psychotic patients is one area of psychiatry in which the therapist can do harm if he does not act with restraint. Then we shall look at initial intervention in various psychotic conditions.

Mistakes to be Avoided

Basically the therapist must avoid making the same kinds of mistakes with the psychotic patient that the patient has made with himself. Just as the psychotic patient may resort to paranoid, disorganized, excited, and intropunitive methods of coping with uncertainty, the emergency therapist may find himself tempted toward the comple-

mentary responses of (1) false structuring of the situation (paranoia), (2) inappropriate refusal to put a basic treatment plan together (disorganization), (3) maneuvers that exceed his own executive limits (excitement), and (4) unnecessary guilt over his own inadequacies in the treatment situation (being intropunitive).

False Structuring of the Situation. In spite of the complexity involved in reaching a diagnosis, many therapists, out of anxiety, turn to labels and drugs before they have clarified what is wrong with the patient. In Example 5-1, such a false structuring occurred when the therapist gave the patient chlorpromazine to drink and wrote "acute schizophrenia, suspected" on his admission note. Such rote behaviors tend to reinforce each other in a sort of delusional logic: "I gave her chlorpromazine, so she must be schizophrenic; I've called her schizophrenic, so I must give her chlorpromazine." Then "evidence" for the diagnosis may take on the quality of a delusional perception: "I saw her sniff the chlorpromazine and not mind the smell; in fact she drank it—only schizophrenics do that—she *must* be schizophrenic!"

In this particular case the emergency therapist should have written, "acute psychosis, characterized by mutism, withdrawal, disorganization, and possible disorientation." These are not indications for immediate drug treatment but for further evaluation, and he should have withheld drugs. If the patient appeared to be grossly agitated, the best drug would be injectable diazepam, which acts for a short duration, does not block autonomic responses, and does not confuse the diagnostic picture. Thus the patient's treatment would have been appropriate for the many kinds of psychosis she might in fact have had.

Refusal To Make a Treatment Plan. This is the opposite of false structuring. The therapist in Example 5-1 did not fail his patient in this area. Even though the therapist could not have known from the evidence at hand the exact type of psychosis the patient demonstrated, there was considerable evidence of poor judgment and inability to fend for herself: mutism; a shallow, labile affect; and above all, being picked up at night while attempting to hitch a ride along a dangerous stretch of road. Thus, putting this patient on a seventy-two-hour hold until she could demonstrate her ability to take care of herself was a reasonable, caring action.

Therefore some treatment can begin before the diagnosis is clear. Provision always should be made for the acutely psychotic patient's safety. Like the suicidal patient, the psychotic patient need not be hospitalized if others, through crisis support, can arrange for his care. Members of the ecological group can avoid his hospitalization by providing limit setting, administering drugs, and supporting reality with the help of occasional visits by a crisis intervention team. But when no ecological support system exists, the therapist cannot allow a grossly disorganized patient to refuse treatment and walk out of the emergency room unless it is evident that he retains enough ego strength to avoid major mishaps. Involuntary detention is the next logical move.[85] If the therapist decides not to use involuntary detention, he must find a safe alternative: he cannot just let his patient go.

Often a good middle way to work with patients who are not so disorganized that they should be detained automatically but who seem on the verge of losing control is to share concern with the ecological group. It is entirely appropriate to say to a disorganized patient, "I'm concerned for you; I think you need help, and I'm going to tell the others that I want you to come into the hospital." To the others, the therapist can say, "I'm not sure what is wrong, but I'm afraid this situation will get out of control if he continues on the outside." Usually this honesty will bring the therapist, the patient, and the ecological group together in the attempt to find out what is wrong. Even if the patient does not enter treatment immediately, he usually returns to the setting and the therapist who has offered to help him find his way.

Exceeding One's Executive Limits. It has been said that one way to become psychotic is to try to control a situation one cannot in fact control. The

same therapists who are able to assert themselves in the face of psychotic disorganization may fail to recognize that borderline patient whose ambivalence prevents any immediate resolution.

Example 5-7. A woman in her early 30s who had been in analytically oriented treatment for years came to the emergency room and announced that she had terminated with her therapist and was about to walk out of her marriage. Almost immediately she said that this wasn't what she wanted to do, she wanted to try couple therapy. She agreed to be seen with her husband. He was called and said he would be right over. Immediately after the therapist had placed this call, the patient said she didn't really want to face her husband, she was going to go off alone.

She started to walk out of the emergency room, then came back and said, "I'd better tell you that I made a suicide attempt when I left my first husband eight years ago."

The therapist asked her about suicide and obtained a strong suicidal history. She had talked frequently with her former therapist, who was now on vacation, about killing herself.

The husband arrived, and the patient's ambivalence mounted. He turned out to be a patient, boyish young man who tried to reason with her to no avail. She could not decide whether to come home or go off and kill herself.

Finally the therapist decided to place the patient on a hold. He learned that there were no involuntary holds at his facility and he would have to arrange transportation to the nearby county hospital if he wanted to detain her. Arranging transportation was a nightmare: the ambulance would have to cross a county line, which it could not do with an involuntary patient. It was a Saturday night, and the police and sheriff's office were tied up with criminal work. The therapist was afraid to send her alone with her husband.

Assuming his presence would be authoritative enough, the therapist agreed to go with the patient and her husband in their car. She jumped out of the car into the traffic on a main highway and screamed for help. Her husband honked his horn, to signal a police car to stop. Because the couple's car was over the county line, the police were able to flag down a county ambulance, which took her to the facility.

A more experienced clinician at the county hospital diagnosed pseudoneurotic schizophrenia and sent her home to a friend with a return outpatient appointment to him. (She kept the appointment.) In retrospect, the first emergency therapist should have accepted his inability to reach quick closure.

Often the inexperienced therapist overreacts to the borderline patient. Careful history taking of such patients usually reveals latent psychosis and often suicidal or homicidal potential. The conscientious therapist may overstep his bounds in trying to deal with the potential for crisis, forgetting that it is a *chronic* potential in such patients.

If the patient's first responses to offers to help seem ambivalent or help-rejecting, it is often better for the therapist to listen to the patient, and to avoid the temptation to engage him in treatment. Frequently the pattern of a paranoid personality or a hysterical character appears in what the patient tells about his life, and the personality diagnosis will be more appropriate than the soft signs of psychosis, such as ambivalence, restlessness, and poorly controlled rage. It is essential not to try to do more for the patient than can be done and to let the movement for treatment come from the patient. An appeal to listen to ambivalence is not a request for intensive treatment, but a need for attention. It is emphatically not a signal for active, self-defeating crisis intervention.

In many more serious crisis situations, especially those involving manic patients who have not yet

started to "crash," the therapist must also wait for the right moment to intervene actively.

Unnecessary Guilt. Psychotic patients are particularly skilled in making therapists feel inadequate. They do this by taking advantage of the fact that there is no good way for the therapist to establish contact with a patient whose ego is not in control.

Example 5-8. A young therapist was asked by a patient to see a friend who was becoming disturbed. The friend turned out to be a large, bearded, sensitive young man who was disturbed by the emergence of paranoid feelings. After he had begun to tell these to the therapist, he stopped. The therapist asked, "How long have you been feeling this way?"

The patient said, "You can't help me," and walked out of the office.

The therapist wondered what he had done wrong. Had his stiff, clinical questions driven the sensitive patient away? He worried about what the patient who had referred the young man would think.

A month later the young man called the therapist, apologized for "putting you up tight," and explained that he hadn't had the courage to ask for a letter recommending exemption from the military draft because he feared he would be turned down.

No therapist, no matter how experienced, is able to understand the meaning of everything a patient says. Rather than assuming he is defective in his powers of comprehension, the therapist is better off to say, "I'm afraid I don't follow you. Can you try explaining that to me again?"

Provoking guilt can be a way for the patient to rid himself of it by passing along a "bum rap." The schizophrenic person often has been made to carry the guilt for an entire family.[86] The therapist sets an example for his overburdened patient by showing that it is possible to refuse such undeserved guilt.

Steps to be Taken: Initial Intervention in Various Psychotic Conditions

This section illustrates various interviewing techniques and procedures that may be used to approach paranoid, disorganized, excited, and intropunitive patients. The problems posed by working with a psychotic patient's ecological group are described in detail in Chapter 10. If psychosis is a response to crisis within the group, the process of crisis intervention is as described in Chapter 1. Detailed specific treatment of the separate syndromes is beyond the scope of this book.

Initial Intervention with Paranoid Patients. The therapist must be firm and emphatic in standing up with common sense and realistic medical authority to his patient's psychotic attempts to maintain control. The following case of Enelow's[87] illustrates this stance:

Example 5-9. Mr. B.G. was a 25-year-old old engineer who was first seen in the emergency room at the community hospital. The patient had attempted to purchase a Cadillac in the middle of the night. On finding the automobile agency locked up, he attempted to force an entry. The police overpowered him and they took him to the emergency room for treatment of his wounds. Here the intern found him to be suspicious, sullen, and delusional. He spoke of having been hypnotized by someone he was unable to identify. He felt that he was being secretly groomed for the presidency of the engineering firm at which he worked. He was offered hospitalization on the psychiatric ward and refused. A psychiatrist was called; he made a rapid examination and then in a friendly but firm way, said: "I want you to come into the hospital and to take some medication." "On what basis?" Mr. G. inquired suspiciously. "On the basis that I am a doctor and know you need it," the psychiatrist replied. "Oh!" said

Mr. G. and quietly signed the admission sheet. Phenothiazines were begun at once. One week later, Mr. G. was discharged, free of psychotic symptoms, to outpatient care.

Initial Intervention with Disorganized Patients. Often the most helpful approach is to *talk to the patient's affect.* For acutely disorganized patients, a suppressed affective issue is often behind the shift from the cognitive to the symbolic mode.

Example 5-10. Perry[88] has described a woman in her early 30s, a nurse who was admitted to the hospital with a diagnosis of acute catatonic schizophrenia. She was often wildly excited and would draw furiously during her therapy sessions. One drawing revealed an "archetypal" symbol, a serpent hung upon a cross. For several days Perry sought to find what connection this archaic symbol might have to her present life. During this time his patient was especially turbulent.

Finally, realizing that the serpent resembled a caduceus, Perry asked his patient if the drawing had anything to do with her feelings about her profession. "I hate it!", she exclaimed, and explained that her widowed mother, who depended on her for support, ironed her uniforms as if she were her husband. The patient had begun to feel she had no life of her own. Expressing this, she cleared.

To help a disorganized and confused patient make sense out of what is happening, the therapist often has to do much of the talking.[89, 90] The therapist should tell the patient why he makes his statements so he does not reinforce the fear that he or others can read the patient's mind ("thought broadcasting"). The therapist may say, "From the way your hands are trembling and the scared look on your face, I would guess you're feeling pretty frightened" (rather than "You're feeling pretty frightened"). The therapist can state facts he *does* know, e.g., "It looks as if you've been having a pretty rocky time recently," or "Your husband says you haven't been getting much sleep," or "From the way you're looking all around the room, it must be difficult to concentrate on what I'm saying."

Often such reflections provide the bridge the patient has been looking for to enable him to engage with the therapist. If the patient makes symbolic references or uses unlabeled metaphors, the interviewer should listen most attentively. This does not mean that he shakes his head in understanding if he does not or that he agrees with delusions that he does not agree with, but rather that he tries to enter into the patient's experiential world, that he is willing for the time being to hear "crazy talk," and that he wants to hear about feelings which, however symbolized, are real and important to the patient. By doing so, the therapist can begin to establish rapport and start treatment.

Example 5-11. A 32-year-old chemist was picked up by the police on a freeway where he had been carrying a placard with a political slogan. He was unkempt, wore a long beard, had a messianic gleam in his eye, and told the emergency therapist that he had been instructed "by the forces of God" to campaign for this candidate. He also said he had been instructed by such forces in the past, that he had been locked up in a mental hospital with a diagnosis of schizophrenia, and that he wasn't going to talk with this therapist further if he were going to do the same.

The therapist said he'd have to know the patient better before he'd say or do anything and asked him to describe what had been going on in his life recently. The patient described an increasing preoccupation with political and religious matters, racing thoughts, inability to concentrate on his work, and loss of sleep and weight (all brought about by his efforts to get his candidate elected).

The therapist told the patient that he didn't think his political tactics were as effective as

those a candidate of this stature deserved. Because his thoughts were racing and his concentration poor, the patient couldn't give good, coherent speeches. Because of his unkempt appearance, he would put off those who might be favorably disposed to the candidate, and so on.

This criticism made sense to the patient. The therapist asked him if he would take some medication to slow his thoughts and improve his concentration. The patient asked if this meant the therapist thought he was schizophrenic. The therapist said he hadn't reached any diagnostic conclusion (he hadn't, although he was thinking of paranoid schizophrenia, schizoaffective disorder, and manic-depressive illness, manic phase, as possibilities), but that he thought the medication would help, whatever the diagnosis might be. The patient accepted the medication and returned for regular visits. Hospitalization was avoided as his psychosis was treated and cleared.

Not every success in connecting the patient's affective response to a dynamic issue in himself or the ecological group means that a psychosis is resolved.

Example 5-12. A 52-year-old woman was brought into the emergency room by her husband and two teenage daughters. She had had radical breast surgery for carcinoma and was receiving large doses of steroids as part of her treatment for metastasis. She had not seen her doctor for two months; her next appointment was a month away. Her husband reported numerous wild behaviors, including failure to take her steroid medications.

The therapist learned that her surgeon and her husband had agreed not to tell her of the recurrence of the cancer. Feeling that this was a pseudosecret, the therapist obtained their permissions to tell the patient the truth. She seemed almost relieved to hear the painful news, and her mood improved and her erratic behavior diminished.

Nevertheless, she continued to ramble, and her husband found it exhausting to care for her. On a return trip to the emergency room, a consultant examined her with the therapist. Noting her lability, the consultant said he strongly suspected organic factors were involved and recommended that she be admitted. The final diagnosis turned out to be steroid psychosis, secondary to her antitumor medications. Only when these medications were changed did she improve for good.

Initial Intervention with Excited Patients. Medications and restraints must often be used with this group of patients. Often the patient will be brought in by the police, who should be asked to escort him to a locked room. Before they leave they should give full documentation of what he has done, how he was picked up, any threats, concealed drugs or weapons, and the names of significant others. Often the interview with the police (who may be in a hurry to leave) is the best information that will be available for days or hours and provides the basis for a working diagnosis.

A significant portion of these patients will have been drinking, but this does not exclude manic-depressive disease, acute catatonic schizophrenia, or chronic schizophrenia in exacerbation, all of which may lead to heavy drinking. Barbiturate intoxication may also unleash psychotic excitement. (The treatment of drinking and addicted patients is discussed in Chapters 6 and 9.)

Having obtained all available history and determined (if possible) the presence or absence or intoxication (not discounting the mimic, hypoglycemia), the therapist must proceed to calm the patient. Often this means the involuntary administration of tranquilizing drugs.

The *way* these drugs are offered to excited patients is important. The nurse or doctor emphatically should *not* go to the patient's room alone with a loaded syringe or medication cup. This practice is a form of "exceeding executive limits." The sudden relaxation of controls by recent captors in favor of a benevolent expectation of cooperation invites the patient to overstep his limits and may cause him to panic.

Instead, it seems wisest to demonstrate control by entering the room with five strong men who are prepared to hold down the patient. This procedure is called "show of force" and is meant to be appreciated by the concrete patient. A choice is offered to the patient's remaining healthy ego: he can take the medication voluntarily or be held down and injected. (These issues are discussed further in Chapters 10 and 25 to 28.)

Initial Treatment of Intropunitive Patients. We discussed in Chapter 3 the unambivalent, firm style of caring behavior that is most effective in dealing with intropunitive patients. Evaluation of the suicidal risk and protection of the patient from himself are the overriding concerns in initial management. Antidepressant medications (or, in manic-depressive illness, lithium) should be started as soon as possible.

ECT should be available wherever the psychotically depressed individual is hospitalized. Patients with recurrent depressions may show benefits only from this method of treatment, and hospitalization should be arranged with ECT in mind.

Not all intropunitive patients need to be hospitalized. Much depends on the quality of interpersonal resources in the ecological group. Many patients will be hospitalized on a milieu ward (see Chapter 10). A locked ward may be safer for very suicidal (often bipolar) depressive patients. The patient and his family should be given realistic hope: most depressions respond to treatment.

SUMMARY

Psychotic problems, which are met with in every aspect of psychiatric work, require difficult treatment decisions and a specialized vocabulary. Treatment is most effective when the therapist does not flinch from sharing the psychotic patient's uncertainty and when he defines the reasons for the steps he takes. To accomplish these goals, the therapist must be able to define for himself what he means by psychotic difficulties. When the therapist has a working understanding of psychosis, he will not mystify himself or his patient.

REFERENCES

1. Freedman, Alfred M., Harold I. Kaplan, and Benjamin J. Sadock: *Modern Synopsis of Comprehensive Textbook of Psychiatry*, Williams & Wilkins, Baltimore, 1972, p. 788.

2. Szasz, Thomas: *Law, Liberty, and Psychiatry*, Macmillan, New York, 1963.

3. Cooper, David: *Psychiatry and Anti-Psychiatry*, Ballantine Books, New York, 1971.

4. Spensley, James, James T. Barter, Paul H. Werme, and Donald G. Langsley: "Involuntary Hospitalization: What For and How Long," *Am. J. Psychiat.*, 131:219–222, 1974.

5. Lorr, Maurice, C. James Klett, and Douglas M. McNair: *Syndromes of Psychosis*, Pergamon, New York, 1963.

6. Lorr, Maurice (ed.): *Explorations in Typing Psychotics*, Pergamon, New York, 1966.

7. Perry, John W.: *The Far Side of Madness*, Prentice-Hal', Englewood Cliffs, N.J., 1974.

8. Grinker, Roy R.: "Changing Styles in Psychoses and Borderline States," *Am. J. Psychiat.*, 130:151–152, 1973.

9. American Psychiatric Association: *Diagnostic and Statistical Manual of Mental Disorders*, 1st ed., Washington, D.C., 1952.

10. American Psychiatric Association: *Diagnostic and Statistical Manual of Mental Disorders*, 2d ed., Washington, D.C., 1968.

11. Freedman et al.: op. cit., pp. 202–215.

12. Menninger, Karl A., Martin Mayman, and Paul Pruyser: *The Vital Balance*, Viking, New York, 1963, pp. 260–261.

13. Ibid.

14. Lorr et al.: Acute Psychotic Types," chap. 4, in op. cit., pp. 33–75.

15. Freedman et al.: op. cit., pp. 250–251.

16. Bellak, Leopold (ed.): *Schizophrenia: a Review of the Syndrome*, Logos Press, London, 1958, p. 157.

17. Freedman et al.: op. cit., p. 249.

18. Tyhurst, James C.: "Paranoid Patterns," in A. H. Leighton, J. A. Clausen, and R. N. Wilson (eds.): *Explorations in Social Psychiatry*, Basic Books, New York, 1957, p. 31.

19. Schneider, Kurt: *Clinical Psychopathology*, M. W. Hamilton (trans.), Grune & Stratton, New York, 1959, p. 133.

20. Mellor, C. S.: "First Rank Symptoms of Schizophrenia," *Brit. J. Psychiatry*, 117:15–23, 1970.

21. Rosenbaum, C. Peter: *The Meaning of Madness: Symptomatology, Sociology, Biology and Therapy of the Schizophrenias*, Science House, New York, 1970, p. 37.

22. Schneider: loc. cit.

23. Bleuler, Eugen: *Dementia Praecox, or the Group of Schizophrenias*, J. Zinkin (trans.), International Universitites Press, Inc., New York, 1950, p. 213.

24. Carlson, Gabrielle A., and Frederick K. Goodwin: "The Stages of Mania: a Longitudinal Analysis of the Manic Episode," *Arch. Gen. Psychiat.*, 28:221–228, 1973.

25. Kraepelin, Emil: *Manic-Depressive Insanity and Paraphrenia*, R. Mary Barclay (trans., ed.), E. S. Livingston, Edinburgh, 1919.

26. Carlson and Goodwin: op. cit., p. 224.

27. Taylor, Michael Alan. and Richard Abrams: "The Phenomenology of Mania," *Arch. Gen. Psychiat.*, 29:520–522, 1974.

28. Rosenbaum: loc. cit.

29. Grinker, Roy R.: "An Essay on Schizophrenia and Science," *Arch. Gen. Psychiat.*, 20:1–24, 1969.

30. M. L. Simmel (ed.), *From the Reach of the Mind: Essays in Memory of Kurt Goldstein*, Copyright 1968 by Springer Publishing Co., Inc., 400 Park Ave. S., New York. By permission of the publisher.

31. Grinker: "An Essay on Schizophrenia and Science," op. cit., p. 14.

32. Bateson, Gregory, Don D. Jackson, Jay Haley, and John Weakland: "Toward a Theory of Schizophrenia," *Behav. Sci.,* vol. 1, 1956.

33. Deikman, Arthur: "Bimodal Consciousness," *Arch. Gen. Psychiat.,* 25:481–489, 1971.

34. Buss, Arnold H., and Peter J. Lang: "Psychological Deficit in Schizophrenia: I. Affect, Reinforcement, and Concept Attainment," *J. Abnorm. Psychol.* 70:20, 1965.

35. Ibid.

36. Callaway, Enoch: "Schizophrenia and Interference: An Analogy With a Malfunctioning Computer," *Arch. Gen. Psychiat.,* 22: 193–208, 1970.

37. Bowers, Malcolm G.: "Pathogenesis of Acute Schizophrenic Psychoses," *Arch. Gen. Psychiat.,* 19:348–355, 1968.

38. Arieti, Silvano: "An Overview of Schizophrenia from a Predominantly Psychological Approach," *Am. J. Psychiat.,* 131:241–249, 1974. Copyright 1974, the American Psychiatric Association.

39. Ibid., p. 245.

40. Whitmont, Edward: "Prefatory Remarks to Jung's 'Reply to Buber,'" *Spring,* 188–195, 1973.

41. Hoch, Paul: "Differential Diagnosis in Clinical Psychiatry," in Margaret O. Strahl and Nolan D. C. Lewis (eds.), *The Lectures of Paul H. Hoch,* Science House, New York, 1972.

42. Perry, John W.: "The Messianic Hero," *J. Anal. Psychol.,* 17:184–198, 1972.

43. Levinson, Fritz: "Religious Delusions in Counter-Culture Patients," *Am. J. Psychiat.,* 130:1265–1269, 1973.

44. Laing, Ronald: *The Divided Self,* Tavistock Publications, London, 1960.

45. Herjanic, Marijan: "Schizophrenia: Pieces of the Puzzle," *Medical World News, Psychiatry* 1972, Eli Robins (ed.), pp. 75–77.

46. Ibid.

47. Rosenbaum: loc. cit.

48. Donlon, Patrick T., and Joe T. Tupin: "Rapid 'Digitalization' of Decompensated Schizo-

phrenic Patients with Antipsychotic Agents." *Am. J. Psychiat.,* 131:310–312, 1974.

49. Bleuler: loc. cit.

50. Ibid.

51. Rosenbaum: op. cit., p. 10.

52. Rosenbaum: ibid.

53. Perry: "The Messianic Hero," loc. cit.

54. Freedman et al.: op. cit., pp. 268–311.

55. Ibid., pp. 268–269.

56. Engel, George L., and John Romano: "Delirium, a Syndrome of Cerebral Insufficiency," *J. Chron. Dis.,* 9:260, 1959.

57. Freedman et al.: op. cit., p. 270.

58. Ibid., p. 271.

59. Ibid., p. 272.

60. Ibid., pp. 272–273.

61. Grinspoon, Lester, and Peter Hedblom: "Amphetamine Abuse," *Drug Therapy,* 2: 83–89, 1972.

62. Spencer, D. J.: "Cannabis Induced Psychosis," *Brit. J. Addiction,* 65:369–372, 1970.

63. Slater, E., A. W. Beard, and E. Glithero: "The Schizophrenia-like Psychoses of Epilepsy," *Brit. J. Psychiat.,* 109:95–150, 1963.

64. Feighner, J. P., Eli Robins, S. B. Guze et al.: "Diagnostic Criteria for Use in Psychiatric Research," *Arch. Gen. Psychiat.,* 26:57–63, 1972.

65. Janowsky, David S., Melitta Leff, and Richard S. Epstein: "Playing the Manic Game: Interpersonal Maneuvers of the Acutely Manic Patient," *Arch. Gen. Psychiat.,* 22: 252–261, 1970. Copyright 1970, American Medical Association.

66. Ibid., p. 253.

67. Rosenbaum: op. cit., pp. 30–31.

68. Ibid., p. 31.

69. Ovesey, Lionel: *Homosexuality and Pseudohomosexuality,* Science House, New York, 1969.

70. Woods, Sherwyn M.: "Violence, Psychotherapy of Pseudohomosexual Panic," *Arch.*

Gen. Psychiat., **27**:255–258, 1972; quote is on p. 257. Copyright 1972, American Medical Association.

71. Ibid., p. 257.

72. Lorr, Klett and McNair: op. cit., pp. 254–255.

73. Raskin, David E.: Akathisia: A Side Effect to Be Remembered," *Am. J. Psychiat.*, **129**: 345–347, 1972; quote is from p. 345. Copyright 1972, the American Psychiatric Association.

74. Kline, Nathan S.: "18 Years on Chlorpromazine," letter to the *Am. J. Psychiat.*, **113**: 228, 1974.

75. Winokur, George: "Diagnostic and Genetic Aspects of Affective Illness," *Psychiat. Ann.*, **3**:6–15, 1973.

76. Winokur, George: "Depression: The Clinical Perspective," *Pract. Psychiat.*, **2**:2, 1974.

77. Guze, S. B., R. A. Woodruff, and P. J. Clayton: "Secondary Affective Disorders: A Study of 95 Cases," *Psychol. Med.*, **1**:426–428, 1971.

78. Winokur: "Diagnostic and Genetic Aspects of Affective Illness," loc. cit.

79. Ibid.

80. Ibid.

81. Kaplan, Harold I., and Benhamin J. Sadock: "An Overview of the Major Affective Disorders," *Psychiat. Ann.*, **4**:31, 1974.

82. Ibid.

83. Feighner et al.: loc. cit.

84. Kessler, David: "Preventing Psychiatric Hospitalization: A Crisis Intervention Approach," talk given at Pacific Medical Center, San Francisco, Calif., Mar. 8, 1973.

85. Spensley et al.: loc. cit.

86. Stabenau, James R.: "Schizophrenia: A Family's Projective Identification," *Am. J. Psychiat.*, **130**:19–23, 1973.

87. Enelow, Allen J., and Murray Wexler: *Psychiatry in the Practice of Medicine*, Oxford University Press, New York, 1966, p. 263.

88. Perry: *The Far Side of Madness*, op. cit., chap. 12.

89. Gendlin, Eugene T.: "Research in Psychotherapy with Schizophrenic Patients and the Nature of That Illness," *Am. J. Psychotherap.*, **20**:4–16, 1966.

90. Rosenbaum: op. cit., chap. 14.

Evaluation and Treatment of the Drinking Patient

THE DIFFICULTIES

Drinking patients appear frequently in emergency rooms. They are dealt with in a variety of ways, depending on how their physicians view drinking and alcoholism, but the pattern reflects a major prejudice. Studies conducted by a group led by Morris Chafetz[1] show that patients with jobs, family, and insurance are likely to be admitted to a medical service with a medical diagnosis, and even though the drinking problem is recognized, no psychiatric referral is given.[2] The diagnosis of alcoholism and referral to an alcohol treatment program is reserved for "skid row" persons without signs of social competence who are the poorest treatment risks. The referral is made in a cold, disinterested manner, with little attempt to instill motivation.[3] The poor follow-through of patients who are referred in this manner is used to justify the idea that drinking problems and alcoholism cannot be treated. Thus the best candidates for treatment of such problems are protected from treatment, and the patients who are hardest to treat are pushed toward alcohol treatment programs in a way that greatly reduces their chances of successful entry into therapy.

Thus the emergency therapist who receives a drinking patient on referral must fight hard against a medical stereotype: the alcoholic patient is a childish pest who has brought all his problems on himself and little can be done for him. The psychiatric version of this stereotype is that drinking patients do very poorly in psychiatric treatment too, and therefore any extensive contact with them is wasted professional time. This moralistic approach begs the real question, which is to find the *right* treatment for a drinking patient and to offer it to him in the right way.

Indeed, patients who drink do tax the emergency therapist to develop skills in many areas of competence. Drinking presents a continual challenge to many levels of the patient's existence—biological, spiritual, marital, vocational—all demanding expert attention, some later, some at the moment. Particularly demanding is the acute problem of a drug-induced syndrome that involves a change in state, shifting rapidly over a short period of time, with quick variations in the kind of distress felt and the kind of intervention required. The beginning therapist needs to develop a feeling for the ways patients change in response to chemical stress. This is not an easy skill to master. Almost as difficult is to "open" treatment, not only to members of the patient's ecological group, but also to other health professionals—the internist, the vocational counselor, the social worker at the family service agency, and the visiting public health nurse—whose skills may be required to master particular problems. The therapist almost always has to share the drinking patient with other professionals. It becomes obvious why problem drinkers have been rejected so often: they need (as well as demand) more than average therapeutic skills.

This chapter, which presents basic information, attempts to bridge the distance between the general therapist's skill and the problem drinker's need. First, it will survey the vexing problem of the classification of emotional problems that involve alcohol use and will examine kinds of problem drinkers and criteria for the diagnosis of alcoholism. Next, it looks in detail at the biological effects of alcohol use, examines the organic response to alcoholic intoxication and withdrawal, and suggests methods of treatment for this pharmacologic crisis and its complications. Finally, it presents major psychological considerations in the therapeutic management of patients with drinking problems.

Throughout, two emphases will be apparent. One will be upon the appraisal of the patient's acute state, whether biological or psychological. The second will be upon using a multidisciplinary approach to the resolution of chronic problems. Once the therapist has mastered these difficulties and the different time frames to which they apply, he can offer considerable help, even to those who appear to be the most unpromising candidates.

CLASSIFYING ALCOHOL PROBLEMS

A Matter of Definitions

Not everyone whose psychological difficulties are associated with alcohol should be classed as an alcoholic. In 1967 the Cooperative Commission on the Study of Alcoholism[4] specifically rejected the use of alcoholism as a "collective term for a family of problems correlated with alcohol," or to describe "any use of alcoholic beverages that causes any damage to the individual or society or both." [5] Instead, the Commission's report suggested that the term *alcoholism* be reserved for "a condition in which an individual has lost control over his alcohol intake in the sense that he is consistently unable to refrain from drinking or to stop drinking before getting intoxicated." [6]

Additionally, the Commission's report noted that the term "loss of control" usually includes two phenomena. The first is the inability to do without alcohol or to manage personal tensions without drinking, often called the "inability to abstain." The second is the inability of the individual to stop drinking after he has started. These phenomena are consistent with the conception of alcoholism as a disease characterized by a "pathological dependency on ethanol," which is how alcoholism is classified by the American Psychiatric Association. [7] This latter definition set the stage for the first presentation of uniform criteria for the diagnosis of alcoholism by the National Council on Alcoholism in 1972.

Problem drinking is now the term preferred to refer to "a repetitive use of beverage alcohol causing physical, psychological, or social harm to the drinker or to others." [8] This term makes it possible to discuss persons with alcohol problems without classifying them as suffering from the disease alcoholism, an approach that can all too easily lead to a stereotyped, inflexible approach to evaluation and treatment. At the same time, some problem drinkers are indeed alcoholics.

Kinds of Problem Drinkers

Kissin[9] says that the population of problem drinkers is "completely heterogeneous," ranging from the skid row type (less than 5 percent) through the inner-city dweller (20 percent), the blue-collar worker (40 percent), the middle-class citizen (30 percent), to the upper-class executive (more than 5 percent). In the United States there are thought to be 9 million alcoholics and problem drinkers, as opposed to only 250,000 "hard drug" addicts.

This section offers some impressionistic profiles of the different kinds of problem drinkers who may seek help and gives some preliminary guidelines for intervention. Each one presents a different psychodynamic picture and requires a different kind of psychiatric help. Any given patient, however, may have the characteristics of several profiles. Nevertheless, experience has shown that definite types do exist; the following text introduces some of the common ones. The section ends with current information about the drinking problems of women and the young, both of whom are still poorly defined groups.

The Reactive Drinker. Some people, when faced with emotional stress, turn reactively to alcohol for relief of emerging anxiety and depression. When the stress is resolved, the excessive drinking ends.

> *Example 6-1, Andy.* Friends bring a drunken Andy to the emergency room. He is a good-looking man in his 30s. The friends report that his drinking has increased noticeably in recent months and that tonight he tried to set fire to a wedding picture on the mantel. Andy spills out the story of having been separated from his wife and children for six months, of the sexual difficulties he and his wife had while they were together, and of the loneliness of his recent life. The scene borders on bathos, but the pain is real. The emergency therapist sets an appointment for two days later, asks the friends to take Andy home, put him to bed, and remind him about the appointment when he is sober.
>
> Andy shows up, sober and well-groomed, for the appointment, and remembers only vaguely what he said in the emergency room. The therapist tells Andy what he remembers from the session, and Andy quickly enters into brief psychotherapy to grieve the loss of his wife and to start building a new life for himself.

> After six sessions these goals have been accomplished; he has a new girlfriend and his drinking is no longer excessive.
>
> Six months later he requests a single therapy session to discuss a possible new marriage and some potential in-law problems. The session helps him to obtain a better perspective on these problems; his drinking has remained under control. The therapist last hears from him a year later, when Andy happily reports the birth of his first child in the new marriage.

Reactive drinking frequently appears when a love problem or a crisis at work cannot be resolved. Not all reactive drinkers are as easily or successfully treated as Andy, but most experience a similar process. Once psychotherapy uncovers the underlying life issue, the patient usually decides on his own that excessive use of alcohol affords poor relief and is in fact adding to his problems. (This is in marked contrast to the course of psychotherapy with patients who habitually manipulate their lives into crisis, to have an excuse to drink.)

Reactive drinking sometimes is an attempt to reduce the tensions felt in developmental crises (adolescence, the end of early youth in the late 20s, the onset of mature middle age in the early 40s). Patients who turn to alcohol at these times may be using it (wrongly) as an antidepressant. Indeed, successful psychotherapy for them may require the adjunctive use of an antidepressant drug as they approach the deep problematic issue. It is as if the patient needed to switch from alcohol to a more effective medication while he works out the problems of his life.

The Schizophrenic Drinker. Some schizophrenic patients use alcohol as a tranquilizer to mask the disquieting symptoms of chronic anxiety, sense of unreality, threatening hallucinations and delusions, and so forth. In other instances, marginal or poorly compensated borderline characters drink, and the ensuing loss of psychological and physical defenses allows the emergence of frankly psychotic ideation and behavior. Some nonschizophrenic persons suffer from an aftereffect of chronic drinking called alcoholic hallucinosis, which may be difficult to differentiate from paranoid schizophrenia. Finally, many schizophrenic patients stop taking phenothiazines when they start drinking.

Example 6-2, Bill. Police have picked up Bill, a 35-year-old veteran, for assaulting union pickets outside a movie theatre. There was no discernible motive.

The emergency therapist learns that Bill lives alone on a VA pension of 100 percent psychiatric disability and that he has been in and out of VA psychiatric hospitals since his separation from the service for psychiatric disabilities. His last outpatient visit was three months ago. He evades the interviewer's glance, grimaces when asked a question, and gives largely evasive answers until, in a single rush of breath he says, "Yeah, the voices told me to do it—why don't you get it done?" At this point he is willing to be hospitalized. He later reveals that he had started to drink heavily a week before, when the voices had first started to get louder, and that he had tried to keep them under control by drinking a quart of gin a day. At that time he had discontinued the chlorpromazine which had been prescribed for him. On the day he had been picked up, the main voice had gotten particularly loud, insisting he "Go beat up that picket!"

The diagnoses of schizophrenia and alcoholism are often used by federal and local health facilities as much for administrative purposes as for medical ones. Public funds may be available for the treatment and support of patients with one diagnosis but not the other. The emergency therapist should make his own, independent judgment rather than rely too heavily on records from VA, state, and local hospitals. Some schizophrenic patients are also alcoholic, but most alcoholic patients are not schizophrenic. In either event, withdrawal from alcohol (often in a hospital) is

the first order of business. After that, schizophrenic patients can be returned to a safer and more effective tranquilizer. Alcohol interferes with the judgment of a schizophrenic patient as much as it does with anyone else's, and the rate of violence and crime for schizophrenic patients is much higher when they have been drinking than when they have not been.

The Cyclothymic Drinker. There is a small but highly memorable group of people who seem extraordinarily dependent on the praise and esteem of others to feel good about themselves. The external reassurances must be many and constant; these people are exquisitely vulnerable to narcissistic injury and often expend prodigious energies in manipulating others to meet their needs. Their moods go up and down; their lives seem to be muted forms of a manic-depressive cycle, hence the term "cyclothymic." Sober, they often appear to be charming extraverts; when they are drinking, their charm may become pathetic and irritating.

Example 6-3, Cal. Cal has just awakened from a night during which he had slept off a drunk in a holding bed in the emergency room. He is past 40, but he pushes his weather-beaten face into the puckish grin of a 9-year-old child. He asks you your whole name and proceeds to call you by your first name from the first minutes of the interview. He inquires where you went to medical school (especially if you are not a physician) and proceeds to name various doctors in the city where you say you studied. Anything you reveal about yourself may become the focus of Cal's next sentence.

During the interview, Cal has more history than you can possibly assimilate: he seems to have done everything, lived everywhere, met everyone. The names of people, places, and jobs pour out of him.

Finally exasperated, you ask Cal what is troubling him now, and he starts to cry. His pain is genuine: he has no resources, his friends have deserted him. Only you can help him.

You ask him what you can do. "I'm not sure," Cal says, "I have no place to stay." He implies he will talk more about treatment plans *after* he has been admitted; it is beneath his dignity to discuss plans when he has no roof over his head. He tightens the yellow scarf around his neck and winks at you, behind his tears. "You doctors have a tough time," he says, and smiles kindly. Treatment? It's your move.

In such patients alcohol is part of the up-and-down cycle of ego inflation and deflation. The vicissitudes of the drug effect, its joys and miseries, its anxious highs and depressed lows, have become integrated into the lifestyle of the patient. Would he be less cyclothymic if he abstained from alcohol? Probably, but one of the functions of his drinking is to keep him on the exciting roller coaster of mood swings that follow the rhythm of alcohol intoxication and withdrawal. Indeed, other drugs such as LSD, marihuana, cocaine, amphetamines, and barbiturates are used along with alcohol to exaggerate the ever-shifting pattern of highs and lows such patients seem to require. The increased use of alcohol by frankly manic-depressive patients during the manic phase has recently been reported.[10]

In treatment, the underlying mood disturbance, the problem of self-esteem, and the need for a cycle of success and defeat must be recognized. Alcoholics Anonymous (AA) may provide such patients a model program. Bateson[11] notes that for the grandiose, power-loving person who insists on his ability to master every situation, AA tends to do what alcohol does: it reduces his inflation. The "first step" for the individual in AA is to admit that he is powerless with regard to alchohol. When he takes this step and admits weakness, he is given much attention, praise, and peer support; indeed, he will be criticized for proclaiming any strength in being able to hold his liquor. This paradox undercuts the power motivation and places the individual in a more realistic position vis-à-vis others and his own instincts.

The Heavy Drinker under Pressure. Some persons start drinking heavily and steadily during high school, college, or military service. They are able to handle their drinking relatively well for many years; perhaps they even take perverse pride in never missing a day's work. Although they are not terribly happy at how inefficient their hangovers make them, they pride themselves on being able to hold their liquor and dismiss the protestations of their wives and the curious glances of their supervisors. The years catch up with them. The iron constitution starts to rust, and the ravages of chronic alcoholism, even while the drinker tries to deny them, become increasingly apparent to families and employers.

Example 6-4, Don. Don is 38, married and has children of ages 8 and 4. He has worked as an airline mechanic for fifteen years. His wife Diane leads him firmly to the psychiatrist's office in the emergency room. He is tremulous and red-eyed. Her upper lip quivers, but she has a determined look. She announces that Don wants to enter the hospital for treatment of alcoholism.

The psychiatrist asks Don what he feels, and Don says, "If you think that's what I should do, Doc." The psychiatrist asks Don what *he* wants to do, and Don says, "You're the doctor."

Diane says pleadingly to the psychiatrist, "We hoped you'd admit him. It's taken a lot to get him here." She mentioned that she has told Don that if he doesn't get treatment for his alcoholism, she is going to leave him. Additionally, he is under the threat of suspension from work unless he participates in an alcohol treatment program. Don hands the psychiatrist the name of the airline doctor who wants to be called after a decision has been made.

The patient who likes to drink appears for treatment only when the drinking problem poses a threat to another vital need. When this crisis is the threat of the loss of a job, a marriage, or a lover, an involved person may bring the patient in. The therapist may well be tempted to try to stand between the patient and this outside pressure, noting that when the others "lay off" the patient becomes less anxious because his is not the motive force for change. The therapist should consider the positive value of the pressure and the anxiety it engenders. Without it, would the patient realize anything was wrong? Thus the wise therapist often *supports* the ecological group when it applies pressure to the patient. He reminds the significant others that the patient's tentative entry into therapy is not a signal for them to reduce this pressure: the ambivalent patient will continue to need outside insistence on change if his own motivation to abstain from drinking is to persist.

On the other hand, scapegoating the drinking person for all work and family problems should not be supported. As part of the pressure toward health, the others should be encouraged to enter treatment along with the patient and avail themselves of consultation or therapy to work toward an understanding of roles they have played in producing the alcoholic solution to conflict. When the patient is well into mastering his drinking problem, members of the ecological group may try to maneuver him into "being to blame" because of his past behavior. These attempts usually reflect difficulties on the part of the others in looking at their own contributions to family conflicts. A patient's alcoholic "slip" after a long period of remission is a particularly good time to observe and identify such scapegoating behavior. Often it will develop that the family has literally pushed the patient into drinking again. Family members can be helped to see their destructive influence when the effects of it on the patient's drinking are immediate rather than long-range.

Generally, when a drinking person is brought in for help by someone else, it is a good idea to evaluate whether the other person desires to motivate or to scapegoat the patient. Usually, provoking anxiety is motivating and provoking guilt is scapegoating. Much progress in treatment depends upon the therapist's ability to recognize

when to side with, and when to question, outside pressure. For patients who have been drinking heavily for a long time, outside pressure to stop, however brusquely presented, is almost always caring behavior and a motivation for change. Such pressure should be supported.

The Heavy Drinker without Funds. Some heavy drinkers run out of money and need food and shelter. County jails have served as semisatisfactory halfway houses for such patients; hospital emergency rooms are another portal of entry to institutional care. Hospitals are not hostels, and inhospitable doctors are often hostile to patients who do not present an interesting set of medical or psychiatric symptoms. Some alcoholic patients have become expert at playing the roles of "interesting patients."

> *Example 6-5, Earl.* Earl is a man in his early 50s. His hair is still blonde, and he dresses eccentrically in toga and sandals. He wears a look of benign philosophical understanding. There is alcohol on his breath. When asked what is wrong, Earl gazes through an open window and says, "Young man, my spirits have sunk down." Asked to explain, he responds condescendingly, "Young man, have you ever heard of the planet Venus?" He explains that he is in daily contact with higher intelligences from the cloudy planet, and that he has single-handedly saved the Earth from invasion. Now he feels too weak to continue without rest. It is the twenty-second of the month, and he must be strong when the first comes.
>
> Earl is admitted with a diagnosis of chronic paranoid schizophrenia in acute exacerbation. His airy imperviousness resists therapeutic efforts for eight days. On the first of the month, Earl's pension check arrives, and he asks for discharge. When asked what he has got from being hospitalized, he finally confides, "A place to crash, you fool."

Many alcoholic patients have learned how to con

a hospital into a free ride while they wait for their disability checks. It is wise to confront their lack of financial resources directly. Helping the alcoholic patient without funds to find temporarily safe shelter is a wholly appropriate task for the emergency therapist. The hospital is an inappropriate "hotel."

A penniless patient may still want treatment. Often a good test of motivation is to ask the patient if he is willing to take disulfiram (Antabuse®) after detoxification is effected. If he is, the patient is probably motivated to participate in an alcohol treatment program. Another approach is to refer the patient to a public hostel but to invite him to return for inpatient treatment after the first of the month, when definite detoxification can be undertaken. In either case, the therapist reserves the hospital setting for those who seriously desire treatment.

The Middle-aged Alcoholic in Crisis. Many middle-aged drinkers manage to keep functioning over the years until, because of an accident, malign fate, or physical deterioration, they cannot cope any longer. They turn to alcohol even more until a single event or a succession of events makes life a burden, and a self-destructive or suicidal crisis builds.

Example 6-6, Fritz. Fritz is 57 years old. He comes to the emergency room with a stricken look; his chart contains many previous diagnoses of problem drinking and alcoholism. Earlier in the evening he developed chest pains and came to the hospital to be checked. His EKG shows no change; indeed, the surgical intern suggests he may have a hyperventilation syndrome. He refuses to leave the hospital; psychiatric consultation is requested.

He says, "Doc, I think I may be killing myself." He tells you that lately, since the death of his wife from cirrhosis ("We both drank a lot, Doctor"), he has been drinking even more. Two days ago he accidentally set a fire in his apartment. Tonight, he had chest pain that lasted an hour. He admits to being depressed, and when asked about suicide, he starts crying and says, "I bought a gun today. I figured if I got drunk enough, I'd have guts enough to pull the trigger." He had tried to fire the gun at himself, but missed. He hoped that his heart reading would be "just off enough" to ensure his admission to the hospital for a few days. "But I know, Doctor," he concludes to the therapist, "that it's your department I need."

The diagnosis of alcoholism does not preclude other diagnoses. The therapist should probe especially deeply for suicidal and homicidal concerns because this is the population in which both suicide and homicide occur most frequently. A visit to the hospital is often a "cry for help," as is the case with Fritz. His need for shelter and emotional support should be respected: he is asking for a lifeline. It is sometimes difficult to distinguish Fritz from Earl. Despite Fritz's alcoholism, his appeal for help is typical of the proud, compulsive, widowed older man who is high-risk for suicide. The crisis of his depression may be the springboard for treatment that was impossible before. Often, older patients will be willing to give up alcohol for health reasons when in younger, healthier years they could not be persuaded to do so. As one man in his 50s put it, "It finally caught up with me."

The Woman Problem Drinker. In this country women who drink have been far less numerous than men. According to Verdery,[12] the ratio of women to men who drink excessively is 1:5; in England, 1:2; and in Norway, 1:23. Many observers feel the United States ratio is increasing because women are growing less inhibited about drinking in public.

The woman problem drinker is frequently divorced, in the crisis of middle life, has grown children, and no future career to inspire her. She may be very hard to engage in treatment, harder than a man, possibly because most treatment programs are predominantly oriented to male needs. Frequently another sympathetic woman can be the bridge to treatment. The visiting public health nurse can perform this service.

> *Example 6-7.* In one such case it took seven years of a growing and deepening relationship, punctuated by help given in a variety of critical family events, for a mother of many children, a capable and very worthwhile person with a long alcoholic history, to ask the nurse to go with her to a treatment clinic. Up until then she had refused any such suggestions and had reacted to a meeting of Alcoholics Anonymous with scorn and revulsion. She stuck with the treatment, which was reasonably successful, though it involved quite a few backsliding incidents. [13]

The case of Alice (Chapters 2 and 3) is a sustained description of a woman with a drinking problem who faces the crisis of middle life. She is in a state of almost total psychosocial disruption yet is attempting to achieve the dignified married role traditionally required of noncareer women. Her story also points up the high suicide risk present in all problem drinkers.

The Young Drinker. A burgeoning alcohol problem is appearing among the young. A recent review article [14] notes that

> The National Parent-Teacher Association estimates that of the 75% high school students who drink, more than one-half have a serious alcohol problem. Alcoholics Anonymous (A.A.) reports that 10% of its membership of 400,000 is currently under 21 years old, and one 10-year-old member recently marked his first anniversary with Alcoholics Anonymous, capping a drink-free year.

No one personality profile typifies these young problem drinkers, although sexual identity conflicts and parental alcoholism seem to play important roles.

The Diagnosis of Alcoholism

Which of these problem drinkers are alcoholic? In the past there has been a tendency to overdiagnose alcoholism once the problem of alcohol use has been uncovered. To qualify as a *disease*, alcohol use must have been sufficient to lead to transient or permanent deterioration of psychosocial and/or physiological function. (These changes may occur within two years after the individual has started to drink, and in early adolescence.) Isolated episodes of inebriation, however unfortunate their consequences, cannot be considered as evidence of the disease of alcoholism.

A major contribution in the definition of the physiological and behavioral criteria of alcoholism came in 1972 with the simultaneous publication of a system developed by the National Council on Alcoholism in the *American Journal of Psychiatry* [15] and the *Annals of Internal Medicine.* [16] Some of the tabular data of that system has been adapted in Table 6-1. We strongly encourage those who are going to work with alcoholic patients to read the original article.*

In the Council's system, signs and symptoms of possible alcoholism are grouped into two tracks: Track I is a list of physiological and clinical indicators, and Track II consists of behavioral, psychological, and attitudinal indicators. Each track is subdivided into major and minor criteria, and each of these is assigned a diagnostic level. A criterion with a diagnostic level of 1 is clearly associated with alcoholism; a level of 2 is highly suggestive of alcoholism, and a level of 3 indicates possible alcoholism or an incidental finding.

For example, see Track I, Major Criteria, Item A1, physiological dependency: physiological dependence as manifested by evidence of a *withdrawal syndrome* when the intake of alcohol is interrupted or decreased without substitution of other sedation: (*a*) gross tremor; (*b*) hallucinosis; (*c*) withdrawal seizures; (*d*) delirium tremens. Each

---

*Reprints are easily obtainable from any local office of the National Council on Alcoholism.

Table 6-1: Major and Minor Criteria for the Diagnosis of Alcoholism
[National Council on Alcoholism] [15]

MAJOR CRITERIA

Criterion	Diagnostic Level	Criterion	Diagnostic Level
TRACK I. PHYSIOLOGICAL AND CLINICAL		Pancreatitis in the absence of cholelithiasis	2
A. Physiological Dependency		Chronic gastritis	3
1. Physiological dependence as manifested by evidence of a withdrawal syndrome when the intake of alcohol is interrupted or decreased without substitution of other sedation.		Hematological disorders: Anemia: hypochromic, normocytic, macrocytic, hemolytic with stomatocytosis, low folic acid.	3
(a) Gross tremor	1	Clotting disorders: prothrombin elevation, thrombocytopenia	3
(b) Hallucinosis	1	Wernicke-Korsakoff syndrome	2
(c) Withdrawal seizures	1	Alcoholic cerebellar degeneration	1
(d) Delirium tremens	1	Cerebral degeneration in absence of Alzheimer's disease or arteriosclerosis	2
2. Evidence of tolerance to the effects of alcohol. (There may be a decrease in previously high levels of tolerance late in the course.)		Peripheral neuropathy (see also beriberi)	2
		Toxic amblyopia	3
		Alcohol myopathy	2
(a) A blood alcohol level of more than 150 mg. without gross evidence of intoxication.	1	Alcoholic cardiomyopathy	2
		Beriberi	3
		Pellagra	3
(b) The consumption of one-fifth of a gallon of whiskey or equivalent daily for more than one day, by a 180 lb. individual.	1	**TRACK II. BEHAVIORAL, PSYCHOLOGICAL AND ATTITUDINAL**	
3. Alcoholic "blackout" periods	2	All chronic conditions of psychological dependence occur in dynamic equilibrium with intrapsychic and interpersonal consequences. In alcoholism, similarly, there are varied effects on character and family.	
B. Clinical: Major-Alcohol-Associated Illnesses, in a person who drinks regularly. In such individuals, evidence of physiological and psychological dependence should be searched for.		1. Drinking despite strong medical contraindication known to patient.	1
		2. Drinking despite strong, identified, social contraindication (job loss for intoxication, marriage disruption because of drinking, arrest for intoxication, driving while intoxicated).	1
Fatty degeneration in absence of other known cause	2		
Alcoholic hepatitis	1	3. Patient's subjective complaint of loss of control of alcohol consumption.	2
Laennec's cirrhosis	2		

Table 6-1 (cont'd):   Major and Minor Criteria for the Diagnosis of Alcoholism

MINOR CRITERIA

Criterion	Diagnostic Level	Criterion	Diagnostic Level

TRACK I. PHYSIOLOGICAL AND CLINICAL

Criterion	Diagnostic Level	Criterion	Diagnostic Level
A. Direct Effects (ascertained by examination)		3. *Minor* — Indirect	
		Results of alcohol ingestion:	
1. Early: Odor of alcohol on breath at time of medical appointment	2	Hypoglycemia, hypochloremic alkalosis	3
2. Middle:		Low magnesium level	2
Alcohol facies	2	Lactic acid elevation, transient	
Vascular engorgement of face	2	uric acid elevation, potassium	
Toxic amblyopia	3	depletion	3
Increased incidence of infections	3	Indications of liver abnormality:	
Cardiac arrhythmias	3	SGOT elevation	3
Peripheral neuropathy	2	SGPT elevation; BSP elevation;	
3. Late (see Major Criteria, Track 1, B)		Bilirubin elevation; Urinary urobilinogen elevation; Serum	
B. Indirect Effects		A/G ratio reversal	2
1. Early:		Blood and blood clotting:	
Tachycardia	3	Anemia: hypochromic, normocytic, macrocytic, hemolytic	
Flushed face	3	with stomatocytosis, low folic	
Nocturnal diaphoresis	3	acid	3
2. Middle:		Clotting disorders: prothrombin elevation, thrombocytopenia	3
Ecchymoses on lower extremities, arms or chest	3	ECG abnormalities:	
Cigarette or other burns on hands or chest	3	Cardiac arrhythmias, tachycardia: T waves dimpled, cloven,	
Hyperreflexia, or if drinking heavily hyporeflexia (permanent hyporeflexia may be a residuum of alcoholic polyneuritis)	3	or spinous; atrial fibrillation; ventricular premature contractions; abnormal P waves	2
3. Late: Decreased tolerance	3	EEG abnormalities:	
C. Laboratory Tests		Decreased or increased REM sleep, depending on phase	3
1. *Major* — Direct		Loss of delta sleep	3
Blood alcohol level at any time of more than 300 mg/100 ml	1	Other reported findings	3
2. *Major* — Indirect		Decreased immune response; Decreased response to Synacthen test; Chromosomal damage from alcoholism	3
Serum osmolality (reflects blood alcohol levels): every 22.4 increase over 200 mOsm/liter reflects 50 mg/100 ml alcohol	2		

Table 6-1 (cont'd): Major and Minor Criteria for the Diagnosis of Alcoholism

	MINOR CRITERIA (cont'd.)		
Criterion	Diagnostic Level	Criterion	Diagnostic Level

TRACK II. BEHAVIORAL, PSYCHOLOGICAL AND ATTITUDINAL

Criterion	Diagnostic Level	Criterion	Diagnostic Level
A. Behavioral		B. Psychological and Attitudinal	
1. Direct effects		1. Direct effects	
Early: gulping drinks	3	Early: When talking freely, makes frequent reference to drinking alcohol, people being "bombed," "stoned," etc., or admits drinking more than peer group	2
Surreptitious drinking; morning drinking	2		
Middle: Repeated conscious attempts at abstinence	2	Middle: Drinking to relieve anger, insomnia, fatigue, depression, social discomfort	2
Late: Blatant indiscriminate use of alcohol	1	Late: Psychological symptoms consistent with permanent organic brain syndrome (see also Major Criteria, Track I, B)	2
Skid Row or equivalent social level	2		
2. Indirect effects		2. Indirect effects	
Early: Medical excuses from work for variety of reasons; Shifting from one alcoholic beverage to another; Preference for drinking companions, bars, and taverns; Loss of interest in activities not directly associated with drinking	2	Early: Unexplained changes in family, social, and business relationships: complaints about wife, job, and friends	3
Late: Chooses employment that facilitates drinking; Frequent automobile accidents; History of family members undergoing psychiatric treatment; School and behavioral problems in children; Frequent change of residence for poorly defined reasons	3	Spouse makes complaints about drinking behavior, reported by patient or spouse	2
		Major family disruptions: separation, divorce, threats of divorce	3
		Job loss (due to increasing interpersonal difficulties), frequent job changes, financial difficulties	3
Anxiety-relieving mechanisms, such as telephone calls inappropriate in time, distance, person, or motive (telephonitis)	2	Late: Overt expression of more regressive defense mechanisms: denial, projection, etc.; Resentment, jealousy, paranoid attitudes; Symptoms of depression: isolation, crying, suicidal preoccupation	3
Outbursts of rage and suicidal gestures while drinking	2		
		Feelings that he is "losing his mind "	2

of those four manifestations of withdrawal carries a diagnostic level of 1; a patient showing one or more of them should be considered alcoholic.

By similar logic, patients satisfying other clinical or behavioral *major criteria* are at a diagnostic level of 1 alcoholic. Patients satisfying several *minor criteria* are most probably alcoholic, especially if those criteria are drawn from one track. Note that a blood alcohol level of greater than 300 mg/100 ml is a major criterion, even though it may be associated with several minor criteria of a clinical nature. In many cases the minor criteria categories also help differentiate between early, middle, and late stages of alcoholism. The presence of only minor criteria indicators at a diagnostic level of 3 is probably *not* diagnostic of alcoholism.

In short, these criteria (described in greater detail in the original publication) afford the therapist a set of relatively easily determined physiological and psychosocial standards by which he can assess a patient's degree of alcoholism at the initial evaluation. The therapist can reassess the patient's condition as treatment progresses to document improvement, stability, or deterioration. Proper use of these criteria can protect the overzealous therapist from the pitfall of diagnosing alcoholism when only a few level 3 criteria are satisfied. They can aid him in properly making the diagnosis when one or more level 1 features are present.

In estimating daily consumption, the whiskey equivalent chart (Table 6-2) is useful. Alcoholic patients are notorious for underestimating their consumption with statements such as, "Oh, I only drink a couple of beers or so." The interviewer should ask specific questions; for instance, ask the patient to examine a typical day's drinking. Does he drink in the morning; at lunch; before, during, or after dinner? What does he drink at each of those times (whiskey, gin, wine, beer)? How much at each juncture? How many shots go into each hard drink? How big are the shots (one ounce, doubles?) And so on. When totaled, even the patient may be surprised at the quantity of ethyl alcohol he consumes in its various guises during a twenty-four-hour period. Often, however, it is quite difficult to obtain an accurate drinking history from the actively drinking patient, and he must be questioned about other criteria.

Table 6-2: Whiskey Equivalents of Consumption of Wine and Beer

Equivalents are based on:
0.8 quart = one-fifth gallon
32 ounces = 1 quart
Whiskey contains 43 percent ethyl alcohol
Fortified wine contains 20 percent ethyl alcohol
Table wine contains 12 percent ethyl alcohol
Beer contains 4 percent ethyl alcohol

Person's Weight (pounds)	Whiskey (quarts)	Fortified Wine (quarts)	Table Wine (quarts)	Beer (quarts)	(12-oz. bottles)
220	1.0	2.0	3.6	11.0	29
200	0.9	1.9	3.2	9.7	26
180	0.8	1.7	2.9	8.6	23
160	0.7	1.5	2.5	7.5	20
140	0.6	1.3	2.2	6.5	17
120	0.5	1.0	1.8	5.4	14

THE PHARMACOLOGY OF ALCOHOL

We turn from the identification of alcoholism in the problem drinker to the specific effects of the drug alcohol on the central nervous system. Both its enormous appeal and the great capacity of this drug to do harm can be traced to its specific pharmacology. Additionally, patients appear at various stages of intoxication or withdrawal, and it is necessary to develop skill in recognizing the various states that are produced during these pharmacological stages.

Acute Alcohol Intoxication

It is easy to believe that the experience of being drunk is so universal that no description is necessary. In fact, drunkenness is a great mimic of other psychiatric syndromes, and a great deal of time is wasted by the beginning emergency therapist in gathering "psychiatric" data from patients in the drunken state. The intoxicated person, for his part, is all too eager to bend the listener's ear and can be quite skillful at impersonating hysteria, schizophrenia, depression, or whatever seems to be required to hold his psychiatric audience.

A survey of the stages of intoxication is in order. These resemble the stages of anesthesia, from excitation to depression. The best description of them is an old one: verbose, jocose, lachrymose, bellicose, and comatose. A classic description of alcohol intoxication shows how these stages progress:

> In a mild state of intoxication there are unnecessary vocal efforts, pathos which is incongruent in view of the unessential content of conversation, exaggerated expressions of affect, laughter, and exaggerated motorics. With this comes an increase in the subjective feeling of well-being. After larger alcohol intake there is impairment of sensory function, the thought processes become superficial, and conversation becomes flatter. There is a tendency towards flight of ideas. Judgment is clouded and self-criticism, especially [recognition of the] disproportion between the increased ego feeling and the objective ability to produce. This contrast is sometimes vaguely felt by the intoxicated person and results in a feeling of insecurity. On the basis of this mood tone then develop symptoms of irritability and readiness to paranoid reactions. In a severe state of intoxication there is ataxia, staggering gait, slurred speech and finally, severe impairment of perception. The intoxicated person becomes apathetic and falls into a deep sleep. Although some personality characteristics break through into the picture of intoxication it is not possible to construct a law of relation between type of alcohol reaction in personality, especially if the picture may change on different occasions in the same person. The degree of drunkenness is related to the alcohol concentration in the blood only in a very broad way.[17]

Others have pointed out the disruption of perception, as did the philosopher Kant, who wrote that "Drunkenness is the unnatural state of inability to organize sense impressions according to the laws of experience." Psychiatrists are fond of noting that "Conscience is that portion of the personality which is soluble in alcohol."

All these observations make it clear that a person who is acutely intoxicated may show disorders of thought, affect, perception, or judgment and that an observer may be led into thinking the drunken patient is schizophrenic, manic-depressive, organic, or antisocial, depending on his state at the initial evaluation. The important clue to intoxication, when breath odor or history are not diagnostic, is the extreme lability: no other condition involves such dramatic changes of state over so short a period of time.

Pathological Intoxication

In some individuals, dissociative, rage, or psychotic reactions appear after only minimal amounts of alcohol have been consumed. Following a period of grossly disruptive behavior, the patient may fall into a profound sleep. This untoward response to alcohol should not be confused with similar reactions appearing after large quantities of alcohol have been consumed. Sufferers from this condition often have explosive (or "epileptoid") personalities. They need to abstain from alcohol altogether.

Limitations of Interviewing the Drunken Patient

The therapist should guard against making any psychiatric diagnosis while the patient is still in the drunken state; base-line ego functioning can be appraised only when the patient is sober. Similarly, the therapist must be cautious about the significance he attaches to alcoholic monologues. Although these can be extremely meaningful, even beautiful, to the listener who has not heard them before, the patient may not derive much benefit from what he reveals when drunk. The deep material is analogous to the material obtained through amytal interviewing. Many of the ordinarily repressed emotional conflicts rise to the surface with refreshing immediacy, but the same material sinks down again without a trace when the patient is fully conscious. The meaning, as well as the content, is again repressed; along with it goes the feeling of rapport with the listener. All that is left for the patient may be a vague sense of uneasiness at having somehow exposed himself against his will.

However, what is observed about the patient's personality and behavior during the drunken state is valid for predicting how the patient is likely to behave the next time he is drunk. Therefore, the therapist should take careful note of the kind of pathology that belongs to the patient's drunken state, not as a psychiatric diagnosis in itself, but as a means of determining how alcohol influences his potential for suicide, homicide, psychosis, and antisocial behavior.

Acute Alcohol Withdrawal

The emergence of disturbing symptoms upon withdrawal is the proof of dependency on any drug. In alcohol-dependent patients, withdrawal symptoms appear forty-eight to seventy-two hours after the intake of alcohol is abruptly stopped or sharply reduced. The main symptoms are (1) tremor, (2) convulsions, (3) hallucinosis, and (4) clouding of the sensorium. (When the fourth is of sufficient degree, it is called delirium tremens, which is the most serious stage of alcohol withdrawal. In the past it has had a 15 percent mortality.) It must be pointed out that these symptoms may appear even though the patient continues to drink: withdrawal symptoms may appear when the rate of intake is *reduced* (with a consequent dip in the blood level of alcohol); absolute cessation of intake is not required.

Some withdrawal symptoms are direct effects of depriving a dependent nervous system of alcohol, others indirect effects of the nutritional disturbances that also affect the brain. Therefore it is important to realize that symptoms of *acute intoxication*, symptoms of *withdrawal*, and symptoms of *nutritional deficiency* may all be present at the same time, contributing to impairment of brain function and to the "alcohol withdrawal syndrome."

By the time a drinking patient comes to the emergency room his brain function may be seriously compromised. Most of the early indications that this crisis is developing are subjective: he feels awful and cannot organize his thinking properly. It is imperative that the significance of his subjective discomfort be grasped so appropriate treatment can be instituted before the crisis results in death or permanent brain injury.

Milton Gross[18] has defined the withdrawal syndrome as advancing through a series of stages: early, prodromal, and advanced. This outline will be followed to present basic information about the course of alcohol withdrawal.

Early Phase. Not every alcoholic bout ends in withdrawal symptoms. Usually there is a severe depressive reaction involving a loss of appetite and sleep disturbance, which leads to a great intensification of the desire to drink. Alcohol intake becomes extremely heavy, but the patient may not feel his drinks as much as usual. They only seem to cancel the major depressive symptoms. This is the point at which the person finds himself drinking around the clock yet feels sober much of the time. Alvarez[19] describes such depressive drinking:

Mostly, I'm a social drinker. Like everyone else, I've been drunk in my time but it's not really my style; I value my control too highly. This time, however, I went at the bottle with a pure need, as though parched. I drank before I got out of bed, almost before my eyes were open. I continued steadily throughout the morning until, by lunchtime, I had half a bottle of whiskey inside me and was beginning to feel human. Not drunk: that first half-bottle simply brought me to the point of calm where I usually began. Which is not particularly calm. Around lunchtime a friend—also depressed, also drinking—joined me at the pub and we boozed until closing time. Back home, with our wives, we kept at it steadily through the afternoon and evening, late into the night. The important thing was not to stop. In this way, I got through a bottle of whiskey a day, and a good deal of wine and beer. Yet it had little effect.

The culmination of Alvarez' drinking was a suicide attempt on Christmas Day. The holiday drinking obscured his own marked increase in intake. Although treatment of withdrawal is not indicated at this stage of drinking, recognition of the pattern of depressive drinking and evaluation of the suicide risk is imperative. (Alvarez called his old therapist on Christmas Eve and was given an appointment for the day *after* Christmas, on the face of Alvarez' statement that it could wait.) This is the phase of withdrawal in which the prompt cessation of alcohol intake and transfer to an antidepressant drug can avoid major physical and psychiatric complications. Without prompt intervention, progression to a stage in which withdrawal symptoms will appear is almost certain—unless, as in Alvarez' case, another self-destructive act supervenes.

Prodromal Phase. The patient begins to experience (in addition to intoxication) the toxic organ effects of prolonged excessive drinking, disturbances secondary to nutritional deficiencies, and the early effects of alcohol withdrawal called "impending DTs." This phase involves gastrointestinal, perceptual, motor, vegetative, and sleep disturbances. It need not lead to frank delirium tremens.

The gastrointestinal symptoms include nausea and vomiting. "Dry heaves" appear when the patient awakes, presumably because of relative alcohol withdrawal during sleep. There may also be gastritis and an increased loss of appetite, leading to still further dependence on alcohol for caloric needs.

Perceptual disturbances are found in auditory, visual, and somesthetic disturbances. The most common auditory symptom, according to Gross, is *tinnitus*, a ringing, blowing, or whistling sound in the ears. Some patients experience clicking, popping, or shotlike sounds. (These have been related to spasms of the tensor stapedius muscle in the middle ear and are considered by some to be the basis for the later appearance of frank auditory hallucinosis, as the organism attempts to integrate the unfamiliar input.) Visual symptoms are spots, flashes of light resembling falling rain, and blurring of vision. Bodily sensations include paresthesias and numbness. Motor disturbances include marked tremulousness, weakness or severe cramps in the extremities, and impairment of gait.

Massive autonomic (vegetative) nervous system discharge is marked by a rapid pulse, fever, hypertension, and profuse night sweats accompanied by itching and increased tremulousness. Sleep disturbance is great, starting with insomnia (which eventually cannot be relieved by alcohol) and leading to brief periods of restless sleep punctuated by nightmares.

At this stage, intellectual functions start to become impaired, and the first signs of confusion appear. This is the stage at which many authorities recommend hospitalization and at which many alcoholic patients seeking help experience professional rejection.

Advanced Symptoms. The next stage is the appearance of frank psychotic symptoms and autonomic reactions that can lead to death in as many as 15 percent of those treated.

Gross[20] calls this stage the *Walpurgisnacht* of the actual acute withdrawal. Serious failure of mental functions and hallucinatory manifestations occur. Delusions may be present. Recent memory, concentration, integrative and synthetic functions, and orientation to time and place are all impaired. As stable internal points of reference for contact with reality disappear, patients are driven to seek cues from external sources. When these are absent (as at night when the patient lies alone in the dark, afraid or unable to sleep), psychotic manifestations emerge.

Because a certain percentage of the alcoholic population is schizophrenic, it becomes important to distinguish organic psychosis in the phase of alcohol withdrawal from paranoid schizophrenia. Both conditions involve delusions and auditory hallucinations. In schizophrenia, however, the voices appear before other signs of toxicity (such as disorientation) and persist after the toxic effects of withdrawal are gone. Moreover, the voices are more plausible in cases of withdrawal psychosis, and their statements are exclusively in the third person. ("He did that; look at him," and so on.) Finally, suspiciousness and hostility are usually present in withdrawal psychoses only when the physician is not identified as a professional, whereas in paranoid schizophrenia the physician may be seen as an enemy even when his medical role is fully grasped.

Convulsions are another advanced symptom, occurring in as many as 60 percent of patients treated at this stage. Electroencephalographic evidence shows multiple disturbances in sleep. In addition to rebound of fast-wave rapid-eye-movement (REM) sleep, there seems to be an interruption of deep, dreamless delta-wave sleep. Recovery from the withdrawal accompanies the reestablishment of delta-wave sleep, experienced subjectively by the patient as "the first good night of sleep." Anxiety and confusion may also play a role in lowering the seizure threshold, pointing to the need for good environmental support.

The autonomic discharge of the prodromal period is intensified, with a pronounced rise in fever over 100°F in dangerously ill patients. Usually the term delirium tremens is reserved for cases that show *both* marked clouding of sensorium *and* this massive, life-threatening autonomic discharge. Lesser degrees of withdrawal psychosis, characterized primarily by tremulousness and auditory or visual hallucinations, are not as serious and are usually spoken of as "acute alcoholic hallucinosis."

TREATMENT IN THE PHASE OF ALCOHOL WITHDRAWAL

Management of Uncomplicated Alcohol Withdrawal

Properly treated, alcohol withdrawal usually runs its course within five days. Convulsions may appear forty-eight to seventy-two hours after treatment has begun and yet be directly related to the withdrawal. Fevers and hallucinations appearing twenty-four to thirty-six hours after treatment has begun often point to a complicating medical or psychiatric condition. We shall discuss complications later in this chapter.

It is helpful to learn a standard method for handling withdrawal. The following list of procedures was adapted from Gross, [21] then modified by suggestions taken from O'Briant: [22]

1. *Vitamins.* On first contact, the patient is given an injection of 100 mg of thiamine. Thereafter he is given 50 mg of thiamine three times a day orally, and vitamin-B complex three times a day.

2. *Aluminum hydroxide gel and a bland diet.* It is wise not to feed the patient until half an hour after the thiamine is administered: severe thiamine deficiency blocks the body's ability to metabolize foodstuffs, and deaths from pyruvic acid poisoning after patients have eaten have been reported.

3. *Fluids.* Until recently it was thought that the therapist should "force fluids" with alcoholic patients on the premise that alcohol (a diuretic) causes dehydration. Recent research[23] has shown that overall a relative retention of fluid occurs after heavy drinking, so fluids should be administered moderately during the first twenty-four hours. In well-nourished patients, the total body water level should decrease to

normal in about four days, with no specific fluid or electrolyte therapy. [23]

4. *Environmental support.* The setting may be an alcoholic rehabilitation center, a recovery home, or a general hospital ward. The purpose is to help the patient maintain contact with reality by keeping the light on at night, talking with him, reminding him where he is, to whom he is talking, and why he is there.

Often it is best not to accomplish this work in a medical setting but in a social treatment setting where the caretakers are committed to the long-term rehabilitation of the alcoholic person. The detoxification ward should be reserved for severely ill patients with frank DTs. A rehabilitation unit with medical back-up support is ideal, but the earliest contacts should be with alcohol treatment workers, not with nurses and doctors who are committed only to easing immediate bodily pain. [26]

In any setting *talking down alcoholic hallucinations* can be accomplished easily. The patient may be asked, "Do you see something?" ("Yes.") "Where?" (The patient indicates that the vision, often an animal, is by his bed or chair.) "Close your eyes." (The patient does.) "Do you still see it?" (The patient indicates that he does.) "Then you know it isn't there!" [22]

Contact with people experienced in alcohol rehabilitation at this time of greatest fear and need may well facilitate a *religious conversion* to the ideal of abstinence, one of great benefit to the marginally motivated, despairing patient.

5. *Psychopharmacological treatment to end and reverse the acute withdrawal state.* In a sense, this is replacement therapy, and in some specific situations the most practical solution will be to have the patient return to alcohol. Or, the therapist may use a sedative-hypnotic drug that can be interchanged with alcohol (such as a barbiturate). However, the clinical challenge has been to find a drug that will

"cover" for alcohol without posing the same toxic and addictive risks.

Currently, three agents are preferred: chlordiazepoxide (Librium®), paraldehyde, and hydroxyzine (Vistaril®). Chlordiazepoxide has the advantages of being nonodorous, easily palatable, and pleasantly sedative. It has the disadvantages of having no effect in restoring terminal delta sleep, or not reaching sufficient terminal delta sleep, of not reaching sufficient stration) to cover the severest forms of withdrawal, and of becoming part of an addictive cycle. Chlordiazepoxide by injection is a rapid and effective means of bringing patients in the prodromal stage of alcohol withdrawal under control.

The following regimen has been found to be effective. At first contact with a tremulous, nonpsychotic patient, administer 100 mg of thiamine and 100 mg of chlordiazepoxide intramuscularly in the same syringe. If the patient is hungry, give him something to eat after half an hour. After giving the drugs an hour to take effect, continue the evaluation. During the first twenty-four hours of treatment, repeat oral, 100-mg doses of chlordiazepoxide every six hours if the patient is not vomiting, or give it by injection if he is. On the second day, continue 25 mg of chlordiazepoxide every six hours; on the third day continue it at the 10-mg level. If more sedation is needed, 1 gram of chloral hydrate can be given and the dose repeated once or twice an hour as necessary. Such a program is effective and does not produce undesirable oversedation.

Paraldehyde is often touted as the drug of choice for patients in advanced alcohol withdrawal. Although it is addictive, it is decidedly effective. Experienced alcoholic patients and ward nurses prefer it: it produces good, delta-wave sleep, which mimics natural, terminal sleep. It is therefore a rational treatment for withdrawal. Unfortunately, its chemical structure resembles that of ethyl alcohol, and its degradation uses the same enzyme system in the body. Accordingly, it may cause stress to the diseased liver and add a new risk of toxic injury. Its use is being increasingly questioned. [22]

When paraldehyde is used, it should be given on a regular schedule. It is malodorous and produces vomiting in sensitive patients. Previous administration of aluminum hydroxide greatly increases its chance of being held down. Injections of paraldehyde sting, and they may cause sterile abscesses. It is hard to find a rationale for their use. A standard schedule is 10 cc orally every four hours (every six hours in patients past 45 to avoid cardiac arrythmias) during the first twenty-four hours; 10 cc orally every six hours during the next twenty-four hours; and 10 cc only at bedtime on the third and fourth days. If there is an acute infectious or inflammatory process, the dosage schedule of the first twenty-four hours is maintained until the complicating condition is brought under control. If there is hypersomnolence in response to paraldehyde, the dose should be reduced and the possibility of Wernicke's encephalopathy (which responds to thiamine) or other brain syndromes (including trauma) should be explored.

Currently, hydroxyzine (Vistaril®) is coming into favor with clinicians such as Dr. Robert G. O'Briant. [22] He reports success with the following schedule: 100 mg of hydroxyzine is given intramuscularly (IM) initially, together with 100 mg of thiamine. The 100-mg hydroxyzine IM is repeated as needed every two to three hours for two doses. Then 75 mg is given as needed every four to six hours. Chloral hydrate, 1 gram, is used for sleep. This regimen is effective for about 95 percent of withdrawing alcoholic patients and is conducted with their immediate participation while they are still in the withdrawal phase and under a program of social treatment aimed at alcoholic rehabilitation. Only the most severe cases require admission to an intensive care detoxification unit. For them, injectable diazepam can

be used, 10 mg IM as needed every three to four hours until the most severe stage of withdrawal is under control.

This hydroxyzine regimen avoids the potential dangers of both paraldehyde (possible stress to diseased livers) and chlordiazepoxide (a new habit-forming drug). Moreover, it is not oversedating. (Patients do not becomed "spaced" on hydroxyzine, and later they do not seek to obtain mellow "highs" by combining it with alcohol. Patients who have experienced a pleasant withdrawal on chlordiazepoxide sometimes do try to achieve later highs from that particular combination.) Hydroxyzine also controls vomiting.

Only after the patient has gone for twenty-four hours without psychotic manifestations or medication is he ready for release from all medical management of the alcoholic withdrawal.

Common Complications and Their Management

We shall discuss the most commonly found complications of excessive drinking; descriptions of others can be found in standard medical texts. The syndromes to be presented are the Wernicke-Korsakoff, infections, and gastrointestinal and psychiatric complications.

The Wernicke-Korsakoff Syndrome. The various manifestations of this syndrome have been called Wernicke's encephalopathy, alcoholic cerebellar degeration, Korsakoff's psychosis, and "the alcoholic psychoses." It is the result of prolonged B-vitamin (especially thiamine) deficiency often found in patients who drink but do not eat.

Victor, Adams, and Collins[24] have traced the progression of symptoms. Initially the sensorium is mildly clouded, followed by global confusion, dullness, and apathy. When the confusion clears, there is a severe memory deficit marked by (1) loss of past memories, invariably coupled with an inability to form new memories or to learn; (2) relatively minor but definite impairment of perceptual and conceptual functions; and (3) diminution in spontaneity and initiative. Often the patient will *confabulate*, that is, make up a past he cannot remember, and in the past this colorful symptom was taken as a hallmark of Korsakoff's psychosis, even though it is not always present. If the condition is severe or treatment has been withheld, a permanent deficit, without confabulation, may remain; this deficit is called "alcoholic dementia."

The first indications of the disease are eye signs and incoordination of gait, ataxia. The eye signs include paralysis of ocular muscles (reported as double vision) and nystagmus on fixed lateral gaze. Ataxia suggests cerebellar dysfunction. If thiamine is administered to patients who manifest only ocular and cerebellar symptoms, improvement occurs in hours or days, and Korsakoff's psychosis is prevented. The amnesic psychosis responds to thiamine in 80 percent of the cases; its continued administration for days and weeks will cause marked improvement in many of the others.

> *Example 6-8.* A 50-year-old man brought himself for his first emergency room visit. He seemed tired, listless, superficially in contact with his surroundings, and only marginally attentive. A careful mental status examination revealed the degree of his memory deficit. Of the last six presidents, he could name only Kennedy, Truman, and Roosevelt. His eyes showed paralysis of conjugate gaze and nystagmus. He spontaneously reported seeing double images. He was given a shot of 100 mg of thiamine. An hour later the patient reported that his vision was clearing and that he was feeling much better. Asked again to name the last six presidents, he said, "Nixon, Johnson, Kennedy, Eisenhower, Truman, Roosevelt" without hesitation.

Infections. Alcoholic patients in withdrawal often have fevers. In the absence of other signs of autonomic hyperactivity (such as sweating, tachycardia, and dilated pupils), fever must be regarded as the result of infection. Pneumonia is the most common; often tuberculosis must be ruled out. Consultation by an internist is virtually mandatory when fever, gastrointestinal complaints, or other medical complications are present.

Gastrointestinal Complications. During alcohol withdrawal, bleeding episodes from severe gastritis, a duodenal ulcer, or esophageal varices are not uncommon and require immediate medical consultation. Additionally, pain and risk to life from acute pancreatitis may be present. Finally, severe acute alcoholic hepatitis, which is the probable precursor to cirrhosis of the liver, may cause nausea and jaundice. It is a reason for prolonged hospitalization, as continued drinking in the presence of this condition will surely produce cirrhosis. All alcoholic patients should have complete liver profiles on the third or fourth hospital day to check for hepatitis. If it is present, strenuous measures should be taken to see that the patients do not have opportunities to drink again soon.

Psychiatric Complications. According to Gross,[25] 14 percent of the alcoholic population are also schizophrenic. Chronic schizophrenic patients may also discontinue phenothiazines when they start drinking. Alcohol withdrawal may trigger a full-blown psychotic break in a usually borderline individual, who must then be treated as for a functional psychosis. (See Chapter 5, "Evaluation and Treatment of the Psychotic Patient.") Phenothiazines can be given after the second hospital day if the patient's liver function permits, but they will lower the seizure threshold. Because the high-vulnerability period for seizures is forty-eight to seventy-two hours after withdrawal begins,[26] an antiseizure medication such as diphenylhydantoin (Dilantin®), 100 mg, three times a day, should be administered to withdrawing patients who are receiving phenothiazines. An additional problem is posed by the potentiating effects of phenothiazines on other medications with sedating effects; care should be taken not to obtund the patient. Some patients become agitated and depressed after alcohol withdrawal, especially if they regret their behavior when they were drunk. After the patient has been withdrawn from alcohol, the risk of suicide may require his transfer to a psychiatric ward.

MEDICAL PROBLEMS OF ADVANCED ALCOHOLISM

The Therapist's Responsibility

In addition to the problems posed by withdrawal, the drinking person is generally liable to many accidents and infections, as well as to a host of diseases caused either by the direct toxic effects of alcohol on organs or by the nutritional consequences of alcoholic debilitation. These conditions may result in the crisis that caused him to seek psychiatric help: the threat to health. Although not all alcohol-related illnesses can be examined here in detail, it is the therapist's job to take his patient's suffering seriously and to be willing to refer him for careful evaluation. The patient may respond to the health crisis with a sense of narcissistic injury, which is why it comes first to psychiatric attention. The therapist may be the only one who can obtain an adequate history; he must serve as the patient's advocate in bringing key symptoms to the attention of an internist. The therapist's interest is one way of guaranteeing that the patient will receive thorough, thoughtful medical care.

The therapist who is not familiar with the signs and symptoms of the following conditions should become sufficiently knowledgeable about them so he can suspect them when symptoms develop and make the appropriate referral to an internist.

The Medical Problems

Cirrhosis. The most dreaded consequence of alcoholism is cirrhosis of the liver, a variably progressive disease in which fibrous scar tissue gradually replaces vital liver cells and interferes with the vast array of life-promoting functions of the liver. The precursor of this disease is acute alcoholic hepatitis, not fatty liver. During heavy drinking, fatty cells often occupy liver tissue, but this condition is temporary and reversible; the patient can resume drinking without inevitable progression to cirrhosis. By contrast, acute alcoholic hepatitis often leads to dangerous, permanent liver damage and requires hospitalization for about six weeks until the condition is stabilized.

Once cirrhosis is established, the alcoholic patient lives under threat. He will need to stop drinking and be supervised by an internist. From this point on, nutrition will be a paramount problem because he will absorb less fat, calcium, magnesium, and fewer selective vitamins, and he is likely to develop considerable protein deficiency. With this malnutrition, symptoms of depression grow worse, and the energy for life tasks becomes less. Equally, the patient's ability to metabolize alcohol decreases, and his tolerance for alcohol is lowered considerably.

Nutritional Disorders. Besides brain thiamine deficiency, beriberi, pellagra, and scurvy are found in alcoholic patients. Anemias resulting from iron, folic acid, and pyridoxine deficiencies are common. Finally, mineral deficiencies—including potassium, magnesium, and zinc—may appear in the course of advanced alcoholism. Any of these may materially affect the patient's well-being and have major adverse effects upon his heart, muscle, and nerve functions.

Alcoholic Heart Disease. Toxic alcohol effects weaken the muscles of the heart, causing heart failure in relatively young men. Recognition of cardiac failure may produce the anxiety that causes an otherwise well-functioning heavy drinker to seek psychiatric treatment. Reports of physical fatigue should be taken seriously, and a basic examination for heart disease should be arranged.

Accidents. Drinking patients are prone to falls, auto accidents, and fires. Although trauma victims include a large proportion of true alcoholic patients, surgeons often miss this diagnosis. Whenever the psychiatrist is given the opportunity, he should help the surgeon to share the drinking patient. Too often a patient with severe emotional problems is subject to the long confinement of a hospitalization for a fracture without any opportunity to discuss the emotional events that led to the accident. Furthermore, many "accidents" are suicide attempts that have gone unrecognized. A long hospitalization without contact with significant others becomes a semipunitive rest cure, effective for some depressions, wholly detrimental to others. The same hospitalization could be the beginning of a meaningful participation in psychotherapy or an alcohol treatment program.

Summary. Therapists must take the alcoholic patient's medical needs seriously, work with him in his struggle to recover health, help him to realize how alcohol impedes that struggle, and set the stage for discussions of psychological suffering. As one patient put it, "I'm sick and tired of feeling sick and tired." If the psychiatrist neglects these areas, sees them as "the patient's problem" or as "what he gets for drinking," he indicates that he cannot really receive the patient's own experience and discourages him from taking his treatment seriously. For the nonmedical therapist, mastering these areas is similar to entering a foreign country of vaguely hostile intent. He will be repaid for his labors by the knowledge that he is coming much closer to understanding the world in which his patient is forced to live.

LONG-RANGE TREATMENT OF THE DRINKING PATIENT

A description of all aspects of the treatment of the advanced alcoholic patient is beyond the scope of this book. What should be mastered initially, however, is a certain skill at setting the stage for definitive treatment and an understanding of the basic principles of that treatment. For a thorough description of the modern social approach, O'Briant and Lennard's[26] brief, definitive text, *Recovery from Alcoholism,* should be consulted. Hoff[27] has presented a concise statement of some initial principles of alcoholic rehabilitation, and many of his points will be summarized here.

Setting the Stage in the Initial Evaluation

The major task in the initial interviewing of the drinking patient is to keep the patient open to the idea of therapeutic intervention. This task becomes easier if certain ground rules are kept in mind.

Establish That Drinking Can Be Discussed. At first, most drinking patients are chary of revealing too much about their drinking behavior because they anticipate censure. The emergency therapist's first task is to establish that he can stand to hear about drinking. A good way is to inquire about the patient's bodily sensations in relation to drinking: does it make his head ache, his stomach get upset, his vision blur? Almost any drinking person will welcome this opportunity to talk about his body (which is probably suffering), and the therapist has established that he wants to hear about the patient's experience with alcohol.

Mediate Catharsis. Getting drunk is a way of becoming unconscious, which perforce interferes with putting feelings into words. The therapist must expect to do a good deal of the talking at first, helping the patient to articulate his feelings by verbalizing them for him. To the patient who mentions a divorce five years ago, the therapist may say, "And of course you felt extremely low when that came through." A great deal of patience is required to help the patient recapture his lost affect; the therapist should expect repression. Alcoholic patients often forget whole chapters of their lives, and considerable therapeutic patience is needed to obtain this material.

Establish Early the Right to Communicate with Others. Problem drinking is a chronic psychosocial disease; the drinker is rarely the only person involved. Despite the fact that the family knows he has a drinking problem, the alcoholic patient will often try to bind the therapist with pseudoconfidentiality. In such a role the therapist is as therapeutically confined as a bartender. Yet the patient insists on keeping their relationship confidential, claiming it would destroy the family to know that he drinks.

Usually the family knows but has developed a conspiracy of silence. The patient's insistence on confidentiality mirrors a family style of keeping feelings under wraps, as if there were a tacit rule: important emotional facts may not be discussed. The alcoholic family, like many others, adopts a strategy of denial to deal with problems for which no easy solution is at hand. This policy of denial is continued even when it has grown grotesquely ineffective. One of the therapist's first tasks is to counter this policy of denial with his own commitment to talking things out. He starts by making it clear to his patient that effective service means talking with other members of the ecological group. Indeed, it is often effective to work with a spouse *first:* the alcoholic partner will come in later.

Expect Lability. Neither the acutely intoxicated nor the acutely withdrawing patient is in a normal emotional state. He may be alternately excited or depressed. It is often helpful to indicate to the patient, tactfully, that the problem of emotional dyscontrol is recognized and that full control is not expected. Initial interviews should be short; they may often be conducted after an injection of chlordiazepoxide and between interviews with other emergency patients. The full-scale interview can be conducted after he has begun to quiet down.

Watch for Overattachment to the Interviewer. It is an oversimplification to say that all persons with drinking problems are passive-dependent or "oral"

characters. Nevertheless, chronic excessive drinking does occasion regression to more dependent stages of development, not without considerable resentment on the part of the regressing patient. At the same time, the self-isolating (and society-alienating) existence of the confirmed alcoholic patient intensifies his needs for human contact, warmth, and support. A vicious circle is set in motion whereby the patient has intensified dependency needs just when he is most ashamed of himself for being so dependent.

The therapist can unwittingly participate in this vicious circle if he gives the patient too much support, leading to the familiar situation in which the patient is telling him, by a drunken telephone call at 2 A.M., that he is the only person who ever really helped. The patient's alcoholism worsens as it becomes his only way of expressing autonomy (and anger) toward the person on whom he has become so dependent.

In some cases erotic feelings color the picture, particularly if the patient is ashamed of erotic feelings, as is often true of homosexual, hysterical, and "masochistic" patients. Then the patient must punish himself for spoiling the therapeutic relationship with sexual fantasies.

Finally, hostile feelings may reach the level of active homicidal fantasy toward the therapist, especially when the patient is drinking. Threats to the therapist's life are not uncommon from drinking borderline patients who perceive the therapist as embodying all they can never control or attain.

A classical dyadic transference neurosis, for both patient and therapist, becomes intolerable when alcohol enters the picture. The therapist becomes (and feels like) a problem drinker's spouse caught in the bind of protecting a sadomasochistic partner, feeling like a sadomasochist himself. All this undercuts the patient's learning that he can share his problem with a wider group, not focusing all his libidinal energy on one person who seems to promise acceptance.

From the beginning, the therapist should eschew manipulating the patient into accepting individual or other long-term treatment by showing excessive personal interest in him. The interview should be straightforward and matter of fact, directed toward the unexciting but realistic prospect of a conventional alcoholic treatment program involving group and family approaches. If the patient seems uninterested, the therapist should be willing to let him go. He should not appear to promise unlimited dependency gratification. Equally, any attempt by the patient to restrict therapy to a one-to-one, long-term relationship with the initial therapist should be viewed as a resistance to treatment. Beginning therapists (especially those just beginning to prize their own work) must watch for that seduction: "You're the only person I really feel can reach me." The motive, too often, is a desire for access to drugs and hospitals as a means of bolstering, not changing, the addictive process. Yet every inpatient ward has a subpopulation of patients who "cycle" through under the protective custody of doctors who cannot insist that the patient make an effort to change as part of the therapeutic contract.

Determine Where the Patient Hurts and What He Wants. Not all drinking patients can be sold on treatment. Some want only to weather the physiologic crisis of alcohol withdrawal. Others want food and shelter. Others simply want a current physical evaluation. And a few want to be sure they are not losing their minds.

Helping the patient to define his need is therapeutic. It is important that the patient have a major say in the kind of treatment he is offered. The patient should not be "trapped" in a treatment program for which he is not ready. Until the patient has reached a sober and physiologically stable condition, the therapist cannot assess his motivation for further treatment. Often, as Hoff points out, all the therapist can do is admit the patient to the hospital and accomplish a safe detoxification there. This much is surely the patient's right if he is medically ill, and it is most certainly *not* a "misuse of the hospital."

Discuss Matters with Significant Others. When treatment is started, wide communication is extremely important. Often, members of the ecological group are caught up in the conspiracy of silence, afraid to share what they know of the patient's drinking with the patient or with each other. The wife feels bound not to tell the boss; the boss is afraid to tell the wife. Yet both know, and both are concerned.

The therapist can act as a model for the group by sharing freely what he understands of the patient's dilemma. Some therapists make it a rule to interview the patient alone. They secure his permission to bring in a family member to "share with him what they have been discussing." Often the therapist asks permission to call the boss, especially if hospitalization is going to cause the patient to miss work. He may telephone other members of the ecological group who are not present and pass the telephone back and forth to let them talk to those in the office. The therapist shows by his behavior that the problem can be openly and rationally discussed, and that he thinks alcoholic treatment is dignified and effective.

Example 6-9. A man in his early 60s had been admitted to the hospital for detoxification. His wife was also a heavy drinker, and they both believed that they had kept their drinking a secret from the other members of the family.

A conference was scheduled that was to include some close cousins who had consistently expressed concern. Just before the conference was to take place, the patient told the therapist that his cousins had been good to him since childhood and that he couldn't bear for them to find out he was an alcoholic. The therapist replied that it was better if the family knew, and finally the patient said, "You tell them."

In the presence of the wife and the cousins, the therapist told about the patient's serious drinking problem, explaining that it had caused the current admission. Immediately they revealed that they had known about it for several years but had never felt free to bring it up. In a very moving way, they expressed their willingness to help.

The patient seemed relieved. He said he hadn't realized that they had known. His wife then revealed she hadn't known what to tell the patient's employer and that she had finally reported that her husband had suffered a heart attack. The patient described great affection for his boss of twenty years, and great fear of losing his job.

The therapist asked permission to talk to the boss by telephone. Perhaps because the interview with the cousins had gone so well, the patient gave his consent.

The boss was greatly relieved to learn that his employee had not had a heart attack. This "saving" lie had, in fact, been the cause of considerable pressure from others at work to terminate the patient's employment, which involved heavy lifting.

When he learned that the patient had a drinking problem, the boss expressed interest in participating in the patient's treatment. The therapist asked if he would be willing to have his secretary administer a daily tablet of disulfiram (Antabuse®) so the patient would not have to depend on his wife or himself to remember. The boss was delighted to help in this way.

Upon hearing that his boss was willing to help him, the patient readily agreed to start disulfiram. Two weeks later he was back at work, and at the end of three months was still abstinent, for the first time in twenty years. He and his wife had begun attending AA meetings.

Make Referrals Personally. Morris Chafetz'[28] research has shown a marked increase in follow-through on referral suggestions by drinking patients when the referral is made in a personal way. His method is to set up the initial appointment in a concerned manner and then send the patient a follow-up letter reminding him of the appointment.

When the telephone is used, it is good to make the referral in the patient's presence so he can hear what is said about him. (This will also make it easier for him to open up to the next therapist; it is a way of "passing the mantle.") It helps if the therapist knows the person he is calling; he can introduce the patient to the new therapist over the phone and let the patient set up his own appointment. But even if he must look up the phone number of a local alcohol treatment program in the telephone book, he can do that in the patient's presence and share the problem of "breaking the ice" with him. Again, after the therapist makes contact he hands the telephone to the patient to set up an appointment.

With experience, therapists become familiar with people who work with alcoholic patients. The referral to the internist, the AA group, or the halfway house can be made with greater confidence and more genuine personal feeling, and the patients tend to follow through.

Principles of Treatment[27]

If the emergency therapist belongs to the team that offers long-range treatment, he will want to come to an agreement with the patient. This agreement is often described in therapeutic circles as a "contract," or "covenant of treatment."[27] In it the goals of treatment, and the therapist's expectations and limitations, should be spelled out clearly. This agreement is negotiated, like a labor contract, and the bargaining that takes place between the patient and therapist is an essential part of the treatment process. As the initial stages of bargaining take place in the emergency room around the issue of hospitalization, the therapist will want to keep certain principles in mind.

What Therapy Can Offer. The patient should be given a realistic picture of what therapy can give him. For instance, every patient can be given medical attention, even if he elects to refuse psychiatric help. The patient whose drinking is symptomatic can be offered conventional psychotherapy and the reasonable hope that his depression can be treated. The confirmed alcoholic patient should be given a description of the multidisciplinary approach, with stress on the necessity for open communication. It is proper to offer the opinion that modern treatment can help.

Privilege of Abstaining from Drinking and Therapy. The therapist should make it clear that only the patient can exercise the choice of changing his drinking habits. Although the therapist has the right and responsbility to limit the patient's freedom to hurt himself or others, the ultimate decision to abstain rests with the patient. The patient should be told he must come to terms with making this choice.

The patient may balk at further therapy. The therapist must make it clear what the alcoholic prognosis is. All drinking holds a potential for addiction and organ damage. Even reactive drinking may acquire a life of its own, apart from the original conflict alcohol had been selected to treat. The patient's rationalizations should be met with a statement of what he may expect if he continues to drink excessively, whether or not he enters treatment.

What Will Be Asked of the Patient. Many psychiatric units have prerequisites to admission. Some insist on a trial of disulfiram after detoxification. Others make a rule of strict abstinence during the ward stay, and the patient who fails to comply is subject to dismissal. Still others insist upon intensive family interviewing. It is not fair to spring these demands on the patient *after* detoxification has begun. He needs to know before, when he has some choice about whether or not to surrender to treatment.

Meeting the demands of a treating institution before treatment begins can be a kind of initiation for the recalcitrant alcoholic patient. As AA has stressed repeatedly, it is not beneficial to offer too much help to drinkers who are not "ripe." It is better to give them essential medical treatment when withdrawal symptoms appear and to hold

firm on the ground conditions to be met before the doors to a long-term supportive program are opened.

Informing Significant Others. From the beginning, the family should hear that its involvement will be an essential part of the patient's treatment. Family members should be told to expect the first months of abstinence to be rocky. The patient will miss alcohol, will be in a depressed, irritable, and joyless state, and will be even more difficult to live with than when he was drinking. They should expect to find themselves wishing him back on the bottle, even subtly encouraging that solution.

They should recognize that such reactions are normal but that they will be expected to talk about their feelings with a professional. It should be made clear that therapy for them means working on their own emotional problems, not just supplying moral support to the patient in his struggle to remain abstinent. The step of defining the family members as being in need of therapeutic help in their own rights is best taken before extended treatment is planned. The family can be refused as a unit until everyone is ready to participate.

Involving the employer from the beginning, as in Example 6-9, is often strikingly effective. The timing of this intervention is a difficult matter and requires individual judgment. Often the therapist must set as a goal of treatment the patient's ability to share his difficulty with those in positions of authority. He should be told that those who get better make a strict policy of frankness: it makes it harder for them to deceive themselves, as when they call in sick for alcohol-related illnesses.

Resources for Drinking Patients

The overlapping network of treatment resources for drinking people can seem like a morass to the beginning therapist. The manipulative patient will make the most of the therapist's confusion, so it is helpful to keep in mind a structured overview of the resources available in this area. As in all psychiatric referrals, the therapist should try to avoid culture shock by matching up the patient and the program. For a merchant seaman, a recovery home run by other merchant seamen who hold AA meetings on the premises may be the ideal resource. For a lower middle-class industrial worker, the alcohol treatment program run by his own company may be ideal. An upper middle-class person may insist upon a private psychiatrist, and one skilled in the treatment of alcoholic patients is mandatory. Detailed descriptions of specific resources are found in Fox.[29]

Organizations. *The National Council on Alcoholism* offers pretreatment evaluations as a public service at most of its 125 affiliate offices in major and smaller cities throughout the fifty states. The patient may be seen on his own direct request or on referral from a professional. The National Council on Alcoholism is listed in the regular listings of the telephone directory, not as a governmental agency. No files with patient names are kept, and efforts are made to keep the consultation strictly confidential. The patient is not treated but is evaluated for treatment, and the evaluators are skilled in making the best possible referral for the patient at his stage of drinking. The therapist who is uncertain about how to proceed in making recommendations to a given patient should not hesistate to use this resource.

Alcoholics Anonymous has developed and grown during the past ten years. No longer is it a monolithic, quasi-religious organization committed to reciting the twelve steps and indulging in long monologues at its meetings. Nor is it beneficial only to lonely extraverts and cyclothymic individuals and not to other kinds of problem drinkers. It is a many-faceted, flexible organization, with as many kinds of meetings as there are subcultures of alcoholic people. In the San Francisco area there are 130 AA groups, including young people's, black, Chicano, and gay groups. A suburban AA meeting may resemble a PTA meeting. In short, it is a good place for persons like those who used to drink together to meet together without drinking.

Also, AA members often devote a certain amount of time to providing information, transportation, and moral support to persons who are becoming serious about alcohol treatment. They visit hospitalized patients on medical and psychiatric wards.

One good way to become knowledgeable about alcoholic treatment programs in individual communities is to develop a rapport with AA members who are, by and large, quite gregarious, eager to help interested persons. When he suggests the patient avail himself of AA, the therapist can call an AA member known personally to him. Simply saying to a patient, "Go to AA" is so rejecting that the therapist should hardly expect a follow-through. (A special use of AA is made by the schizophrenic alcoholic person, ambivalent about intimacy, who finds through his alcoholism a reason to socialize with others in a way both close and impersonal enough to meet his conflicting needs.) Sometimes hospitalization can be avoided during the stage of alcohol withdrawal by referral to an AA-connected recovery home. The experience of being cared for by AA members at the time of greatest need may facilitate "conversion" to an AA-based, abstinent lifestyle.

Example 6-10. A man in his 50s had been drinking for twenty-five years. He was a merchant seaman with a boisterous, extraverted personality. He came to the hospital because he was frightened by visual hallucinosis during the withdrawal phase of his most recent heavy drinking spree. He had experienced mild alcohol withdrawal symptoms many times previously without psychotic manifestations; the psychosis scared him. He seemed to be in generally good health, and his vital signs and physical examination were essentially normal.

He was given chlordiazepoxide and thiamine as an outpatient and referred to a halfway house for alcoholics run by merchant seamen belonging to AA. The empathy he found with the others in that environment permitted a dramatic conversion to abstinence. He later attributed his change to the anxiety caused by the visual hallucinosis and the support of the AA members. A year later he had continued to remain abstinent and was very active in AA. Admission to the psychiatric unit would probably have interfered with the experience of salvation that this man found in the supportive AA environment, for which he was obviously ripe.

AA is not for every problem drinker. Those persons particularly who are reactive drinkers or deeply depressed should not be encouraged to see all their problems as resulting from alcohol use and requiring only conversion to an abstinent style and membership in AA to effect a complete cure. Overemphasis on symptomatic alcohol use with such an individual may lead him to select (often masochistically) the mask of chronic alcoholism to hide from confronting an acute life situation that could be resolved. For him psychiatric treatment aimed at the specific life conflict is indicated.

Alcohol treatment programs vary in quality from city to city, county to county, and state to state. Patients who have actively concerned family members do very well in programs that have a team of psychiatrists, social workers, psychologists, and vocational and rehabilitation workers. Such programs are offered primarily by large hospitals and community mental health centers. Special mention should be made, however, of industrial programs open to those who work for specific companies. Usually treatment is combined with a period of job probation. Participation in such a program by individuals whose frequent absences from work are alcohol-related is often made a condition for continuing employment.

Residental Settings. The patient without funds who is withdrawing from alcohol needs food, shelter, and environmental support. The *recovery home* is often found in cities and is a good setting for the socially damaged alcoholic person to become motivated toward a less self-destructive life style. Such settings are no longer skid row flop houses. (In fact, there is evidence that skid row is disappearing in many cities.) AA meetings are often held on the premises. Treatment is encouraged by the banning of alcohol from the premises and the insistence on abstinence in return for admission to a program of longer-term stay and vocational rehabilitation. Personnel are not highly trained, and conditions vary.

The *alcoholic rehabilitation center*, similar to the recovery home, usually has provisions for sleeping, eating, and group meetings, as well as for intensive care detoxification. Usually a doctor will be on the premises and will provide a certain security during the withdrawal phase. Personnel are usually highly skilled in alcoholic rehabilitation. However, the medical focus can place too much responsibility on the caretakers instead of on the patients. Insistence on a social treatment model is the hallmark of the advanced rehabilitation center. It can be a center for referral to other resources. The stay at the Garden Hospital Jerd Sullivan Rehabilitation Center in San Francisco lasts three weeks, during which the patient is helped to establish a "social support system" aimed at overcoming his urge to drink. Group therapy and one-to-one counseling are offered. Members of the ecological group are involved.[26]

The *halfway house* is for alcoholic patients who require extensive residental support, often six months or longer. It provides an alcohol-free environment to come home to after work or, for some persons who work on the premises, a frank shelter from the world at large. Often there are separate halfway houses for men and for women. The directors of such houses are frequently persons with great sensitivity and skill at managing the crucial long-term problems of alcoholic people. This resource should not be the *first* step in recovery, but a choice made by the patient after he has gone through withdrawal and a period of preliminary rehabilitation. The criteria for admission to such houses usually is an authentic commitment to the goal of abstinence. As the housing cost is low, some of the patients will agitate to obtain entry to such houses without being authentically committed to change. They bring their addictive patterns with them, only to cause havoc in the house and guilt in themselves. Occasionally the therapist will find himself pressured by a patient of this type into helping him gain admission to a halfway house before he is ready for it. In this case, a pretreatment evaluation by a National Council on Alcoholism affiliate may give an official recommendation for the kind of treatment that is appropriate for the patient at his particular stage.

Outpatient Clinics. General hospitals and family service agencies offer individual, group, and family therapy to the public at large, often without specific provision for the needs of alcoholic patients. Patients whose drinking is not their primary problem may benefit from conventional evaluation and treatment. Prominently alcoholic people should not be steered toward resources that cannot provide for them simply because these resources are available.

Individual Resources. These include clergymen, internists, therapists who specialize in the treatment of alcoholism, and visiting public health nurses.

The *clergyman* is an underutilized resource. Catholic families still rely on the priest, and often he has a fund of information about the family. Usually clergymen are extremely willing to discuss their parishoners' drinking problems with interested doctors.

The *general practitioner* or *internist* is an essential resource for the patient with a drinking problem. Nowadays there is a return to the practice of home visiting and an increasing sophistication about psychological problems. Many internists in private practice have a large group of alcoholic patients whose problems they manage quite well. Often internists like to work with therapists; they turn to the therapist for help at crisis points and handle the major part of the support by themselves.

Not all internists are effective with alcoholic patients, and indeed, some perpetuate an un-

healthy dependency, contributing to the addictive pattern. Nevertheless, increasing numbers of the medical profession have become interested in the treatment of alcoholism. With consultative help from the therapist, this resource can be very useful.

An *individual therapist* is in general *not* a good referral source for drinking patients unless he specializes in alcohol problems or unless the drinking is clearly of a reactive character. Reactive drinkers generally do well in individual or group therapy with a conventional focus on interpersonal conflicts and their resolution. A few therapists specialize in the treatment of drinking people and seem to know how to proceed. Individual therapy with a skilled specialist is often the referral of choice for problematic patients who do not fit the usual referral options. A word must be said against the assumption that individual therapy for the alcoholic patient can be done only by psychiatrists because they alone can admit patients to hospitals. Frequently it is better to have this medical power *out* of the therapeutic contract so that the patient can concentrate on which he can do for himself. He has the option of referral to a supportive environment if he cannot manage with outpatient therapy.

The *visiting public health nurse* can be crucial in the treatment of the woman problem drinker. Public health nurses can be contacted to provide regular home follow-up for patients who are not ready to come in regularly to an alcohol treatment program. For older, house-bound, and marginally motivated patients, this supportive resource can be of inestimable value. It is all too infrequently called upon by therapists, usually because they do not know the service exists.

Other Issues of Treatment

Quite often a drinking patient has legal problems. He may resist voluntary treatment even though he endangers himself and others. The role of disulfiram (Antabuse®) in his treatment is controversial. He often uses other drugs concomitantly. These matters will be considered in this section.

The Law. If a drinking patient is facing legal charges, the best procedure is to take care of his immediate medical needs for physical evaluation and detoxification and to insist that he settle his problem with the law before he starts lengthy rehabilitation. Otherwise, the rehabilitation program becomes part of his defense and prolongs his uncertainty about the future.

The patient should know that he can participate in the treatment program both during the legal process and after his release but that he must deal with his legal problems. Occasionally a patient will misrepresent himself as being too mentally ill to stand trial. The patient past the stage of detoxification should not be allowed to use the psychiatric treatment setting in this fraudulent way.

Involuntary Treatment. Drinking patients need involuntary restraint when they pose too great a threat to themselves or others. In acute cases, the treatment is the same as for any homicidal or suicidal patient. (See Chapters 2 to 4.) Some professionals argue that the confirmed alcoholic patient should be kept from destroying himself by drinking. In the case of very debilitated, ill, alcoholic people, involuntary treatment may precede a trial for mental incompetency. Generally, clinical experience confirms the wisdom of Hoff's[27] position that the patient retain the privilege of abstaining. Unnecessary involuntary treatment may simply intensify resistance. The therapist has to be able to let the patient go if he is not ready to accept treatment.

Disulfiram (Antabuse®). The clinical use of the drug disulfiram (Antabuse®) has staged a return in recent years. Originally it was used to produce a most incapacitating sickness in response to the use of alcohol as part of aversive conditioning. Several deaths were reported, and use of the drug declined. However, in low dosages it produces a distinctly unpleasant but not fatal response to alcohol and discourages the intake of intoxicating quantities. This property has led to its return to favor as a deterrent.

Willingness to take disulfiram can be a test of a patient's motivation to stop drinking. It gives him three days in which to decide to take the next drink. The decision to remain abstinent lies with the patient, not the pill; the patient decides when (and if) to take it. Disulfiram reactions consist of nausea, vomiting, low blood pressure, and rarely, convulsions. At doses of 0.25 to 0.5 mg/day, fatal reactions are virtually nonexistent. Every patient on disulfiram should be cautioned about the nature and duration of its effects on alcohol consumption and told to wait three days after the last dose if he intends to start drinking again. Complete instructions and an identification card prepared by the manufacturer are available and should be given to the patient when he starts to use the drug.

Other Drug Problems. Alcoholic persons often take other addictive drugs, such as marihuana, barbiturates, and amphetamines. Mixed alcohol and heroin addiction is not uncommon in the black community. The great jazz singer Billie Holiday died of complications of alcoholism, although she was famous for her heroin addiction. Alcohol use has cropped up persistently among addicts maintained on methadone: it is one drug not measured by the required urine test. The multiple drug abuser often does well in an environment such as Synanon, where active confrontation techniques are employed to break down rationalizing defenses.

SUMMARY

As Ruth Fox[30] has said, successful treatment of alcoholism is almost always multidisciplinary. Drinking problems involve such a variety of levels of functioning, from the biological to the social, that it is only reasonable to assume their cure will involve a variety of supportive professionals. Helping the problem drinker to enter treatment requires specialized knowledge, tact, and perseverance from the emergency therapist. From the beginning the therapist has to recognize that he is dealing with an acute manifestation of a chronic process and that the care and foresight with which he intervenes will have long-range consequences for the physical health, personal motivation, and social integration of his patient.

REFERENCES

1. Chafetz, Morris E., Howard T. Blane, and Marjorie Hill: *Frontiers of Alcoholism*, Science House, New York, 1970.

2. Ibid., pp. 105–155.

3. Ibid., pp. 33–73.

4. Plaut, Thomas F. A.: *Alcohol Problems: A Report to the Nation*, Cooperative Commission on the Study of Alcoholism, Oxford University Press, New York, 1967.

5. Jellinek, E. M.: *The Disease Concept of Alcoholism*, Yale, New Haven, Conn., 1960, p. 35.

6. Plaut: op. cit., p. 39.

7. American Psychiatric Association: *Diagnostic and Statistical Manual*, 2d ed., Washington, D.C., 1968.

8. Plaut: op. cit., pp. 37–38.

9. Kissin, Benjamin K.: "Alcoholism: Is It a Treatable Disease?", *Mod. Med.*, **14**(20):33, Oct. 1, 1973.

10. Reich, Louis H., Robert K. Davies, and Jonathan M. Himmelhock: "Excessive Alcohol Use in Manic-Depressive Illness," *Am. J. Psychiat.*, **131**(1):83–86, 1974.

11. Bateson, Gregory: "The Cybernetics of 'Self': A Theory of Alcoholism," *Psychiatry*, **34**(1):1–18, 1971.

12. Verdery, Eugene A.: "The Clergy and Alcoholism" in Ruth Fox (ed.), *Alcoholism – Behavioral Research, Therapeutic Approaches*, Springer, New York, 1967, p. 273.

13. Wolff, Ilse: "The Role of the Public Health Nurse in the Treatment of the Alcoholic," in ibid., pp. 296–297.

14. Kissin: loc. cit.

15. The Criteria Committee, National Council on Alcoholism (Frank A. Seixas, M.D., Medical Director): "Criteria for the Diagnosis of Alcoholism," *Am. J. Psychiat.*, **129**(2):127–135, 1972. Copyright 1972, The American Psychiatric Association.

16. Ibid., *Ann. Intern. Med.*, **77**:249–258, 1972.

17. From Bowman, K. M. and Jellinek, E. M.: "Alcoholic Mental Disorders," p. 89, in E. M. Jellinek (ed.), "Effects of Alcohol on the Individual," vol. 1, *Alcohol Addiction and Chronic Alcoholism*, Yale, New Haven, Conn., 1942. Copyright by Journal of Studies on Alcohol, Inc., New Brunswick, N.J.

18. Gross, Milton: "Management of Acute Alcohol Withdrawal States," *Quar. J. Stud. Alc.*, **28**:655–666, 1967.

19. Alvarez, A.: *The Savage God*, Random House, New York, 1972, p. 271. Copyright 1972, Random House.

20. Gross: loc. cit.

21. Ibid.

22. O'Briant, Robert G.: Director, Alcoholic Rehabilitation Program, Garden Hospital–Jerd Sullivan Rehabilitation Center, San Francisco, personal communication, 1973.

23. Beard, James D., and David H. Knott: "Fluid and Electrolyte Balance During Acute Withdrawal in Chronic Alcoholic Patients," *J. Am. Med. Ass.*, **204**:135–139, 1968.

24. Victor, Maurice, Raymond Adams, and George Collins: *The Wernicke-Korsakoff Syndrome*, Davis, Philadelphia, 1971.

25. Gross: loc. cit.

26. O'Briant, Robert G. and Henry Lennard: *Recovery from Alcoholism: A Social Treatment Model*, Charles C Thomas, Springfield, Ill., 1973.

27. Hoff, Ebbe Curtis: "The Psychological and Pharmacological Basis for the Treatment of Alcohol Dependence," in Yedy Israel and Jorge Mardones (eds.) *Biological Basis of Alcoholism*, Wiley-Interscience, New York, 1971, chap. 14.

28. Chafetz, Blaine, and Hill: loc. cit.

29. Fox: op. cit. (Ref. 12.)

30. Fox, Ruth: "A Multidisciplinary Approach to the Treatment of Alcoholism," *Am. J. Psychiat.* 123:7, January 1967.

Acute Inpatient Intervention

INTRODUCTION

The modern inpatient psychiatry ward, with its "therapeutic milieu," can be viewed in two ways: as a treatment *experience*, in which an entire community has been organized to facilitate ego-recovery in individuals whose adaptations have collapsed;[1-4] or as a treatment *context*, in which limits can be set on pathological behaviors and skills taught to improve social functioning.[5]

The *dangers* of hospitalization are a constant theme in the literature on this subject. Many authors express concern with preventing the "social breakdown syndrome" which is found in long-term hospital patients who have lost the social skills that could enable them to adapt to a real outside world.[6] Not wishing to encourage regression, many therapists strive to make the in-hospital experience as brief,[7] crisis-oriented, and hostile to the relaxation of ego-controls[8] as possible. A strong case has been made for *alternatives to hospitalization*, such as day hospitals,[9] family crisis teams,[10,11] and visits to the home.[12]

Others have challenged the *shallowness* of conventional hospital treatment. They feel that opportunities for growth are lost because insufficient attention is paid to the experiencing of the hospitalized patient.[13] They fear that the patient may learn only to make a pseudoadaptation to conform to staff expectations and that he will emerge from his brief hospitalization as basically unfit for life as he was before, still stuck in an unresolved developmental crisis which no one has bothered to examine but to which a pathological label has been affixed.[14] They argue for a relatively unhurried approach to the patient's recompensation, modeled less on the crisis resolutions of healthier persons[15] and more on respecting the personal and social nature of the ego-recovery process.[16]

Holmes has pointed out:[17]

> These are two different ways of relating to patients: one might be called the way of Eros, of unconditional (maternal) love, which cannot be earned, but is freely given, of concerns with the feeling and experience of the patient; the other might be called the way of Logos, of rational thought, cause and effect, reward and punishment, of (paternal) love which can be earned with good behavior, of concern with the control and correction of the patient's behavior.

As does ego development in the child, so too does the full return of ego function in the mentally ill adult require both its father and its mother. The ego returns to an adequate level of functioning both by being given real decisions and tasks[18] and by being heard and supported in resolving inner concerns.[19,20] When the therapist wants to make sure his patient is getting a consistent expectation of adult behavior, he will need to be like a father in defining the demands he would like the treating family to make. Learning how to make wise demands and how to secure the staff's cooperation in carrying them out is an important paternal task of the therapist in inpatient work.

When the therapist is alone with the patient, or listening to the concerns of the staff, he will need the receptive mode of the mother. The maternal task is to make sure he has heard the major concerns so that later demands are informed with an understanding of what the patient and staff are struggling with.

Coordinating these two ways of relating to the regressed patient's need is a major task of the inpatient therapist. He must learn when to use which, and he must guide the staff in finding which mode to use with the patient at any point in the treatment. Often the therapist will have to push the staff to be tougher; at other times he may have to protect the patient from the pressure of too many demands.

Aside from this coordination of his own responses, the hardest skill to master is cooperation with the staff. Even when the therapist has defined his own appropriate response to the patient, he will have to deal with the opinions of others in the milieu. The vast literature on social system aspects of treatment[21] repeatedly emphasizes one principle: treatment proceeds best when the involved individuals can agree about the methods and goals. This consensus must include the patient, his ecological group, the therapist, the ward staff, and the other patients on the ward.

Thus hospitalization itself is a crisis, deliberately superimposed upon the patient's original life predicament, so that treatment, via adequate crisis resolution, can occur. When the therapist admits the patient to the hospital, he effectively changes the patient's ecological group. Now the therapeutic deck is stacked with people who are trained to be helpful and who will do what the therapist wants. The therapist deliberately uses this enlarged ecological group to undercut the power that an isolated patient or a rigid family has used to maintain the pathology.

Thus hospitalization is used when it is the best available way to meet an impasse in treatment, when consultation to the patient and his usual ecological group cannot bring about a resolution. The impasse is then transferred to the milieu, which will be in crisis until the patient's treatment becomes unstuck. The therapist's work with the inpatient staff is similar to that with any ecological group in crisis. He functions as a consultant, helping the system to find its own solution, by using his knowledge of it and the patient.

Such impasses are regular occurrences in the treatment of very ill patients. They may reflect aspects of the patient's inner dynamics (for example, psychotic ambivalence) or of his family's pressure. Once their impact is felt in the milieu, however, treatment impasses are social events, accessible to resolution at a social level.

As Peplau has written:[22]

> This is what milieu therapy is all about: recognizing recurring problematic behavior patterns which had their beginning in the early childhood situations in which the child rearing tactics of the mother or of the other significant adults were not equal to the power maneuvers of the child; recognizing the replications of these patterns in subsequent school, peer group, community, and employment situations; and disrupting such replications within the day-to-day nurse-patient interactions in the ward setting.

Equally, milieu therapy is a *context* for other treatment that may become necessary. If ego functioning is so radically altered by mania, depression, or psychotic process that both psychotherapy and sociotherapy become impossible, drug therapy or ECT will be used.

The milieu can also be used as a setting to stage a massive challenge against entrenched character patterns. Abrams[23-25] has described the inpatient treatment of entire families and severely hysterical characters. He emphasizes hospitalization as a symbolic commitment to radical change and structures the ward experience as basic reeducation.

Sometimes referral to a more specialized residential setting is indicated. Among useful resources are *token-reinforcement wards* for chronic schizophrenic patients,[26] *intentional social systems* oriented to the reemployment of marginally adapted and alcoholic men,[27,28] and *anticriminal societies* that provide alternative lifestyles for previously delinquent or addicted persons.[29] In them, acculturation to a culture and its values becomes all-important, and individual psychotherapy may not even be offered.

This chapter will follow a patient through a standard inhospital experience, starting from the decision to hospitalize him and ending on the day of his discharge, to illustrate the tasks that the therapist meets in hospital work. No one patient is representative of all patients who are hospitalized, but the themes of inpatient work reoccur.

THE DECISION TO HOSPITALIZE

Example 10-1, Jerry. Jerry, a 19-year-old Coast Guard recruit, was taken to the emergency room of the community hospital near boot camp. At the end of the first week of his training, he had been found kneeling by his bunk, begging God to forgive him, and had not attended to a direct order to get up and answer the questions of his worried commanding officer. An accompanying note from the C.O. revealed that during his initial week of training he had shown "poor attention at drills and could not learn to pack his duffel bag. He would gaze into space for long periods and only answered questions the second or third time they were put to him." He had been found when he failed to turn up at the muster held before inspection.

In the emergency room Jerry was interviewed by the psychiatrist on call. He met the first several questions with silence. Finally Jerry said, "I'm with God, can't you let it be?"

Following an intuition, the psychiatrist asked, "Have you died?"

"I think so," Jerry replied. "Is this heaven?"

"Where do you think this is?"

"I think it's heaven," Jerry answered with conviction.

"Do you know who I am?"

"Someone who works for God – I know, an angel!"

Jerry responded carefully to the questions, like a small child.

"Do you know what day this is?"

"Tuesday," Jerry said, and laughed a little. Asked why he laughed, he said, "I didn't know you had time here." (In fact, the day was Saturday.) Jerry did not know the month or the day. His answers were, however, consistent with his belief that he had died and might be in heaven. It became clear that he was not sure where he was, except that he knew God was near him.

The psychiatrist said, "Actually, this is a hospital. You've been brought here because you became emotionally upset in boot camp."

"What's that?" Jerry asked.

"Basic training for the Coast Guard."

"Oh. I remember now."

"What do you remember?"

"I was in boot camp when I died."

"You aren't dead," the psychiatrist said, "so I'd have to say you're wrong about that. You got emotionally upset and had to be brought here to recover. I gather something pretty unusual happened inside you, if that's what you mean by dying. This is a hospital, and I'm a doctor. You'll have to stay here until you feel better."

"I feel O.K.," Jerry said.

"Are you frightened?"

"Yes."

"I think I can help you feel less frightened."

"You *can*?"

"Yes I can. Do you want me to help you?"

"Yes."

"It means doing what I say."

"Yes, tell me what I have to do to feel less frightened."

By relating to the patient's own view of what has happened to him, the therapist can often set up a simple contract with the patient that goes, "You feel upset, and I can help. If you do what I say, you will start to feel better." In Jerry's terror (usually the most upsetting part of an acute psychosis), the therapist found an area in which Jerry welcomed intervention. If something could be done to make him feel less afraid, he would cooperate.

From the very first the therapist started to challenge Jerry's psychotic definition of the situation. A cornerstone of the delusional thinking was the unlabeled metaphor, Jerry's assertion that he had died. The therapist called this assertion wrong and proceeded to label the metaphor: dying was Jerry's way of relating to an unfamiliar internal change. The therapist did not deny the reality of this change, or the drastic nature of it, and he indicated that his own attempts to name it would also be only metaphors.

The delusional elaboration – having died, Jerry must now be in heaven – was corrected by a simple comment on external realities: this was a hospital, and Jerry was seeing a doctor.

Finally, the therapist gave the societal definition of their transaction: Jerry had been brought to the hospital for treatment of an emotional breakdown suffered in boot camp. This statement of public fact countered Jerry's falsely individual, grandiose version of the humiliating events and showed that they could be stated. Finally, the current status of Jerry's power was explained to him. He would be made to stay at the hospital, but he retained the choice of agreeing or not agreeing to treatment.

Of course the therapist knew that Jerry did not yet believe or trust him. But he had set a basis for trust by clearly communicating what would follow when Jerry reached the ward. Then an entire society would insist upon this official version of

reality instead of Jerry's psychotic interpretation of his experience. The therapist also had defined his own role as someone who would clarify reality.

ENTRY INTO THE WARD

The way the therapist arranges the admission, mentions the diagnosis, and transfers authority to the ward setting affects, for good or ill, the later course of treatment. After these procedures have been discussed, initial psychotherapeutic strategies and basic responsibilities of the admitting therapist will be defined.

Arranging the Admission

Having established that the patient needs inpatient care, the next step is to ensure (1) that a bed is available in the inpatient unit and (2) that the patient can afford to stay there. If responsible others accompany the patient, financial details should also be discussed with them.

> *Jerry (cont'd.).* Admitting Jerry was a simple task for the emergency therapist: it was the practice to admit Coast Guard recruits directly to the hospital at government expense. He already knew a bed was available on the inpatient ward, or he would not have been so explicit about Jerry's being hospitalized at this facility.
>
> Nevertheless, he placed a call to the inpatient unit to make sure the ward staff knew that he was planning to admit Jerry, so someone would be on hand to receive them. He placed the call in Jerry's presence, saying, "This is Dr. Michaels. I'm going to bring Jerry Butler to the ward. He is 19 and in the midst of an acute psychotic reaction. He looks tired, and I want to give him some chlorpromazine shortly after he arrives to make sure he gets to sleep."

Making the telephone call in the patient's presence is, of course, optional, and many therapists will prefer to have the patient wait outside while they make the necessary arrangements. With psychotic patients, however, it is often a good idea to do as little behind the patient's back as possible. The therapeutic task is to reinforce a socially shared perception of reality against the seductions of the primary process, and to accomplish it the therapist's behavior must be easy to read. Wherever possible, the therapist should act to minimize the formation of paranoid delusions, which can quickly consolidate to form a hardened front against any therapeutic alliance. When the patient listens to the therapist's way of describing his situation to others, a model is formed on which he can base his own later attempts to explain himself. Also, a certain sharing of the dilemma of explanation takes place when the telephone call is made in another's presence. This sharing of difficult ego tasks is important in the early psychotherapy of schizophrenia.

Mentioning the Diagnosis

The therapist mentioned the patient's diagnosis in the initial telephone call. Note that he did not say "schizophrenia," but rather "acute psychotic reaction." At this point the diagnosis of schizophrenia was far from being proved. The more neutral term has the advantages of saying no more than is already known and of being less frightening. If the patient asks, the therapist can explain that "acute" means of short, recent duration and that "psychotic" means confused thinking. Usually the patient will receive this more general diagnosis as a restatement of what the therapist has already told him. A more specific diagnosis given early in evaluation is sometimes received as a sentence of doom, threatening to extend the immediate confusion into a whole psychiatric career. The more general diagnosis also prevents the ward staff from assuming it knows more than it actually does about this new and still unevaluated person.

Not mentioning the diagnosis to the patient is a poor, and all too common, practice. When the diagnosis is not discussed, the patient quickly assumes that either his condition is too terrible to be revealed to him or that he is in fact not really ill and that his hospitalization is a fraud perpetrated by deceptive persecutors. A simple communication to the patient of the meaning of any terms that are going to be used in describing him goes a long way toward undercutting what Laing has called "the mystification of experience." (The patient begins to grasp that diagnostic statements, like his own psychotic statements, are simply metaphors.) Knowing that he will have to explain what he plans to say about the patient *to* the patient, the therapist will be much more careful to use terms which reflect what he really knows. And the vital relationship of trust will be furthered by the frank communication. (A good rule of thumb should not be made into a callous habit. The communication of diagnosis is always a sensitive matter, and at times the therapist will want to say to the patient only, "I'm not sure. You're certainly emotionally upset. I can't say much more than that right now.")

Transfer of Authority

Jerry (cont'd.). The emergency therapist's next step was to introduce Jerry personally into the social system that was to be his total environment for the next weeks — the acute inpatient unit.

The unit, which was cheerful and bright, resembled a well-designed motel. It was decorated in orange and brown hues. Its front door was left unlocked, but a patient or staff member was usually near the entrance to ensure that only patients with hospital privileges left the ward. The ward itself was an L-shaped wing of the first floor of the hospital and had a screened outdoor porch with a Ping-Pong table on it. A punching bag hung from a beam.

Along one side of the L was a line of patients' rooms. One room held four beds; the other five had two beds each.

The ward staff was visibly young, attractive, and mostly female. The nurses wore street clothes; they were not instantly distinguishable from the patients and volunteers. There was, however, an official-looking desk, with a roll-away Cardex file, and behind the desk was a locked, glassed-in area where medications were kept. A young woman stood inside this enclosure. She looked serious and important and had an unusually large bunch of keys. From these signs of authority, it was obvious she was the charge nurse for the shift.

The emergency therapist brought Jerry to the desk and waited. The nurse came out from her medication cubicle, carefully ensured that the door was locked, and looked at the two of them. Jerry stepped back toward the door. The therapist first introduced himself and then his patient: "This is Jerry Butler. He will have to stay on the ward because he has been extremely upset and his thinking has been confused. I will be talking with you and ordering some medicine for him. Right now, could you introduce yourself to Jerry, show him his room, and explain the ward rules?"

This transfer of authority from the therapist to the charge nurse is an essential step. It should be done quite clearly and concretely, as shown in the example. The therapist gives a ward staff member confronted with the uncertainty of a new psychotic patient essential information about the patient's emotional state and the amount of restriction that will be required. By doing so in front of the patient, the therapist provides a model for the nurse to use in talking to the patient. He also lets the patient see that the ward personnel will be aware, just as the doctor is, of the severity of his emotional and cognitive problems.

Initial Psychotherapeutic Strategies

Including the Patient. The transition from the dyadic communication between the therapist and the patient to the milieu process of the ward setting is a crucial one, and it easy to mishandle. It is possible to imagine the same scene played

differently: the therapist leaves the patient at the desk, with a muttered "Wait here." Then he joins the charge nurse in the medication alcove. The two mental health professionals talk for several minutes. They are seen but not heard by the patient. The two emerge from the alcove, assume mannerisms that appear phony, and address the patient. "Miss Jones and I have just been conferring about you, Jerry, and we've decided to give you some medicine now." In an unctuous voice Miss Jones says, "Here you are, Jerry," and hands him a cup of suspicious-looking liquid she had kept hidden in her hands until the therapist spoke.

It is hard to blame a patient as concrete and confused as Jerry for making a paranoid interpretation of these events. He might bolt and force a power confrontation. Later he might reveal his fantasy that the hospital was a front assumed by agents of the devil who were conspiring to keep him from God. This fantasy would probably cause him to be labeled "acute paranoid schizophrenic," when in fact the paranoid fantasy would represent a stress reaction in this concrete, acutely psychotic young man who had been denied information that would support his fragile reality testing. The "paranoid" label, in turn, could cause the staff to relate to him in a more guarded fashion and thereby reinforce a common vicious cycle that tends to enforce a paranoid solution to the crisis of acute psychosis. Again, it is important to let the patient see and hear when vital decisions about his care are being made.

Defining the Role of Medication. In the example, the therapist introduced medication only after he had attempted to support Jerry's ego with a clear and direct communication aimed at improving his orientation and attention. Jerry heard two reasons given for the medication: it could reduce terror, and it could enhance sleep. It was not offered as the only, or even the major, kind of intervention. In short, Jerry's ego was asked to do all it could before drugs were used.

Many psychotic patients will require tranquilizing medication much sooner, of course, well before an attempt is made to enter them onto an open ward.

Theoretical Considerations Regarding Ego Support. The essence of milieu therapy is still contained in Pinel's dictum: "Treat the insane as if they were sane." When an acutely psychotic individual begins hospital treatment, two rules should be followed:

1. The patient must be protected from receiving the impression that his ego is too diseased to function. (Because he is highly impressionable, the acutely psychotic individual can quickly learn to play a sick role.)

2. The staff must make continuous demands on the patient to orient himself and attend to the social realities of the unit.

Basic Responsibilities of the Admitting Therapist

Patient Should Be under Control When He Enters Milieu. Not every patient is as willing as Jerry to enter into a tentative working alliance. Some patients are already caught in a paranoid interpretation of events or are so hysterical or intoxicated that a calm discussion becomes impossible. *These patients should not be brought to an open inpatient ward until they have been brought under control.* Instead, they should be kept in the emergency room, given medication, and even kept in seclusion or restraints until they are calm enough to accept entry into the inpatient ward without belligerence and panic. Although most severely agitated patients respond to a single injection of 75 mg of chlorpromazine, there will be some patients who will need several doses of 200- to 400-mg liquid chlorpromazine orally every two hours before they have been sufficiently calmed to be safely treated on an open unit. It is best to treat these patients on a locked unit or in the emergency room while the medication takes effect. The reason is simple: access to help,

including the police, is greater on a locked unit or in the emergency room.

The combination of high doses of medication and a firm stance will usually bring a highly agitated patient under control within six to twelve hours; then he can be brought to the ward. If the patient remains seriously agitated, "sky-high," or assaultive, he should remain on a locked unit. Such patients are fortunately infrequent, but they are seen; and a rigidly liberal policy toward the civil rights of frenzied patients can involve taking unnecessary risks with the safety of an inpatient ward staff. Often it is fairer to the patient if the therapist recognizes the patient's inability to contain himself.

Example 10-2. A therapist who had promised himself never to lock up anyone admitted a large, overweight man who called himself Senator Smith but was in fact an unemployed janitor. The therapist's ward was an open, patient-governed unit in a large VA Hospital. From the start, the patient was grandiose and belligerent, often clapping other patients on their backs while wearing a friendly grin that only half-concealed a sadistic sneer.

The therapist responded to each provocation with a crisis interview that included a ward nurse. The urgent conferences and the increasing use of medication seemed only to provoke the patient more. Several staff members asked that the patient be transferred to a locked ward, but the therapist informed them that that was the old-fashioned way. Because he was obviously working hard on the case and his arguments were verbally convincing, the ward staff let him have his way.

The patient began to drop lighted cigarette butts on the floor during community meetings, and finally he started a fire in his room. An emergency meeting of the ward was called.

Several patients were among those who called for a vote on the question of a transfer to a locked ward. The therapist made a last, impassioned appeal for "one more chance." A gruff, older man who had been hospitalized for depression spoke up sourly. "One more chance for what? To burn down the ward?"

Everyone laughed, and the controversial patient grinned at his therapist, who was sitting beside him. "Nice try, Charlie Brown," he whispered, "I've been trying to tell you." The vote was unanimous for his transfer to the locked ward.

A month later, Smith, who was now in control and had grounds privileges, saw his former therapist. "I'm O.K. now," he said. "You should have sent me there sooner; it's the only thing that works when I get high like that." A review of the records revealed that his five previous admissions had all involved stays on the locked unit. The patient had obviously come to expect this means of control. He would not accept any other, no matter how well intentioned or "modern."

The Review of Old Records. Example 10-2 illustrates another aspect of the admitting therapist's responsibility: reviewing the old record. Often what has worked in the past is what the patient expects now. Repetition of former treatment can be miraculously successful. Thus another course of ECT, a stay on the same locked ward, the exact dose of a previously used tranquilizer, can swiftly terminate an acute exacerbation of a chronic psychotic process. It is the therapist's duty to communicate the patient's therapeutic past to the ward staff so that it may replicate former successes.

Setting the Necessary Medical Work-up in Motion. Most hospitals require, and every patient should have, a physical examination when the patient is admitted to the ward. Unless the need for chemical restraint is absolutely pressing, no patient should receive large doses of tranquilizing medication until a physician has obtained vital signs and a brief medical history, and has recorded physical findings of cardiac, respiratory, and neu-

rologic status. The large doses of chlorpromazine used at the outset of the treatment of schizophrenia are sufficient to obtund many patients, and gross irregularities in heart action, circulation, breathing, and neurological function may appear as side effects. Major tranquilizers must be used cautiously in any patient with a history of chronic medical illness.

Additionally, many psychiatric patients have concurrent medical illnesses that need attention. Disturbances such as diabetes, heavy metal poisoning, tumors, infections, anemia, and hidden brain injuries can resemble acute schizophrenia, mania, depression, and character disorder. Thus a competent physician (an internist is ideal) should perform a complete physical examination soon after the patient arrives on the ward.

If drug abuse or poisoning is suspected, the therapist should be sure that the internist is alerted to order the blood and urine samples necessary to make this diagnosis. The therapist cannot assume the internist will find and follow through on any physical causes of impaired mental functioning with grossly disturbed individuals. Because his patient is not communicating normally, and he is a specialist in communication, the therapist will have to make sure that the vital information is delivered to the physician.

Problems in communication often arise between the nonmedical therapist and the nonpsychiatric physician. The therapist should arrange an unhurried time to meet with the doctor to learn about the findings of the examination. He should always ask, "Is there any possibility that a medical illness is affecting the patient's symptoms?" He should be sure to find out about any conditions that may limit his patient's comfort, activity, or employability.

Seriously disturbed patients give poor medical histories. The therapist may have to function as the patient's advocate and translator. Anxious patients often forget to communicate major details at the time of the examination and later tell the therapist, who will have to relay the information to the physician.

Summary

The admitting therapist should introduce the patient to the ward in such a way that the ward can take over the treatment from him. The therapist must see to it that his patient is in a state in which he can accept the ward environment and that the ward knows enough about the patient to make an informed intervention. From this point, until the patient is discharged, the therapist will function in an adjunctive way. He will act as a consultant to the ward and patient and will thereby facilitate their interaction. And indeed, his role will remain pivotal. But the actual healing, the return of adequate ego functioning, will come as the patient rediscovers reality in the context of the ward.

THE PROCESS OF TREATMENT ON AN INPATIENT UNIT

Four very different activities proceed concurrently in an inpatient unit: crisis intervention, milieu therapy, drug treatment, and hospital custody. Each requires highly specialized skills. A ward brings together many ambitious, highly trained people whose diverse efforts are in constant need of refinement and coordination by the ward chief. More than any other person he sets the style of the ward, its overall philosophy and ambience. No two ward chiefs are alike, and no two wards are alike. The tasks that must be accomplished, however, are common to all. The therapist must be familiar with the ward and the ward chief's philosophy of treatment.

The therapist will retain the responsibility for coordinating his own patient's treatment but will subordinate his own style to that of the ward. He will continue to direct the crisis intervention by setting up appointments with significant members of his patient's ecological group. If he is a physician, he will prescribe his patient's medications. He will be responsible for writing progress notes in the patient's record and for the admitting history. He will perform psychotherapy and usually will see his patient every day, if only briefly.

This special relationship to the patient places the therapist between the patient and the ward. He becomes his patient's advocate and, at times, his defense attorney. He will hear complaints about the patient, and he will often be blamed if things do not go right. Equally, often he will have to explain to the patient why ward procedures such as meetings, meals, and medications are important.

Overall, the therapist acts as a *troubleshooter to the treatment process*. He must ensure that his patient gets the most from the rest of the staff. Frequently the therapist will need to turn to the ward chief for advice, and he will also need to listen carefully to the opinions of staff. A good way to begin each visit to the ward is by reading the nursing report on the patient. In addition to giving him needed information, this practice creates the necessary receptive set in the therapist, and it is good public relations.

Crisis Intervention on the Ward

Involving the Ecological Group. We return now to the case of Jerry, which illustrates the therapist's direct work with the patient and his ecological group.

Jerry (cont'd.). The ward nurse took Jerry on a tour of the ward and brought him his chlorpromazine. The therapist stood by as he drank it. After the first swallow, Jerry spat out the drug and tried to run out of the room. The therapist said, "No, you're going to have to remain here." The nurse called two male aides, who entered the room. The therapist told the nurse to get another dose of liquid chlorpromazine and to draw up a syringe of intramuscular chlorpromazine. While she was out of the room, the therapist told Jerry firmly, "You will have to take your medication. You have a choice of drinking the liquid or having it injected. Which will it be?" Jerry remained silent while the therapist and the two male aides watched. (They were deliberately exposing him to a silent "show of force.") Jerry eyed them very carefully. When the nurse returned, Jerry drank the oral medication and also accepted a larger cup of orange juice she had brought him as a "chaser" for the chlorpromazine's bitter taste. Then he asked his therapist, "Is my mother dead or alive?"

The therapist asked the nurse and the two aides to leave the room. "I don't know, Jerry, let's find out."

"How?" Jerry asked, wide eyed.

"Call home."

"You mean call her?"

"Yes."

"Wow."

"Isn't it possible? She had a phone when you entered boot camp, didn't she?"

"Yes."

"Well, then dial it."

"I'm afraid."

"I'll stand by if you want."

"What'll I tell her if she answers?"

"Tell her you are in the hospital, and that I'm your doctor, and that she can call me if she wants."

Jerry dialed his father's, not his mother's number. "Hello, Dad, I'm in the hospital. You want the number? It's 483-1000. Yeah. Dr. Michaels." He hung up; his father called back right away, and the therapist answered.

The therapist told Jerry's father that Jerry had been hospitalized for emotional difficulties. The father, in a crisp, rapid, and demanding tone, wanted to know if this would ruin Jerry's chances in the Coast Guard. The therapist explained that it was too early to tell. When he asked to speak with Jerry's mother, the therapist found out that the parents had been divorced for eight years, and that Jerry had been living with his mother. She had been as dubious about Jerry's entering and succeeding in the Coast Guard as his father had been insistent upon it.

After the call the therapist told Jerry that his father really wanted him to be in the Coast Guard. Jerry responded to this with an unenthusiastic "Yeah." Jerry then called his mother, told her he was in the hospital because he was having a breakdown, and handed the phone to his therapist.

In a tired, lackluster voice, his mother told the therapist that she didn't think she and her husband could leave their store and come to visit. The therapist told her that that wasn't necessary immediately. "You won't keep him in the service, will you?" she asked.

"We don't know."

With a faint trace of humor, she said, "Well, let me know what you decide. I don't think you will."

After telling her he would call the next day, he handed the phone to Jerry, who spoke with her for a minute and wound up by saying, "I'll be *okay*. I've gotta go." He hung up and with a hang-dog expression told the therapist, "She's alive. I thought I killed her."

In this sequence the therapist initiated the process of crisis intervention, which would be a major part of Jerry's therapy on the ward. Jerry was directly involved in the realistic communication that informed his parents of his condition and informed him that his mother was alive. At the outset, a major theme of the crisis became apparent in the conflicting parental views on the outcome of the enlistment: his father's strong desire that Jerry be allowed to continue, and his mother's equally strong doubts.

The therapist set this process of crisis intervention and reality testing in motion before Jerry was clear of psychosis. In fact, the intervention helped undercut the psychosis by showing Jerry that his mother was still alive, and it helped both Jerry and his therapist get the feel of the contradictory parental emotion underlying Jerry's decision to enlist.

It was essential for Jerry's treatment that this real conflict resurface early. It was not pleasant for Jerry to have to face, not God in Heaven, but a real father anxious for success; not a dead mother, but a doubting, live one. The therapist shared the pain of conflict with the patient, but he did not protect him from it. Thus the patient was given a crucial message early: the hospital will not be used as a place where reality can be evaded by psychosis. It is a setting where others help in confronting a difficult situation.

Goals Conference. A second task of crisis intervention is to have the patient and the hospital staff agree about the goals of hospitalization. This goals conference is vital for the ultimate resolution of the crisis. If this step is omitted, the hospitalization may acquire a "life of its own" apart from the needs of the patient's particular crisis, and the maladaptive solution of the "sick role" may supervene over any healthier resolution to the crisis.

The goals conference specifies staff tasks as well as patient goals. Lieb et al.[30] have provided the following tasks to be accomplished during a crisis hospitalization:

1. Completion of the evaluation
2. Clarification of the problems bringing the patient to the hospital
3. Communication of important decisions to significant people
4. Involvement in outpatient therapy
5. Resolution of incapacitating symptomatology
6. Reduction or resolution of suicidal or homicidal ideation
7. Completion of detoxification
8. Acceptance of the realities of the situation
9. Acceptance of structure and medication
10. Finding employment
11. Readjustment to the family system
12. Arranging an appropriate disposition

The goals conference also offers the patient a set of expectations for his inpatient stay: his daily "work" will be to perform the tasks the goals conference decides are expected of him.

Jerry (cont'd.). After he talked with his parents on the telephone, Jerry seemed much calmer, and he was able to sleep without difficulty (undoubtedly assisted by the heavy dose of medication he had swallowed). The following morning, before the community meeting, his goals conference was held on the ward.

The therapist, a nurse, a nursing assistant, and the ward chief were present. As was customary on this ward, Jerry was asked to introduce himself and to state his reason for being hospitalized. Jerry looked to his therapist for support and said, "My name is Jerry Butler. I had a breakdown in boot camp."

The therapist was asked to give a brief history of Jerry's illness. He did so.

At this point, the ward chief, a small quiet man with intense eyes, brought up the question of goals. "Jerry," he asked, "What do you expect to accomplish in the hospital?"

"I want to stop thinking things that aren't true," he said.

"Very good. Anything else?"

"I have to decide whether to stay in the Coast Guard."

The ward chief invited the therapist first and then the nursing staff to state their expectations. A nursing assistant took notes. The therapist wanted to better understand Jerry's and his parents' feelings about his enlistment. He wanted a complete physical examination, and he wanted Jerry to be able to think clearly again so that they could prepare a recommendation to the Coast Guard about his enlistment.

The nursing staff expected Jerry to pick up his medications at specific times, to attend group and psychodrama, to take KP, and to keep his area neat.

The ward chief asked the nursing assistant to read from his notes. The assistant read: "Jerry Butler, age 19, acute psychotic reaction, cause undetermined. Goals:

1. Straighten out errors in thinking

2. Decide whether to stay in Coast Guard
3. Evaluation of home situation"

The assistant enumerated the rest of the ten goals based on expectations that had been stated. The therapist, in answer to the ward chief's question, said he would see Jerry briefly every day and have two therapy sessions a week with him. This was added to the list. The ward chief asked Jerry if he agreed to live up to this contract. Jerry somewhat sheepishly agreed. The ward chief asked that the list be typed, with copies for Jerry and the staff, and said to Jerry, "We agree to hold you to this contract, which is your plan of treatment. If we *all* do what it says, your treatment should go very well."

Of course, not every feature of the goals conference was clear to Jerry at the time of this first meeting with the ward staff. He could hardly avoid receiving the impression, however, that his treatment would be a collective effort. Moreover, the staff began its work with a clear idea of what Jerry's treatment would be.

At such a conference it is important that the therapist be as candid as possible in specifying the problem areas. In Jerry's case, errors in thinking and an important decision were the major areas. Another patient might be struggling with suicidal feelings or with impulse control. The therapist should absolutely not protect the patient's privacy at this conference, but rather share as fully as possible the nature of the distress that the ward is being called upon to help resolve. This conference is similar to crisis intervention with an ecological group outside the hospital except that the ward staff is asked to function as the support system.

Discharge planning is part of the goals conference. Ideally, the discharge begins to be planned on the day the patient is admitted. A patient who does not anticipate completion of his hospitalization invites mental illness to become chronic and self-perpetuating. This is *not* to say that patients must be hurried out of the hospital, nor is it an uncritical endorsement of the current trend of

brief hospitalization. There are cases on record of hospitalizations of six months to a year that have been extremely useful to the later adjustment of highly gifted individuals. The long hospitalization can offer a period of incubation and deliberate respite. However, successful long hospitalizations are usually conducted by therapists with an analytic orientation who know exactly what they are doing and when to reapply the pressure they deliberately remove for a time. Thus even the therapist who decides upon a long hospitalization anticipates the day when the patient once more will have to assume full responsibility for his life.

If the therapist adopts a "wait-and-see" attitude about planning, the patient's pathology will often mount to ensure that the hospitalization will continue. Therefore it is recommended that the therapist always try to project the length of an admission and to reason out its ultimate outcome.

Ecological Group Conferences. The artificial ecology of an inpatient milieu, like an artificial heart, cannot be used indefinitely. (It may have to be used intermittently, like dialysis, for those individuals who fall recurrently into "toxic" emotional states. This, as Lieb et al.[31] point out, is a valid use of the inpatient milieu.) The therapist must continue to deal with the patient's relationship to his own ecological group, and conferences with everyone concerned should be scheduled as soon as is feasible.

Jerry (cont'd.). After the goals conference the therapist called Jerry's family. At the father's home a woman answered. In a pleasant and energetic voice she informed the therapist that she had married Jerry's father five years before, that she thought the problem was Jerry's mother, who had never asked enough of the boy. She agreed to come to a conference in five days, and would discuss it with her husband.

The therapist called the mother. Her husband, Mr. Schiavo, a vague and mild man, answered the telephone and said he didn't know if he and his wife could close down their mail-order business for a day to come to the meeting. He agreed to discuss it with his wife.

The therapist called both families that evening. The Butlers energetically agreed to come. The Schiavos reluctantly said they would close down their business and attend.

In the five days before the meeting, the therapist thought about Jerry's future in the Coast Guard. It seemed likely that Jerry had enlisted over his mother's doubts to please his father. Jerry's initial confusion in boot camp may very well have reflected his lack of clarity about who had the right to make important decisions in his life. He told his therapist that when he was given an order in boot camp to carry out, he didn't seem to know who he was. He had started hearing a man's voice, very much like his father's, that talked so much he could not follow it. It also seemed that no matter what he did, his mother was there, until he thought he had killed her and he had been brought before God for judgment. The therapist thought that Jerry had unwittingly accepted a pathological aspect of his parents' communications: that they could control a part of his life that they actually could not, namely, his Coast Guard career; and that Jerry had transformed this assumption and his resentment about it into the voices giving him orders and the delusion that he had killed his mother.

The therapist's intuition told him that it was now time for the decision about Jerry's career to be made by those involved — Jerry and the Coast Guard — rather than by pseudo-omnipotent forces such as his parents. The therapist knew the Coast Guard was reluctant to have a man who might become psychotic under stress serve isolated duty either on land or at sea. Jerry, who had no interest in the Coast Guard, was relieved to know he could get out, although he was angry with his mother for implying that he wouldn't make it. It was easy to decide that Jerry should be separated from the service. Jerry and the therapist entered the family conference knowing that this key decision had already been made.

In inpatient psychiatry the therapist is often forced to rearrange, sometimes with a degree of manipulation, the "balance of power" in an ecological group. After all, the ecological group's workings have contributed to the psychosis of one of its members. Frequently a judicious use of authority will be necessary to rearrange a malignant network of communications during a family conference on an inpatient ward. Often, aspects of the solution will be "imposed" rather than "discovered" as in outpatient work. Just as the patient is not given the choice of whether to take medication, but only of how to take it, his ecological group is not allowed to decide whether he is ill, but rather how to manage the reality of his illness.

Jerry (cont'd.). The night before the scheduled meeting, Mr. Schiavo called the therapist to say that he doubted whether he could miss business for a day to come to the meeting, and that when he had spoken earlier with Mr. Butler, Mr. Butler had expressed similar doubts. The therapist countered with a firm injunction and pointed out that key decisions involving Jerry's future were involved. Everyone came.

The content of the meeting was not as important as the decision making that took place. Everyone was told that the Coast Guard was going to separate Jerry from the service when his hospitalization was over, that he would need continuing outpatient psychotherapy, and that the group had to consider how to pay for it. The father optimistically wondered if Jerry really would need further treatment; the therapist pointed out that Jerry's diagnosis was now "acute schizophrenia." The mother pessimistically wondered if he would ever get well; the therapist pointed out the good prognosis for this condition. The plan for continued treatment seemed to meet both the father's demand for action and the mother's need to see her son as ill.

The family did manage to disagree on one point, and this was who would pay for the therapy. Jerry's father insisted that part of the cost must come from job earnings (of a job Jerry had yet to acquire), and his mother felt the parents should pay "everything until Jerry gets well; who knows when he can work?" Hearing this dispute, Jerry got quite angry. In a key intervention, the therapist got all five of them to agree to defer this issue until the first consultation with the outside therapist, which was to occur the following week as part of a pass. Relieved, the group adjourned amicably.

In talking with a patient's family, the therapist can make use of the psychosis requiring hospitalization as a metaphor for the developmental crisis they need to help manage. The psychosis can stand for Jerry's previous struggle to enter life, and his treatment can stand for his capacity to grow. The family can support his treatment even if they are unable to support him.

Making conscious use of the "medical model" to rally family support, the therapist can (1) reduce uncertainty (by presenting a "medically indicated" decision to separate someone from the service, a troublesome job, or an impossible home); (2) undercut conflicting demands within the ecological group (by presenting common tasks, such as planning for outpatient treatment, that require cooperation if treatment is to progress); and (3) redefine the problem (in Jerry's case, forget the debate over what he can achieve and become concerned with finding a stable professional figure who can offer him guidance).

If hospitalization can be avoided, it should be. But once it has occurred, the therapist can use it as a trump card to deal with the power struggles and contradictory expectations so often found in the ecological group. He has a powerful tool at his disposal; he should not be afraid to use it wisely.

Goals of Ego Support Via Milieu Therapy

If long-term hospitalization is to be avoided, the patient and his ecological group will have to be convinced that his ego is in touch with everyday realities, at least enough to function on the outside. Most of the skill of milieu therapy involves knowing which ego functions to support and how to go about supporting them.

Improving the Testing of Reality. In reality testing, as elsewhere in psychiatry, the vexing concept of "reality" will need clarification. Patients usually come to the hospital because of major disturbances in their relation to one or more of three aspects of reality: (1) outer physical reality; (2) inner emotional reality; and (3) transactional reality.

In the first instance, the crucial ability is to perceive the physical world as most others do, including in and omitting from sense perception what most others include and omit. Accurate testing of outer physical reality means the perception of persons and places according to social norms. (Grossly delusional states, perceptual disturbances, and "overinclusive" thought disorders fall among the pathologies.)

The crucial ability in maintaining inner reality is the correct identification of the affects and images that make up the "inner world" of emotion. (Obsessive-compulsive personalities who become psychotically depressed, alienated from their own great grief, anger, and loneliness fail in internal reality testing.)

The issue in transactional reality is still perception, but in areas that affect judgment. The crucial ability is to recognize the rules, or power realities, by which interpersonal transactions are guided.

Failure of transactional reality testing leads to speech and actions that exceed the accepted limits within a social context and invite the "insane" label. It is often extremely hard to specify what these limits are until a group member tries to exceed them and finds himself isolated, extruded, or taken to the hospital. Often it is not so much a matter of the actual behavior as it is of the timing of behavior. Many of the "last straw" situations that precipitate a borderline individual's being hospitalized reflect a final erosion of the political sense that recognizes the lines within a social system which one must not cross.

Persons with sociopathic or hysterical character styles show major disturbances in testing transactional reality. They may become grossly unadapted despite an accurate perception of both outer physical reality and their own inner emotional reality. Some hysterical personalities are overcommitted to "affective truth," that is, to being true to their inner feelings, which they usually perceive quite accurately, no matter how much they alienate others or how bizarrely flawed their judgment. By contrast, many persons with major disturbances in the testing of outer physical *and* inner emotional reality avoid social difficulties altogether because they have learned to test transactional reality correctly. They do not openly violate the transactional norms of the persons they know. This usual ecological group may in turn have adapted itself to their gross errors in reality testing in the other areas because they "fit in so well" with the group's most-favored (or most comfortable) ways of social functioning.

An inpatient ward usually includes patients who are schizophrenic, psychotically depressed, and hysterical or sociopathic in character style. The ward must therefore undertake to help with the testing of outer physical, inner, and transactional reality. To understand what goes on inside the hospital it is necessary to realize that a milieu is a place where teaching is constantly occurring. To the nonattuned outsider, the constant pointing out of outer facts, the constant inquiry into emotional states, and the continual "holding responsible" of patients for the ways in which they communicate may appear to be horribly infantilizing, and the ward may seem to be a nursery school for adults. In fact, this teaching is entirely necessary and appropriate when it is directed to a patient's true area of weakness. Recognizing *where* the failure of reality testing occurs is a skill that grows with protracted contact with patients: probably no mental health professional has more expertise of this sort than the experienced psychiatric nurse. Much of the rapid readjustment of patients in modern settings occurs as a consequence of her work.

Setting Limits on Pathological Behaviors. Abroms[32] has described the process of a milieu therapy ward as one of "therapeutic limit setting," and he gives a list of the pathological behaviors that must be limited. This list, his "five D's of pathology," in decreasing order of severity, is

1. Destructiveness
2. Disorganization
3. Deviancy (or rule-breaking behavior)
4. Dysphoria (or disturbance in mood)
5. Dependency

In his view this "hierarchy of severity" is also a "hierarchy of intervention." The ward staff should first limit destructiveness in a given patient, then disorganization, and so on.

Teaching Psychosocial Skills. Abroms sees the milieu as "teaching skills" in four significant psychosocial areas:

1. Orientation
2. Assertion
3. Occupation
4. Recreation

To summarize, the goals of milieu therapy are to (1) improve reality testing, (2) set limits, and (3) teach skills. These goals are accomplished in the myriad of contexts provided by the treatment ward. In all these contexts, a process of ego support is occurring. In the next part of this chapter, we shall take a closer look at how ego support is actually carried out within the milieu.

EGO SUPPORT VIA MILIEU THERAPY

The handling of specific transactions in a therapeutic way is the essence of the milieu approach. We shall look at four ways ego support can be introduced into everyday ward transactions. These will be (1) orientation, (2) expectations, (3) limit setting, and (4) participation in the community.

Orientation

Jerry (cont'd.). Each day, one of the nurses asked Jerry if he knew the date, time, and place. At first he made small errors and acted as if they were unimportant. The nurse would persist, and by the end of the fourth day Jerry could say where he was, what day it was, and what time it was. In the late afternoon, when he tended to "fog out," Jerry would ask a ward attendant what day it was, where he was, and what time it was. He wanted to be sure he didn't forget. Gradually he reincorporated the habit of orienting himself to his temporal surroundings, and as he did so he appeared more alert and his paranoid feelings about the ward lessened.

Some therapists balk at using such a concrete, cognitive approach, preferring to relate to their patients' altered perceptions in terms of their accuracy as existential statements. This phenomenological approach to cybernetic error has a great appeal, but it neglects to notice that often improvement, not alienation, may follow when an "error" is corrected. Just as changes in emotion can affect cognition, so too can changes in cognition affect emotion, and simply telling a patient that "this isn't heaven, it's a hospital" can be as profoundly therapeutic as learning *how* the hospital is, in a metaphoric sense, heaven. Bateson et al.[33] have said that "The peculiarity of the schizophrenic is not that he uses metaphors, but that he uses *unlabeled* metaphors," an idea that was mentioned in the description of Dr. Michaels' initial handling of Jerry's psychotic thinking.

In his private contacts with a patient, a therapist can insist that the patient label his metaphors, or he can discourage their use altogether. Often therapists find that the use of metaphors is an effective way to communicate deep inner states. In the ward context, metaphors hinder the patient's solution of such factual outer problems as knowing where he is, what time it is, and what is going on. Poetic solutions to these problems should be discouraged. For orientation, banal, effort-requir-ing secondary process thinking must be used. Expecting the patient to perform along this dimension (and testing his performance) helps him recover the secondary process, which proves to be of enormous help to him.

Expectations. If there were no chlorpromazine, it would probably be possible to maintain order on an inpatient ward by the judicious use of expectation. We have seen how at the outset of the hospitalization the patient is exposed to a number of transactions that indicate how much will be expected of him. The best approach is to treat the patient as if he is a business client, explaining in detail what will be required of him in the course of his treatment.

Jerry (cont'd.). Before Jerry's goals conference, Jerry's therapist explained, "You're going to be presented by me to the goals conference. You will be asked why you came to the hospital. I will say what I have found out about you. Then the staff will tell you what they expect you to do in order to get well. You can tell them anything you want, but you have to make an agreement with them to do the things that are decided on for you."

"What if I don't?" Jerry asked.

"Then the staff will call you back and ask why you didn't. If they aren't satisfied, they can transfer you off the ward."

"Where would I go then?"

"Maybe the county hospital."

"I better do what they say. I don't want to go there."

In making expectations of a patient, it is well to ask things of him that can be monitored. The therapist should not expect a patient to not make noise, for example, because the patient's degree of control over "noise" cannot be easily gauged. Rather, the therapist can tell a difficult patient, "If you want to speak after the lights go out, you have to come out to the nurse's desk." Thus uncontrollable noises are not mentioned even while the problem of unregulated verbal communication is being addressed. Equally, expectations that are too much for the patient should be avoided.

Example 10-3. A middle-aged Southern seaman insisted he could not share a hospital room with a black patient. Several other patients offered to move. The acting ward chief, an inexperienced therapist who had had much luck with the use of expectation effects in bringing difficult situations under control, said, "You have to find a way of working this situation out." (He ignored the fact that the patient had appealed to the community and it was willing to give him his way.)

Soon after the patient became enraged and had to be secluded. He became possessed by a fantasy of strangling his wife. He had been expected to master an anger for which he had some social support, and he did, indeed, find "a way of working it out" – regression to the level of the psychotic rage for which he had been hospitalized.

Although this incident contributed greatly to an understanding of the patient's dynamics, the therapist had exceeded the patient's limits with his expectation and not helped him to discover a new area of ego control. In retrospect, the therapist should have asked the patient to find a way to spare his black roommate's feelings and acceded to his request for a different room.

Among the expectations that can be made of nearly all patients are attendance at all meals, attendance at ward meetings, daily showers, asking permission to leave the ward, taking all medications, and staying out of bed during specified hours. By insisting from the outset upon these simple rules, the therapist almost always brings the patient's ego into play and prevents him from being entirely "taken over" by feelings of panic, hopelessness, self-loathing, and inertia. Specific problems can be met with more specialized expectations.

Example 10-4. A woman in her early 50s, hospitalized for an exacerbation of her chronic schizophrenia, began to lie in bed whenever the ward staff wasn't looking. Telling her to get out of bed seemed to have only a limited effect, and her behavior seemed to say, "All I can do is lie here by myself." Attempts to involve her with others produced a state of panic. The staff felt frustrated and defeated by her psychosis.

Finally, the therapist hit upon a new strategy. He told his patient, "I expect you to take a walk twice each day, all the way to the hospital gate and one block beyond. Then you can come back and lie down for half an hour."

Within a few days the patient had brightened considerably and stayed out of bed without being told. The walks that "earned" her her right to lie down also demonstrated the intactness of her ability to function.

Limit Setting. After the staff has established that it will do its part to clarify reality and that it has certain expectations of the patient, the staff has earned its right to question, criticize, and prohibit the patient's symptomatic refusal to live by the ward rules. Equally, there are certain rules that can be established only by limit setting.

Example 10-5. A woman in her early 40s was admitted for treatment of an agitated depression. A veteran of a previous admission several years back, she presented herself to the staff as grateful to be receiving treatment again and eager to please. She cried a great deal, and she apologized for crying. Her entire stance seemed to say, "Excuse me for having such a tough time." Her husband, a kind man that the entire staff liked, stayed on the ward her first night, holding her hand and attempting to console her while the tears rolled down her cheeks.

After he left, the patient went to bed, and early the next morning her therapist was summoned out of a ward staff meeting with the news that she had cut her wrist. Without thinking, the therapist said, "That poor woman! I'll be in to talk with her immediately." The ward chief could not restrain himself. "You'll get further," he exploded, "if you tell her we don't allow that sort of thing here!"

Braced, the therapist went to his patient, and told her, "No, that's not appropriate. If you are distressed, you can always find the nurse. But you absolutely are not allowed to cut yourself." The patient attempted to apologize, but he held firm that her behavior was out-of-bounds.

By resisting the temptation to offer sympathy, an error the patient's well-meaning husband had made, the therapist was able to set limits on her capitulation to depression. Not surprisingly, the patient soon began to stand up on her own to her depression and to improve.

Limit setting is necessary when patients make infractions of ward rules or fail the expectations contained within their own "contracts." Specifically, failures to appear at a ward meeting, to take medication, or to eat meals require swift intervention because they signal major resistance to the therapeutic process. For a suicidal patient these behaviors may represent indirect suicidal communications. For a psychotic patient, the same behaviors may herald the beginning of a new regression, or a maladaptive paranoid restitution of ego functioning. For a patient with character disorder, a new bout of antisocial behavior may be warned by these first, seemingly trivial infractions.

The wise therapist will be firm. He will listen to excuses, but he will not accept them. "We expect you to be at your meals," he should say to the patient who has just explained why he "had" to miss one. The point is that these "minor" social norms are exactly those the patient, for idiosyncratic reasons, is failing to meet on the outside. An essential part of therapy is the ability to conform to minimal social requirements.

Participation in the Community. "People need people" is the premise of milieu therapy. The emphasis on orientation, the ward expectations, and the practice of limit setting tend to keep patients in the mainstream of the ward's small society[34] and involved with the staff and with each other. Usually there is a program that occupies the patients with common tasks. It is important to realize that special skills are needed to make the patients more than passive recipients of staff attention, and to get them to assume responsibility for keeping the therapeutic community going.[35]

Different wards have different styles of community participation, just as they have different styles in how they orient patients, what they expect of them, and how they set limits. In highly advanced wards, patients help in the orientation, participate in the goals conferences, function on "rules committees," assign extra work, restrict passes, and recommend transfers for other patients. Such wards work best if the turnover of patients is not too rapid and if the population of patients is somewhat uniform (as is the case with some VA wards that specialize in the treatment of marginally adjusted alcoholic men with stays of three to six months).

The community on the more acute ward usually comes together over business such as introductions, keeping the ward clean, supplying its members with coffee, and discussions of major unsettling events. Indeed, a most common topic of community meetings is how to assure that the coffee fund is kept up so that everyone can be sure of a fresh cup of coffee in a clean cup when he wants it. This seemingly banal topic, which could be decided by fiat if the staff intervened, provides endless fuel for the discussion of community conflicts. Dealing with a community task requires the ego functioning of many individuals, and this exercise of egos (not a prompt solution) is the reason for leaving simple issues to the community process.

When they are engaged together in common tasks, the members of the community will stumble over the major handicaps that a given patient has in living. In this way milieu therapy resembles long-term individual therapy in which chronic neurotic distortions appear during a mutual attempt at understanding. As in individual therapy, the therapeutic hope is that the reappearance of the handicap will be followed by its resolution. Here, most milieux hope for more than is possible; the patient simply does not have enough time to overcome more than his most obvious impediments to social functioning. The high hopes do, however, pressure most patients to the point that the obvious impediments *are* removed after a few days of milieu living.

Specialized Techniques

Techniques are the methods by which the goals and processes of milieu therapy are accomplished. Three kinds of techniques stand out: (1) techniques that improve communication, such as community and staff meetings; (2) techniques that encourage expression, such as psychodrama, small group, and family group; and (3) techniques that modify behavior, such as schedules, contracts, and reinforcements.

Techniques That Improve Communication. Because milieu therapy is a coordinated effort to bring about change, constant discussion of the rules of the game seems to improve both the skill and interest of the participants. An effective ward is one that is constantly examining its own behavior.

The *community meeting* is probably the sine qua non of a milieu ward. On most inpatient wards, it is held every morning for forty-five minutes, five or six days a week. It usually begins with the introduction of newly admitted patients, after which there is usually a silence. Then an issue of general relevance is approached by the group, which is aided by a leader who tries to interpret the veiled ways in which this "theme" was broached. Often the issue is the intolerable behavior of a patient which has upset other patients. Once

this common concern is brought into the open, the patient and the community can face their painful interaction together.

Jerry (cont'd.). Jerry became the topic of the community meeting after he had been on the unit more than a week. It seemed at one meeting, which his therapist attended, that everyone was angry. A young woman, charged with managing the coffee fund, insisted that everyone was forgetting to pay her; a nurse whispered angrily to an aide seated beside her; a stiff-postured new patient dropped a lighted cigarette. It was an atmosphere of diffuse tension. As Jerry sauntered in, late, an oppressive silence fell over the group. He took the only vacant seat, on the ward chief's right.

The ward chief said, "Can anybody explain why we're so tense today?"

A large woman said, "'Cause there's some as think they can fool everybody and some as think they're nobody's fool."

"Can you be more specific?" a young nurse asked.

"I'm as pacific as the ocean," the woman said, and would say no more. There was another uncomfortable silence.

Finally an older man on the ward chief's left spoke. "I'll tell you what you want to know, if it'll do you any good. It's Jerry here. He don't try to get better 'cause he knows he can get out of things if he don't."

It turned out that patients and staff thought Jerry was getting away with murder as far as living up to rules and expectations was concerned. He came late to meals, did not keep his area clean, and so on.

Jerry had even said, "You know I can't do that; I'm a goddam schizophrenic." After this statement, some patients had seen Jerry's mental illness as one big act. They thought Jerry's therapist (who met with him every day) supported this role of being irresponsible and fragile. The staff, too, was angry with the therapist because they felt thwarted by him in their desire to deal more openly with Jerry and his infractions.

When he heard this, the therapist said that although Jerry had indeed had a schizophrenic episode, his diagnosis did not absolve him from taking usual responsibility and that, in fact, he thought Jerry would recover a lot faster if he assumed responsibility like everyone else. This assurance greatly relieved the tension. Finally Jerry asked him, "You mean you can get better if you have schizophrenia?"

The therapist said, "Yes, if you try." At this point the new patient who had held himself so stiff seemed to relax, and suddenly got up and exchanged chairs with Jerry, who considerately gave his ash tray to him. The meeting ended with the new patient reaching over to pat the ward chief on the back, which met with comfortable general laughter.

It is obvious from the description of this community meeting how the specific problem of Jerry's laxity (which had indeed been his life problem before and during his brief try at a service career) had activated general concern. The anxiety seemed to be that the staff would label the patients and excuse them from life, and that despite the official ward ideology, mental illness could not be treated: the mentally ill would stay that way. When such a basic fear infects a ward, a general discussion is necessary to dispel it. In this meeting not only did a specific issue in Jerry's treatment unfold, but the ward itself experienced a renewal of its will to strive for health. This became graphically clear when the sickest patient took that chair to which the leader could extend his right arm in support, and Jerry, who was illegitimately clinging to that protection, gave it up.

In *Social Psychiatry in Action,*[36] Harry Wilmer describes the significance of where patients sit in community meetings. The right-hand chair to the leader's is "the sickest patient's," the left-hand, "the leader's helper's," the chair opposite the leader's, "the challenger's," and so on. Seating

diagrams and Wilmer's intuitive concepts are extremely useful ways to come to terms with the group dynamics that obtain within any ward setting. A community meeting offers a sample of the ward's group process on any particular day; its seating diagram is like a blueprint from which the process may be inferred.

The milieu therapist must always take cognizance of group processes. Otherwise he will never understand some of the puzzling emotions that are unleashed in his direction, such as the anger directed at Jerry's hard-working therapist. Once a therapist sees that a given emotional sequence can be reflective of events that are occurring on a broader social level, he can become skilled at making interventions that influence the social context positively. The community meeting is the best place for such far-reaching interventions. The right communication within this circle helps every patient's treatment. Thus, the therapist was correct in countering the ward pessimism, which seemed to say, "We can't get better and it's all *your* fault," with a firm statement that "Patients can get better," spoken to his patient in a way that everyone could comprehend. Then the ward could work on its resistances to operating therapeutically, on its overprotectiveness, and on its fear of psychotic emotion. This shift enabled the most disturbed patient to enter into treatment and freed Jerry from the pseudosick role he was so good at playing but that threatened to impede his treatment.

It is through the *staff meeting* that the emergency therapist gets to know that subculture of the ward, the treatment staff. Whenever staff members meet, their values and philosophy, their reactions to particular patients and their families, and their internal agreements and disagreements become apparent. The therapist must take the same consultative set to *this* ecological group as to the one that exists for his patient outside the hospital. He must learn to shape his interpretations, observations, and interventions in the language and grammar by which this staff operates, not in one he may have worked with previously. If he does not, he may be playing modern jazz in a Dixieland group: what's good in New York does not go in New Orleans.

The new therapist should expect a period of hostility, both toward him and his patients. Only by regular attendance of those staff meetings at which he is welcome can the therapist dispel suspicion and act effectively as an advocate for his patient's treatment.

Rehash meetings occur on many wards after community meetings, small-group meetings, and goals conferences (after any meeting, in fact, in which the patients and staff have met together). These are important meetings in which staff members discuss the nature of the processes afoot in the ward culture and critically evaluate their own responses to these processes. The staff, in effect, decides how to behave vis-à-vis the ward. It is important to attend the rehash meetings because it is at these that the therapist learns whether or not he is making interventions according to current ward policies.

The purpose of *regular* staff meetings is to generally share information and goals. They maintain the integration of the ward and usually are not for outside therapists. Some wards have regular meetings in which the staff meets with outside therapists to monitor a given patient's treatment. Here a process of mutual consultation occurs. The therapist uses his special relationship with the patient to inform the ward about the major conflict areas with which the patient needs help. The staff, in turn, helps the therapist gain objectivity by pointing out areas in which the intimate relationship has placed him in unconscious collusion with the patient's evasion of part of reality.

The "transference bond," so helpful in the treatment of neurosis, often can keep a therapist from making a necessary demand on a hospitalized patient because he seems to be "coming to grips with an internal problem." It is easy to forget that, unlike the neurotic office patient, the hospitalized patient may be using *all* his energy in trying to confront an unconscious conflict and none in

maintaining himself in the world. The staff's consultation may be invaluable in freeing the therapist from this common bind, which makes him feel that therapy is at last going well when it has only been made ridiculously easy.

Again the occasional patient for whom the pressure is deliberately removed so that he will have enough energy to confront an internal problem should be excepted. In this case, the therapist takes a calculated risk that his patient will not react to the artificial return to a supported state with a permanent commitment to infantile solutions of conflict. Nowadays, a therapist who believes in this "incubating" mode of treatment will have a fairly hard time convincing most acute hospital staffs, who have become leery of hospitalizations that last more than six weeks.

In the event of major staff disagreements about the ward ideology, the formal staff meeting, not the rehashes or the meetings over a particular patient's care, is the place to iron things out. Major philosophic disagreements should *never* be the topic of community meetings or meetings at which patients are present. Of course, this is not to say that the staff cannot openly disagree in front of the patients. Rather, patient care should not be taken over by the process of staff dispute. In meetings in which patients are present, the staff should behave professionally and confine disagreeing statements to the issues immediately at hand, not to general issues of ward philosophy, which can be intensely divisive. For the patients' sake, all members of the staff must try to play by the rules on which it has agreed, even when some would prefer to see these rules changed. A good staff will trust its own ability to make necessary changes, and the patient will not find himself in the middle of a dispute about ideology even if one exists.

Thus the techniques that improve communication are various forums in which the *rules* of the ward communication are discussed. Different kinds of discussions about rules belong to different forums. The community meeting discusses rules that govern the treatment of patients. Rehashes discuss rules by which the staff communicates its values to patients. Staff meetings discuss rules that govern the therapist's behavior and the overall rules that make up the ward ideology. Knowing these rules, and how to discuss rule changes that appear necessary, is an essential task of the therapist who is learning to function in a ward context.

Techniques That Encourage Expression. For many patients, catharsis remains a vital part of treatment. Among the techniques that encourage expression are psychodrama, small group, and family group.

Psychodrama involves role playing of a given individual's conflicts by several persons. Jerry did not engage in psychodrama, but if he had, one patient might have played his mother, another his father, and one him. Jerry could have directed them in what to do. In this way he could see his own conflict more vividly, and he could feel himself taking a direct role in its outcome. Moreover, others could criticize his way of directing. Thus various processes of catharsis, insight, and confrontation come literally into "play."

In a *small group* a few patients meet together to discuss their problems in living. Peer support in confronting problems is probably the primary effect of this time-limited group. This experience brings a sense of individual attention and intimacy to hospitalization, and it enhances the psychological set of problem solving. (Many first-time inpatients are quite unpsychologically minded and need all the help they can get in learning to view themselves psychologically, a necessary prerequisite to the effective use of psychotherapy.)

Family group enables the family to voice its concerns, and also provides an interface between the ward group and the patient's own ecological group. It can be a place where communication is improved, but more often actual change occurs in the ecological group conferences that form a vital part of the crisis intervention. Family group, usually held once a week, is an "open house" in which the family is helped to hear and see that they are not alone, that patients can be helped, and that their positive contributions are welcome. Occasionally a particular family problem will surface with glaring malignity, and the family group will resemble a difficult meeting in an ongoing therapy group. Most often it is a place where staff and family obtain information about each other.

Techniques That Modify Behavior. Increasingly, ward therapists are becoming dissatisfied with relying solely on communications and expressive techniques. Abroms'[37] work with hysterical characters points this new direction, which uses the hospital as a place where intensive reeducation can be undertaken:

> . . .We have operationally defined hysteria as the type of behaviors which emerge when the patient is required to adhere to a schedule that demands responsible self-assertion. We have thus concerned ourselves with deficits, excesses, or misdirected (indirect, displaced) forms of assertion or aggression, such as the expression of suicidal impulses, physical complaints, sarcasm, withdrawal of interest, etc. By arranging a corrective feedback system, we have assisted patients in recognizing these behaviors as unwanted – a big step in gaining control over them. Instead of the symptomatic control of others, the patient moves toward self-control, which in this context means simply the recognition and direct expression of her needs and wishes. Learning these kinds of communicative skills . . . may be approached as a current educational task.

In practice, Abroms assigns his hysterical patients to strict schedules which offer time for grooming, meetings, room cleaning, and so on. The staff then helps the patient recognize the ways in which he gets in his own way when he tries to follow a schedule. This "corrective feedback" enables the patient to eliminate his own "undesired behaviors."

Other techniques that have been used to train

patients are token reinforcements, work schedules, and ward contracts. For example, Jerry had a ward contract he had to follow; the woman who took daily walks was on a schedule. Token reinforcements have been used with severely regressed chronic schizophrenic patients, who receive tokens for socially desired behaviors such as making their own beds, eating with utensils, and so on. These tokens may be used to buy candy. In some wards they are required as payment for meals, permission to take a nap, and other basic needs. Such techniques have in common practicality, efficiency, and specificity in that they focus on definite behavioral objectives rather than on less tangible goals. Such specificity is especially good for concrete patients who cannot relate to abstract goals, and for manipulative patients who misuse abstractions for sociopathic ends.

SPECIAL PROBLEMS IN THE MILIEU

Infractions of Ward Rules

Overpermissiveness undercuts milieu therapy. When a patient acts against a ward rule, he should be told firmly that he may not do so. His first obligation is to get along in the ward society. If the infraction is severe, such as hitting another patient, a meeting of the entire ward may be called to deal with the crisis, which usually centers around whether or not the patient can remain on the ward.

After the processes of limit setting and reintegration into the ward society are complete, reasons for the infraction may be safely deferred to discussions with the therapist. In ward work the expression of hostile feelings must always take second place to limit setting because the dangers and consequences of loss of control are grave.

Minor infractions, as was stated previously, may be preludes to suicide or elopement, as well as indications of a burgeoning paranoid or antisocial attitude. They must be taken seriously.

Staff Splitting

A staff will often find itself in a bitter conflict over a patient's care: the dynamic formulation will be pitted against the organic, the phenomenological against the behavioral, the permissive against the limit setting. This widely recognized phenomenon was first described in Stanton and Schwartz' classic *The Mental Hospital*.[38] It appears that splitting more often originates in the patient's dynamics than in the staff's.[39,40]

Jerry (cont'd.). The rehash meeting that followed the community meeting at which Jerry's therapist was attacked was curious. Most members of the nursing staff stood up for the therapist's behavior, but one nurse said, "Jerry has been sicker than you let on." She felt that Jerry's treatment was going too fast and that everybody was expecting more of him than he could deliver. "I just wonder how he's ever going to put it together when he gets out of here," she finally declared. Most of the staff was incredulous that after the good, energetic resolution to the staff meeting she still voiced the pessimistic view of schizophrenia. Several staff members sought to "correct" her, but an older nurse took her side about Jerry. The therapist reiterated his statements in the community meeting and cited research data that supported his contention that Jerry's schizophrenia had a good prognosis.

Finally the ward chief noted that this conflict between the doubting nurse and the optimistic therapist sounded suspiciously like the argument between Jerry's mother and father. "And you each have your allies, as they do. Isn't it possible that you're both right? Isn't that what Jerry has to put together?"

For the first time the staff could feel what Jerry was up against. For a few minutes the group as a whole felt angry, discouraged, and very confused. Both had to be right, but what then should the staff *do*? "Now I'm confused," the older nurse said, and the tension seemed to lift.

"Well, at least we've seen how impossible it feels to be Jerry," said the therapist, who from this point on approached his patient with a certain seriousness that his work had previously lacked. He seemed less cocksure.

To the ward at large, Jerry had become a bit more real. The "doubting nurse" took pains to make a few demands on Jerry, including one speech to him that ended his failure to make his bed in the morning for once and all. "It's the least you can do," she said, penetrating his resistance as the commanding officer who tried to get him to pack his duffel bag right never could.

"Oh, *okay!*" Jerry shouted, and made the bed.

The recognition and working through of staff splits is one of the most potent aspects of milieu therapy, as the previous example shows. Their nonrecognition can lead to bitter staff battles, as a patient's ambivalent conflict, with its warring halves, is acted out by an entire ward. Such bitter disputes may require an outside consultant, who can better identify them.

Self-destructive Behavior

Minor self-destructive acts can be dealt with by limit setting, as in the case of the depressed woman who cut her wrist to relieve her inner tension in a clear-cut signal for help. Major suicide attempts on the ward constitute a crisis for the ward as well as for the patient. Often an emergency meeting of the ward will mobilize the therapeutic community to act as a lifeline for the suicidal person, who can then be kept on the ward. Repeated suicide attempts, despite mobilization of the community, will require referral to a locked facility with maximum security. Not every patient can make it on an open ward.

An actual death by suicide on the ward is a major trauma for the living who are left behind to wonder if they will be stopped from harming themselves. Often the suicide will produce a con-

tagion of suicidal emotion throughout the ward, as if this solution is seen to be a possible way out of severe emotional conflict. A special community meeting that focuses on the event can serve to "bury" the suicidal solution if patients can see that staff is not going to retreat from its attempts to help patients solve problems because one made death his solution. Nevertheless, the staff can expect to have its ability to take reasonable preventive measures tested within a short time after an actual death takes place.

Example 10-6. A suicide took place on a small ward: an elderly man jumped out of a window one day after being let out of a locked room. Two other patients saw him make the jump. A community meeting was held in which everyone had his say about the event. A few hours after the meeting, one of the patients who had watched the man jump, an adolescent boy who had not previously reported suicidal feelings, informed his doctor that he felt suicidal. He was placed in a locked room at his own request. Shortly after, the other man who had watched the suicide also asked to be locked up. The two did not feel free of suicidal promptings for three days, during which time they remained in locked rooms. Later their treatment proceeded without ill effects; they expressed gratitude for being taken seriously during their time of panic and guilt.

Aggressive Behavior

It is a staff's duty to protect patients from assault. A firm rule against touching other patients is usually necessary with borderline and psychotic patients. It should be remembered that hospitalized patients are usually "mad," and that given the least opportunity their anger is apt to surface in an explosive way.

Example 10-7. An 18-year-old woman was leaving the ward after being hospitalized for a month and a half. Her recurrent problem was learning to control her anger. As she was leaving, she said to the therapist who had achieved good results by holding her responsible for her outbursts, "Gee, I'd like to give you a punch in the stomach."

Caught off guard by her good humor, the therapist said, "Go ahead." The patient proceeded to punch him as hard as she could right in the solar plexus.

This example points out that patients usually *mean* what they say to therapists. A good way to stave off trouble is to hold patients responsible for what they say, and to follow up any verbal cues that suggest an outburst of hostile behavior is being contemplated. Patients usually feel that they are being watched on an inpatient ward, and they expect this kind of careful listening from the ward staff. A ward is a good place for the therapist to learn to remember what patients say, to note down the exact words, and to allow himself to be "haunted" by seemingly trivial communications. By taking such idle remarks up in therapy sessions, the therapist can defuse many bombs.

Hostile Dependency

If a patient is hospitalized longer than he needs to be, he may become hostile and break ward rules. Some patients react negatively to hospitalization and presumably are so full of unmet dependent needs that they must constantly defend themselves with anger to hold onto their independence. If a patient becomes more and more angry the more that is done for him, the best approach is to do less. By doing more the therapist tends to "trap" the patient into the intolerable (for him) position of being indebted. By doing less, even to the point of discharging or referring him to another therapist, the therapist gives the patient the dignified "one-up" position of being able to reproach; the patient will feel less angry. This principle is often useful in the treatment of patients with character disorders.

Example 10-8. A middle-aged alcoholic woman kept pressuring a beginning therapist to admit her to the hospital. Finally he yielded to a drunken telephone call and agreed to come in at 3 A.M. to the hospital emergency room. (Previously he had told her she would have to present herself sober during regular working hours to obtain admission, and he was contradicting his own limit setting.)

The therapist immediately set up a schedule of detoxification designed to make her as comfortable as possible. He carefully explained everything that would be expected of her and thoroughly oriented her to the ward. He saw her every day and did everything to make sure she knew what was being done for her care.

At the end of the third hospital day she flew into a rage at the staff, claimed she had been hospitalized against her will, and signed out against medical advice. She called her therapist from home that evening and promised to kill him if he ever tried to control her again. Her now-frightened therapist, on the advice of a senior clinician, referred her to a long-established alcohol treatment program. After telling several professionals at the program that he had "rejected" her, the patient settled into a program that recognized her need to be in control and let the movement into therapy come from her.

Even patients who do not have severe conflicts over dependency will feel that being in a mental hospital represents a failure in their lives and will resent the "one-down" position of being cared for benevolently. Some extremely successful inpatient wards are run by ward chiefs who have harsh, abrasive styles and who do not present themselves as kind, but rather address their patients in a businesslike way. This stance allows hostile dependent patients to feel that what they do, they do for themselves and obviates their need to provoke the ward staff to find someone to resent so that they can feel better about themselves.

Example 10-9. A chronically regressed schizophrenic patient who had proved refractory to the ministrations of a series of well-meaning therapists finally perked up after a blunt, abrasive therapist took over his care. His improvement was so dramatic that after a few months he was recommended for discharge from the mental hospital where he had spent several years.

The discharge staff committee was interested in this phenomenon, and so they asked the patient, still doing well on his first review of the trial discharge, what had made the difference.

"I was sitting in my corner as usual," said the patient, "When this person suddenly was standing over me. I looked up at his mean face, and I said to myself, 'Here's a son-of-a-bitch who's going to get me well'."

Sick Friendships and Sexual Relationships

Inevitably, patients in the hospital recreate their problems in living with each other. Many therapists will not criticize their patients' relationships because they dislike commenting on the behavior of others. On a therapeutic community ward, with its seductive emphasis on patients helping each other, an uncritical acceptance of all relationships between patients can lead to trouble. Patients will sometimes "team up" to resist therapy, a phenomenon that has been described for adolescent inpatients in love when they become two against the therapeutic community. As in the case of Alice in Chapter 3, patients may live together in mutually exploitative relationships after they are discharged. The inpatient ward is not the place to make friends, but to learn to be helpful in more objective ways. When pairs do form, they should be examined.

Jerry (cont'd.). The large woman who spoke at the community meeting in such a cryptic way ("I'm as pacific as the ocean.") took a special interest in Jerry from the first day of his hospitalization. "Come over here, honey," she bellowed into the day room a little before breakfast. "I can see you're in trouble. Sit by Ruby." Jerry obediently sat beside her.

For a few days Jerry spent much of his free time with Ruby. She claimed to be a palmist, and for long minutes would gaze at Jerry's palm. She never revealed what she saw, but the effect was devastating.

Eventually their relationship was explored in the small group to which they both belonged. It developed that Jerry's mother was active in a spiritualist church, and that she had been unable to get a favorable reading from her minister for his enlistment. Ruby had several children who had been taken away from her by court order, many years ago.

On the one hand, these two were reenacting an unhealthy mother-son relationship. On the other, this very reenactment allowed the ward staff to touch upon material that might have gone unnoticed. The depression behind Ruby's paranoia had much to do with her feelings of failure as a mother: Jerry was the first person in whom she had shown interest in many days on the ward. She had been brought in by police who found her picking trash out of garbage cans and talking incoherently to herself. Jerry, as already shown, was overimpressed by his mother's doubts. The relationship they formed on the ward brought out key issues in the illness of each.

Outside Contacts, Contraband, and Unplanned Departures

Occasionally, a patient will *misuse outside contacts* to conduct his own crisis intervention with members of his ecological group.

Example 10-10. Clare, who had been admitted following a suicide attempt after her husband had found her in bed with another man and walked out, spent much of her time on the ward telephone trying to convince him to come back. At the same time, she refused to let her therapist interview him. Eventually the problem was solved by admitting the husband to the ward. The two continued their attempts at reconciliation, but in a context where professionals could observe and help them to clarify their interaction.

This case illustrates an increasingly common clinical practice of admitting both members of a marital couple together. The therapist who uses this method saves much time in trying to convince the nonadmitted spouse that he is also "the patient," in making necessary communications a second time, and in keeping pace with the unregulated contacts between the partners.

If a member of the outside ecological group cannot or should not be included in a patient's treatment, the therapist should try to regulate their contacts. If they cannot be regulated, the therapist should reconsider whether or not this person has to be left out of the treatment. A good compromise is to have the other person be seen collaboratively by another professional: the "intruder" can be included even while the patient maintains his privacy.

Example 10-11. Lois, who developed a psychotic depression her second year of junior college, could not be separated from her mother, a cheery extraverted nurse who was unconsciously crushing her daughter in her zeal to make her feel better. Mother would appear with bright bouquets of flowers which she would spend many minutes trying to arrange in a manner that would please Lois. Lois would stare quietly ahead. When they were seen together in therapy sessions, Lois would remain withdrawn and her mother would do all the talking, often acting seductively toward Lois' therapist. Following a session, Lois wandered off the ward and onto the hospital roof. She was seen there by a frightened patient on a walk.

Clearly, these joint contacts were antitherapeutic. The therapist asked that Lois' mother be seen collaboratively by the ward social worker, herself a motherly woman who was extremely responsible about not doing too much for her patients. He explained to Lois that her mother would be able to talk to the social worker every day, that she would not be attending any more of their sessions, and that her visits would be limited to fifteen minutes twice a week. Almost immediately Lois' depression began to lift, and therapy aimed at Lois' eventual emancipation got underway.

The patient must be told clearly at the beginning of his stay that he cannot keep personal stores of drugs and weapons, i.e., *contraband.* The occasional patient who uses a ward to "push" narcotics and psychedelic drugs should be discharged. The discovery of weapons and drugs threatens the security of the ward and should be made the subject of a community meeting. If a suicidal patient is found to be stockpiling potentially lethal drugs, the entire ward should be made aware of his presuicidal communication. Usually "exposing" a suicidal patient in this manner tends to undercut the feelings of isolation that lead to such behavior. The homicidal patient who harbors weapons on a ward poses a more difficult problem. The therapist should insist upon the removal and sale of all firearms as a condition of treatment. Often the ward chief will be called upon to set the limit with such patients. Sometimes the patient has to be discharged and the police notified.

Patients may arrange *unplanned departures* and leave the ward for brief periods (AWOL) or for good (elopement) without telling anyone. Or, they may leave against medical advice after having signed the necessary papers. Responsible members of the ecological group should be notified of such departures immediately. If a patient threatens to leave against medical advice, these members should be called to the ward for an emergency conference. If the patient is being held on the ward legally against his will and leaves, the police should be notified. In most other circumstances, the police should *not* be notified. A very large percentage of those who leave the ward without permission get in touch with their therapists within a few days. The ward chief will usually rule that the patient who elopes has to apply to the ward through a new goals conference before his readmission can be considered.

EFFECTING THE PLANNED DISCHARGE

Discharge planning begins when the patient first enters the milieu. If the crisis intervention and the handling of transactions within the milieu have gone well, the discharge follows naturally. Nevertheless, certain problems regularly appear when the patient reenters the world, and they are the subject of the next paragraphs.

Passes

No patient should be discharged from an inpatient unit until he has had at least one short pass to demonstrate his fitness to cope with the stresses of the outside environment. Ideally, there will be a short pass, followed by an overnight pass, and then a weekend pass, before a seriously disturbed patient is considered to be ready for discharge. After each pass the therapist should review the nurse's notes to discover the patient's emotional state upon return, whether he appeared inebriated or "high" on drugs, and the nature of his behavior on the ward on coming back. He should then discuss how the patient handled the pass. *No new pass should be written until the patient's reaction to the previous pass has been thoroughly evaluated.*

Passes should be structured around an activity. Thus a pass can allow time enough for dinner and a movie, a job interview, or a visit to a potential therapist. Long stretches of unstructured time are unwise. Patients who request such long passes without plans are usually trying to avoid the process of therapy on the ward.

Reports of behavior on passes can help the therapist spot potential sources of trouble in the patient's readaptation following his experience with hospitalization.

Jerry (cont'd.). At the end of his first week on the ward, Jerry took a four-hour pass to see a Walt Disney movie. He left and returned on time. He went to sleep immediately.

The following week, after the big conference with the members of his family, plans were made for a two-day visit home, with time also allowed for a visit to the prospective therapist's office. (Jerry's family lived several hundred miles away; the intermediate step of a one-day visit had to be omitted in his case.)

When Jerry returned he explained that he didn't have much to say to the outside therapist. "It's kind of hard to talk about yourself to a complete stranger," he said to his ward therapist, adding, "Wouldn't it be great if you could be my therapist?"

A call to Jerry's father revealed that Jerry had resisted all pressures to engage in activities by saying, "You know I'm a goddam schizophrenic."

Jerry's mother reported that her day with Jerry had gone strangely. "You should ask me to do things," Jerry had told her. She had even asked the therapist, "Do you think I don't expect enough of him?"

The pass revealed a number of problems that had grown evident on the ward: Jerry was attached to the ward therapist, and he tended to use his diagnosis as a "cop out." But it also showed that he had begun some real work in his relationship with his mother, which had been the most difficult issue in his life. The information gained from the pass helped guide the therapist in his final work with Jerry. This work involved termination and a redefinition of the meaning of his mental illness.

Options of Disposition

When a patient is discharged from the inpatient milieu, he (1) returns to his former ecological group, which stays unchanged; (2) goes to an ecological group to which new members have been added, such as a therapist or visiting nurse; or (3) enters a new ecological group (day care center, halfway house, or nursing home). The decision is reached on the basis of therapeutic contacts with members of the original ecological group, assessment of the degree of the patient's social impairment, and the resources at hand.

The general error is to be too grandiose, to try to "save" the patient from an environment that has made him ill, only to introduce him into another environment, supposedly therapeutic, in which he stays just as ill. It is often enough to make slight changes in the original ecological group, such as the addition of a good therapist. Major relocations should be reserved for those patients who are truly without social resources or who have deteriorated seriously.

> *Example 10-12.* Annie, 76, was admitted to the hospital, failing in memory, with a history of soiling herself and setting herself afire by accidentally dropping cigarette butts in bed. After a few days of a strong vitamin regimen, enough memory returned to enable her to care for herself on the ward, although she had a clear-cut Wernicke-Korsakoff syndrome. She was visited every day by a 62-year-old gentleman who had borrowed large sums of money from her during the past year. He usually smelled of alcohol. A cousin who had emergency power of attorney revealed that Annie had confided in her that she thought he was after her money, but she loved him anyway. This man supplied her with alcohol, and it was clear that when she returned home she would quickly revert to her drinking ways.
>
> On balance, recommendation to send her to a nursing home was made, with the cousin serving as conservator.

Discharge as a Trial of Readaptation

Transition has its difficulties for all patients. For psychotic patients, this is a time in which suicidal feelings develop. Depressive patients often experience a reactivation of suicidal intent. Patients with character disorders often become angry to the point that they leave AWOL or against medical advice a day before their planned discharge. It is well to explain to patients that they may find the discharge difficult, that it is expected that they will call the therapist if they feel unaccountably depressed, frightened, or angry, and that a number of patients find that they are not ready after all. The option of planned readmission should always be held open so that the patient does not have to stage a crisis to dramatize his need for continued support.

> *Jerry (cont'd.).* A week after his discharge Jerry made a planned telephone call to his ward therapist at a prearranged time. He had chosen to live with his father, and he was looking for work. He had seen his outpatient therapist twice, and the therapist had seen his family twice. "He's pretty sharp," Jerry said. "He doesn't buy that schizophrenia stuff. I was pretty low for a couple of days, like you said, but everybody's trying to change for me, and I'm keeping my thoughts clear. Tell Ruby I found out I have a real long lifeline."

SUMMARY

Crisis intervention in a ward setting involves the same principles as in outpatient work, but many more people become involved, and much more of the patient's life is opened to the intervention. In using this resource, the basic skill is constant attention to the patient's transactions in the variety of situations that the process of hospitalization makes possible.

REFERENCES

1. Bettelheim, Bruno, and Emmy Sylvester: A Therapeutic Milieu," *Am. J. Orthopsychiat.,* 18:191–206, 1948.

2. Jones, Maxwell: *The Therapeutic Community,* Basic Books, New York, 1953.

3. Wilmer, Harry A.: *Social Psychiatry in Action,* Charles C Thomas, Springfield, Ill., 1958.

4. Rapoport, Robert N.: *Community as Doctor,* Tavistock Publications, London, 1959.

5. Abroms, Gene M.: "Defining Milieu Therapy," *Arch. Gen. Psychiat.,* 21:553–560, 1969.

6. Zusman, Jack: "Some Explanations of the Changing Appearance of Psychotic Patients: Antecedents of the Social Breakdown Concept," *Int. J. Psychiat.,* 3:216–247, 1967.

7. Weisman, Gilbert, Alan Feirstein, and Thomas Claudewell: "Three Day Hospitalization – a Model for Intensive Intervention," *Arch. Gen. Psychiat.,* 21:620–629, 1969.

8. Engle, Ralph P., and Elvin V. Semrad: "Brief Hospitalization, the Recompensation Process," in Gene M. Abroms and Norman S. Greenfield (eds.), *The New Hospital Psychiatry,* Academic, New York, 1971, chap. 5, pp. 67–81.

9. Herz, Marvin I., Jean Endicott, Robert L. Spitzer, and Alvin Mesnikoff: "Day Versus Inpatient Hospitalization: A Controlled Study," *Am. J. Psychiat.,* 127:1371–1381, 1971.

10. Langsley, Donald G., David M. Kaplan, F. S. Pittman et al.: *Treatment of Families in Crisis,* Grune & Stratton, New York, 1968.

11. Langsley, Donald G., Pavel Machotka, and Kalman Flomenhaft: "Avoiding Mental Hospital Admission: A Follow-up Study," *Am. J. Psychiat.,* 127:1391–1394, 1971.

12. Kessler, David: "Preventing Psychiatric Hospitalization: A Crisis Intervention Approach," talk given at Pacific Medical Center, San Francisco, March 8, 1973.

13. Holmes, Marguerite J.: "Influences of the New Hospital Psychiatry on Nursing," in Gene M. Abroms and Norman S. Greenfield (eds.), *The New Hospital Psychiatry,* Academic, New York, 1971, chap. 6, pp. 83–100.

14. Levene, Howard I.: "Acute Schizophrenia: Clinical Effects of the Labeling Process," *Arch. Gen. Psychiat.,* 25:215–222, 1971.

15. Beck, James C., and Kathy Worthen: "Precipitating Stress, Crisis Theory and Hospitalization in Schizophrenia," *Arch. Gen. Psychiat.,* 26:123–132, 1972.

16. Perry, John W.: "Reconstitutive Process in the Psychopathology of the Self," *Ann. NY Acad. Sci.,* 96:853–876, 1962.

17. Holmes: op. cit., p. 85.

18. Cumming, John, and Elaine Cumming: *Ego and Milieu,* Atherton, New York, 1963.

19. Levene: loc. cit.

20. Perry: loc. cit.

21. Polsky, Howard W., Daniel S. Claster, and Carl Goldberg (eds.): *Social System Perspectives in Residential Institutions,* The Michigan State University Press, East Lansing, 1970.

22. Peplau, H.: "Psychotherapeutic Strategies and Its Discussion," *Perspect. Psychiat. Care,* 6:264–286, 1968.

23. Abroms: "Group Methods in the Milieu," in Gene M. Abroms and Norman S. Greenfield (eds.), *The New Hospital Psychiatry,* Academic, New York, 1971, chap. 9, pp. 133–146.

24. Kass, David J., Frederick M. Silvers, and Gene M. Abroms: "Behavioral Group Treatment of Hysteria," *Arch. Gen. Psychiat.,* 26:42–50, 1972.

25. Abroms, Gene M., Carl H. Fellner, and Carl A. Whitaker: "The Family Enters the Hospital," *Am. J. Psychiat.,* 127:1363–1369, 1971.

26. Ullman, Leonard P.: "A Theoretical Overview of Behavior Modification Techniques with Schizophrenics," in Gene M. Abroms and Norman S. Greenfield (eds.), *The New Hospital Psychiatry,* Academic, New York, 1971, chap. 16.

27. Daniels, David N., and J. M. Kuldau: "Marginal Man, the Tether of Tradition, and Intentional Social System Therapy," *Community Ment. Health J.,* 3:13–20, 1967.

28. Daniels, David N.: in C. Peter Rosenbaum: *The Meaning of Madness: Symptomatology, Sociology, Biology and Therapy of the Schizophrenias*, Science House, New York, 1970, chap. 13.

29. Yablonsky, Lewis: *Synanon, The Tunnel Back*, Macmillan, New York, 1965.

30. Lieb, Julian, Ian Lipsitch, and Andrew Slaby: *The Crisis Team: A Handbook for the Mental Health Professional*, Harper & Row, New York, 1973.

31. Ibid.

32. Abroms: "Defining Milieu Therapy," loc. cit. cit.

33. Bateson, Gregory, Don D. Jackson, Jay Haley, and John Weakland: "Toward A Theory of Schizophrenia," *Behav. Sci.*, vol. 1, no. 4, 1956.

34. Caudill, William A.: *The Psychiatric Hospital as a Small Society*, Harvard, Cambridge, Mass., 1958.

35. Ludwig, Arnold M., and Frank Farrelly: "The Code of Chronicity," *Arch. Gen. Psychiat.*, 15:562–568, 1966.

36. Wilmer: loc. cit.

37. Kass et al.: loc. cit.

38. Stanton, Alfred H., and M. S. Schwartz: *The Mental Hospital*, Basic Books, New York, 1954.

39. Burnham, D. L.: "The Special Problem Patient: Victim or Agent of Splitting?" *Psychiatry*, 29:105–122, 1966.

40. Main, T. F.: "The Ailment," *Brit. J. Med. Psychol.*, 30:129–145, 1957.

Organizing Emergency Work

PART 1: A FLOWCHART SYSTEM OF EVALUATION AND DISPOSITION OF PSYCHIATRIC EMERGENCIES

The preceding chapters presented ways to order, evaluate, formulate, and apply information in intervening with persons caught in crisis. Observing the patient in his particular situation, responding intuitively to the patterns inherent in the dilemma, allowing appropriate feeling to emerge from the confusion of emotion, and reasoning out possible solutions with the participants are requisites for good crisis intervention. A final skill involves the ability to take command, to orchestrate the elements of intervention into a smoothly executed plan of action. Here the emergency therapist must use his executive abilities, even if only to lend his authority to a solution he has helped the participants to find for themselves. This chapter is a kind of executive training for therapists and includes a test of mettle at its end. It is an approach to that most difficult of executive functions, *organization.*

At this stage of his work, the emergency therapist must establish relations with the patient's *ego.* He must ensure that there is enough ego functioning present to avert catastrophe. If there is not, the therapist must support the patient's ego with his own. One aspect of ego functioning is internal and external control over the expression of sexual, aggressive, and dependent impulses. The patient must be able to avoid detrimental action as he attempts to meet his needs. One method of increasing control is through the use of environmental support; another is through the use of tranquilizing and sedative medication.

If loss of control is the major consideration, a true psychiatric "emergency" is said to exist, and Salamon[1] lists three principles of basic management: (1) deal with the healthy part of the patient's ego, (2) establish controls, and (3) use medication.

As Salamon points out, there is almost always some healthy ego to appeal to in even the most disturbed patient. The therapist must make it clear to this healthy ego that he will not tolerate uncontrolled behavior and that he will take control until the patient is able to exert his own controls again. The therapist should present medication as an aid in achieving the return of self-control.

These three principles draw heavily upon the medical model, but emergency therapists coming from a nonmedical background should avail themselves of them. (Much of the mystique attached to psychiatrists as medically trained therapists amounts merely to *comfort* in using the medical model when it is appropriate in therapy.) A psychologist or social worker should, as a mental health professional, be able to take command of a deteriorating situation with a disturbed patient, talk to the healthy ego, be able to interpose his own ego-controls, and make sure an available physician furnishes the appropriate medication. (In contemporary crisis teams, a physician need only countersign the medical prescription and the admission order; the decisions to use these modes of intervention are made by the mental health professional.)

It follows that the nonmedical therapist will have to train himself in the areas of medicine that apply to emergency psychotherapy, specifically those concerning the nature and effects of psychotropic drugs. He will also need a good working alliance with the physician who countersigns his plan of management. Indeed, unless the lines of authority and responsibility are clearly drawn, the nonmedical therapist should not accept an assignment to do emergency psychiatric work. Usually if he has demonstrated a basic ability to assume responsibility for managing the patient and seems comfortable with the medical model, he will have no trouble in his relationship with the medical man who legally supervises his emergency work.

CHOICE POINTS AND DECISION MAKING

Assuming responsibility means more than taking control; it also involves the formulation and defense of a treatment plan (in emergency work, sometimes called "the disposition"). In making decisions concerning the final plan, a series of choice points emerge, questions that must be answered before the next step in decision making can be pondered.

It helps the therapist to do his job if he asks himself a series of yes and no questions. Suppose, for example, that he is confronted with a patient who is threatening suicide, who has no interpersonal resources, and who is threatening to walk out of the emergency room. He asks himself:

1. Is the patient dangerously suicidal? Yes.

2. Is involuntary hospitalization legal in this state under these circumstances? Yes.

3. Do I have the means and facilities available to hospitalize the patient involuntarily? Yes.

The answer to each question leads to the next, and the final answer to the final question is the disposition: hospitalize the patient involuntarily.

Much psychiatric emergency work can be organized in this fashion. Each of the kinds of patients — the suicidal, homicidal, drinking, and so on — described in the preceding chapters operates under a particular set of conditions, often unique to the particular condition under consideration, which recur and which the emergency therapist must keep in mind. He must consider conditions A, B, and C for the suicidal patient; resultant choice-points may be A^1, B^1, and C^1, and so forth.

We have tried to present the most important questions that must be asked and answered by the therapist, and the logical choices that flow from their answers; these choices for several kinds of patients are presented in the flowcharts that follow. Later we shall provide an analysis in a similar form on how to organize knowledge about disposition resources.

FLOWCHART ANALYSIS FOR SPECIFIC CONDITIONS

Evaluation and Disposition of Psychiatric Emergencies: General Considerations

The most serious considerations in evaluating a psychiatric emergency center around severe incapacitation, the potential danger of the patient to himself or to others, and the degree of risk of further serious medical or psychiatric disabilities. If the death or severe disability of a patient or someone else is possible if appropriate intervention is not taken, hospitalization (involuntary if necessary) should probably be effected. Less severe probable outcomes may call for less drastic measures. The major evaluations that must be made and the decisions that result from them are shown in Figure 11-1. Table 11-1 is to be used in conjunction with this figure.

Can patient function without serious risk to himself or others?

Yes   No, or in doubt

Evaluate complaint further.
Is it psychiatric?

Yes   No

Determine which modalities of
psychiatric intervention are
appropriate, and attempt to
initiate treatment.

Refer (if
necessary) to
appropriate
resource.

Evaluate nature of problem after examining
patient and interviewing collaterals. Hold
for 12 to 24 hr if necessary for further
evaluation. Initial formulation should
include evaluation for both *social* and
psychiatric-medical diagnoses associated
with severe incapacitation.

*Social diagnoses associated with
severe incapacitation*

1. Suicide attempt or risk
2. Homicide attempt or risk
3. Gravely disabled
4. In medical straits, e.g., DT's
5. Environmental crisis or other
   danger to self or others

*Psychiatric-medical diagnoses associated
with severe incapacitation*

(See Table 11-1.)

Does patient fit one or more such diagnoses; if so,
is his functioning seriously compromised?

No   Yes

Is hospital treatment for a medical condition mandatory?

No   Yes

Is hospital treatment for a social-
psychiatric condition mandatory?

Arrange for admission to medical
service.*

No   Yes

Arrange for admission to psychiatric
service.*

Is hospital treatment for medical, psychiatric, or social condition
highly desirable but not mandatory?

No   Yes

Strongly encourage patient and collaterals to accept
voluntary hospitalization; do they accept it?

No   Yes

Arrange voluntary hospitalization.

Complete evaluation and offer outpatient
treatment and/or referral to community
resources where appropriate.

* Many patients for whom hospitalization is necessary will voluntarily agree to transfer to the
appropriate facility only to change their minds en route. Whenever this is a possibility, be
willing to make use of involuntary, "hold" procedures to preclude it.

Figure 11-1   Evaluation and disposition of psychiatric emergencies. 1: general considerations.

TABLE 11-1: Psychiatric-Medical Diagnoses Associated with Severe Incapacitation

(Diagnoses often occur in combination. Once all diagnoses are made, go to the sections in this chapter that outline needed evaluation and treatment decisions in greater detail.)

Talking with collaterals can often be far more profitable than spending much time with a patient who is delirious or suffering from impaired reality testing. Always get the old chart as soon as possible; this may be a "repeat performance." Descriptions of earlier episodes may provide the guide to the treatment of this one.

I. Acute or chronic complications of medicosurgical conditions: NB: Whenever these are present to a significant degree, they must be treated adequately on a medical-surgical service *before* the patient is transferred to a psychiatric hospital where diagnostic and treatment facilities are often inadequate. Psychiatric consultation should be freely available to the attending internist or surgeon.

    A. Organic brain syndromes associated with

        1. Primary (CNS) pathology, such as

            (a) Space-occupying cranial lesions, intrinsic or the result of trauma (e.g., gunshot wounds, subdural hematoma, etc.)

            (b) Ictal and postictal confusional states

            (c) Hypertension

        2. Toxic states associated with

            (a) Alcohol

            (b) Psychotropic drugs, e.g., sedatives, especially barbiturates, glutethimide (Doriden®); methaqualone (Quaalude®); major and minor tranquilizers

            (c) "Street drugs" and "bad trips," including those from ingestion of LSD, marihauna, amphetamines, belladonna compounds, DMT, STP, cocaine, etc.

            (d) Opiate addiction

            (e) Carbon monoxide

            (f) Other poisons

        3. Metabolic and infectious diseases, especially those that may mimic functional illness

            (a) Possible mimics of anxiety and manic states: hyperthyroidism, pheochromocytoma, tertiary syphilis, hypoglycemia

            (b) Possible mimics of schizophrenia, alcoholic delirium: diabetic coma, systemic lupus erythematosis, corticosteroid reactions, Cushing's disease

            (c) Possible mimics of depression: hypothyroidism, Addison's disease

    B. Physical trauma: lacerations, stab and gunshot wounds, etc.

II. Primarily psychological states

    A. Depression and suicide (NB: Suicide risk found also in other conditions in which depression may not be significantly present)

    B. Homicide (often in conjunction with alcohol, other drug use)

C. Psychotic states
 1. Schizophrenia
 2. Depressive psychoses, unipolar and bipolar
 3. Manic states
 4. Paranoid states
D. Miscellaneous other states, including fugues, amnesias, multiple personality, and other dissociative reactions

Depression and Suicide

The major choice-points of depression and suicide center around self-destruction, by either a recent or a highly possible future overt attempt, or by "chronic suicide" (e.g., continued heavy drinking when known liver damage is present, or chronic heavy drinking in combination with barbiturate addiction), and around the recurrence of suicidal emotion after the initial intervention has taken place and treatment has been instituted (see Figure 11-2).

Homicide and Violence

The choice-points for evaluating the potentially violent patient should include his potential for violence *now*, his potential for violence *later* (especially if drinking or drug taking is not presently a problem but may be in the future), reducing the personal and social forces that may be building to a violent explosion, exerting control over the potentially violent person, and protecting the safety of potential victims (see Figure 11-3).

Psychotic States in General

Psychosis denotes only a serious impairment in the ability to perceive or respond appropriately to external and internal reality. Psychosis can result from a variety of organic states, including alcohol and other drug ingestion, brain disease, and so on, and from several kinds of so-called functional states, such as the schizophrenias, manic-depressive illness, and so on.

Once the general diagnosis of psychosis has been made, certain interventions, largely aimed at preventing the patient from doing harm to himself or others, can be made. Specific treatment (including administering drugs and ECT) depends on making specific diagnoses, and these in turn may demand that additional hours and days be spent in obtaining a history from the patient and members of his ecological group, in making observations, and in preparing a psychiatric formulation. Guidelines for pursuing both general and specific diagnostic and treatment possibilities are given in Figure 11-4.

The Schizophrenias

The basic issue in the emergency treatment of schizophrenic patients is whether the psychosis is likely to result in destructive behavior or incapacitation, not whether schizophrenia per se requires hospital treatment. There are large numbers of obviously schizophrenic people living peacefully in society, in whatever idiosyncratic ways, who constitute no threat to others and who are able to provide for their own food, shelter, and personal needs. Many such patients require help in managing their lives *outside* the hospital, which they cannot learn *inside* (see Figure 11-5).

Alcohol and its Complications

The choice-points to be considered for patients with alcohol problems almost always involve at least one other health professional in addition to the emergency therapist. (This is true whether the therapist is a psychiatrist, psychologist, or other mental health professional.) The person most frequently called upon is an internist or general physician who can help evaluate and treat the patient medically; but representatives of many social agencies (including the police) may be involved. The first major choice is that of evaluating and treating concomitant serious medical illness that may accompany the drinking. The second is the treatment of acute intoxication, and the third is treatment of the underlying psychiatric and social problems (see Figure 11-6).

Street Drugs and Bad Trips

The major question in treating a patient who has taken a street drug or is having a bad trip is, "Does the treater know what he is treating, i.e., does he have highly reliable information as to which drug(s) the patient has taken?" If he does, he can often, in addition to supportive treatment (e.g., talking the patient down), use a specific antidote. If he does not (which is usually the case), he must restrict himself to using minor tranquilizers or sedatives, such as diazepam. He must also rule out an underlying functional psychosis which may be masked by acute drug intoxication. All these possibilities are represented in Figure 11-7.

Opiate and Sedative Addictions

First the therapist needs to know whether the patient is suffering from an overdose or a withdrawal syndrome, and second whether the patient has been taking opiates, barbiturate sedatives, nonbarbiturate sedatives, or some combination of these (see Figure 11-8).

Is the patient depressed?

No   Yes

Complete usual psychiatric evaluation.

Has there been a recent suicide attempt, or is there current serious risk of one?

No   Yes

Is there concurrent serious medico-surgical problem, e.g., sequelae of alcohol, barbiturate, other drug ingestion or habituation; physical trauma such as laceration, gunshot wounds, and so on?

No   Yes

Hospitalize on *medical-surgical* ward until physical condition treated and stabilized; provide psychiatric consultation. Then: is suicide still a serious risk?

No   Yes

Hospitalize on psychiatric ward. Observe suicidal precautions; obtain drug-free baseline state. Start antidepressants or ECT as indicated. When ready for discharge:

Start appropriate outpatient treatment, e.g., individual, couple therapy; anti-depressants; involvement of family, and so on.

Is there recurrence of serious suicidal risk?

No   Yes

Continue outpatient treatment.   Reconsider psychiatric hospitalization.

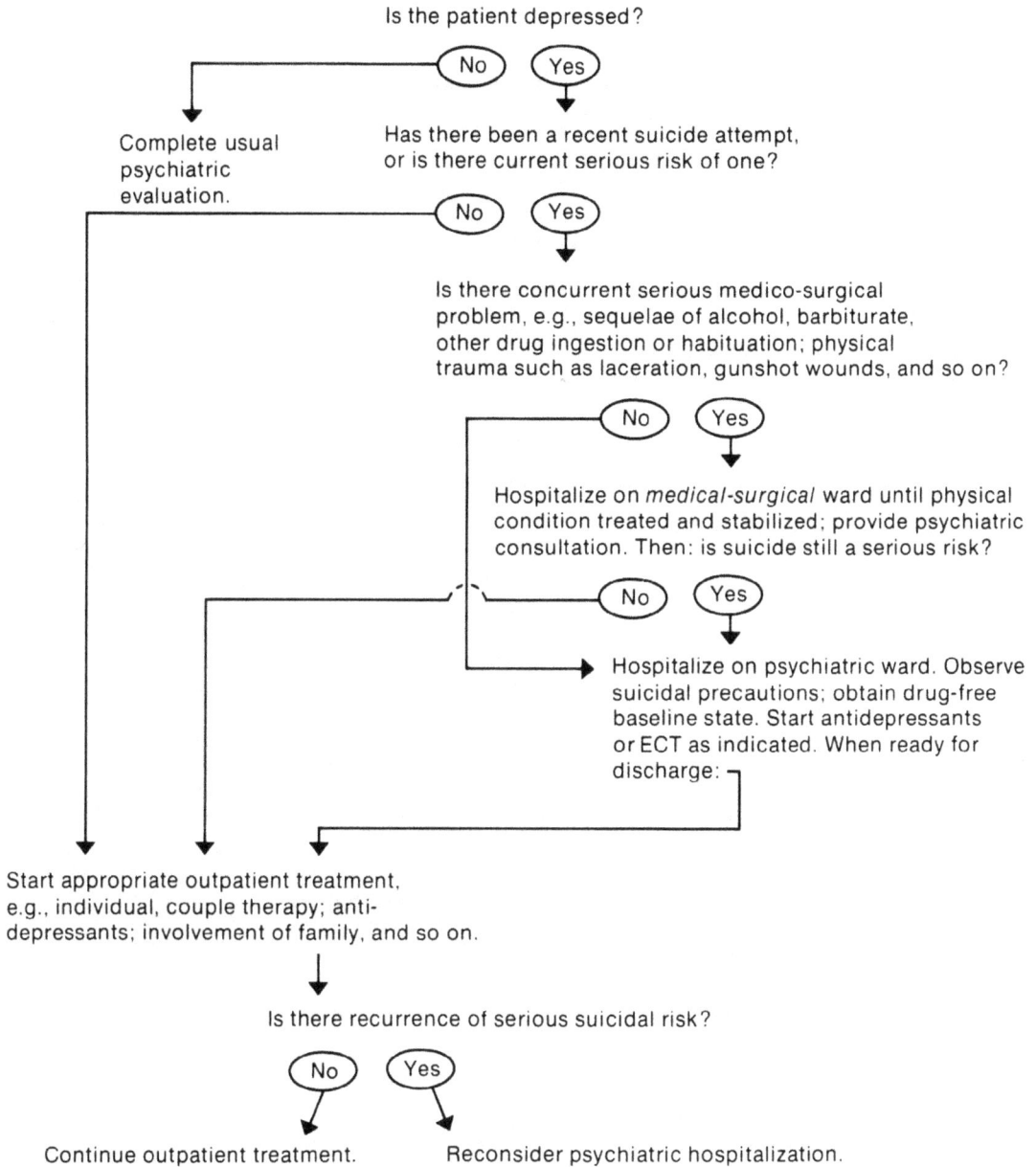

Figure 11-2 Depression and suicide.

Does patient show signs of being in a preassaultive
state, e.g., one or more of the following:

1. Feeling of unbearable tension, that he might "blow".
2. Rage toward known other, often family member, with
   conscious thoughts of violence.
3. Recent increase of assaultive behavior, e.g., fights.
4. Toxic decrease of self-control, as with alcohol.
5. History of past violent behavior; parental brutality
   in past; triad of youthful bedwetting, cruelty to
   animals, and firesetting.
6. Arrest and prison record for violent crimes.
7. Arrest or convictions for dangerous auto crimes, e.g.,
   speeding, hit-run driving, and so forth.
8. Well-formulated paranoid plan to "get him (them),"
   often in response to voices.

(No) (Yes)

A. Further evaluation

Complete usual   1. Discuss with patient and collaterals the difference between
psychiatric   thought and action; the need to exert control that psychiatrist
evaluation.   cannot substitute for.
                      2. Evaluate temporary separation of warring parties, from moving
                         in with family or friends, to motel, to psychiatric hospitalization.
                      3. Evaluate and discuss possible role of potential "victim" in
                         promoting homicidal escalation.
                      4. Appeal to patient's narcissism, that violence on some level is
                         "not very smart for a bright guy like you," i.e., is self-destructive,
                         no matter how sweet the revenge. Appeal to his pride and sense of
                         strength and control.

B. Decision making. Even with supportive psychotherapy, is the
    situation still high-risk for violence?

(No) (Yes)

Continue treatment.   Advise potential victim of personal and legal
                                           rights for self-protection; use whatever pro-
                                           fessional and legal restraints (including incarceration)
                                           are necessary to control patient until acute potential
                                           for violence subsides. Patient may be more willing to
                                           accept *medical* rather than *psychiatric* hospitalization
                                           to avoid "crazy" or "psycho" label; service chief
                                           more likely to agree if psychiatrist says he will take
                                           complete responsibility for managing patient; can
                                           get neurological evaluation there if he suspects
                                           neurological basis for dyscontrol.

Figure 11-3 Homicide and violence.

Is the patient psychotic? (Is his ability to perceive reality or respond appropriately to it seriously impaired?)

No   Yes

Complete usual psychiatric evaluation.

Institute general level of controls which are necessary to proceed with next steps of medical and psychiatric evaluation.

Perform preliminary physical examination, looking especially for evidence of an organic brain syndrome, fluctuating levels of consciousness, delirium, intoxication by alcohol, other drugs. Are such signs present to a significant degree?

No   Yes

Try to determine general major type of disturbance (paranoid, disorganized, excited, intropunitive). See Figure 11-4, part 2, for guides on making such differentiations and for general and specific treatment interventions in each type.

Evaluate further and treat. Does organic condition respond fully to treatment with no psychiatric residual?

No   Yes

Is patient still psychotic?

Complete treatment.

Yes   No

To Figure 11-4, part 2

Refer for further psychiatric treatment.

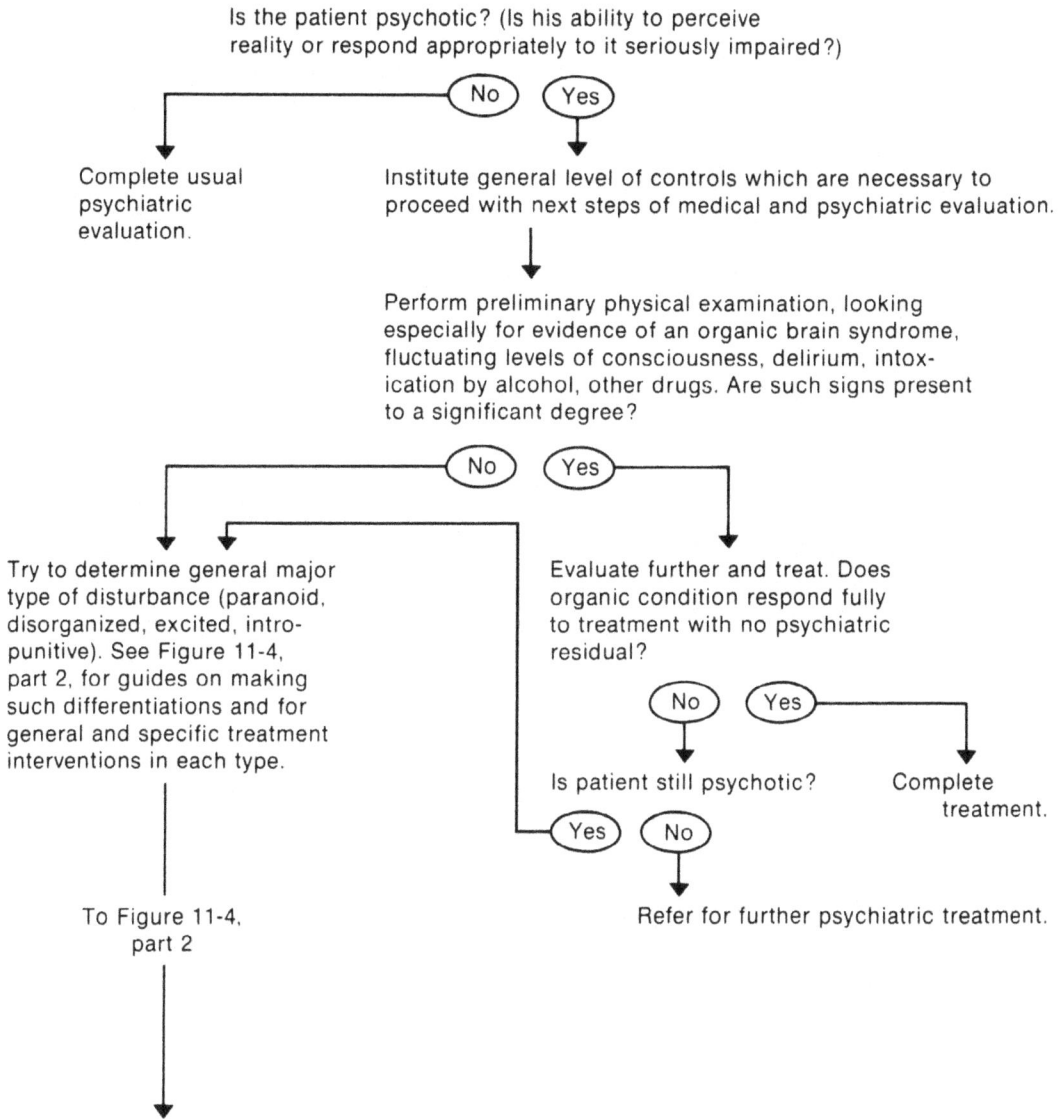

Figure 11-4   Psychotic states in general.

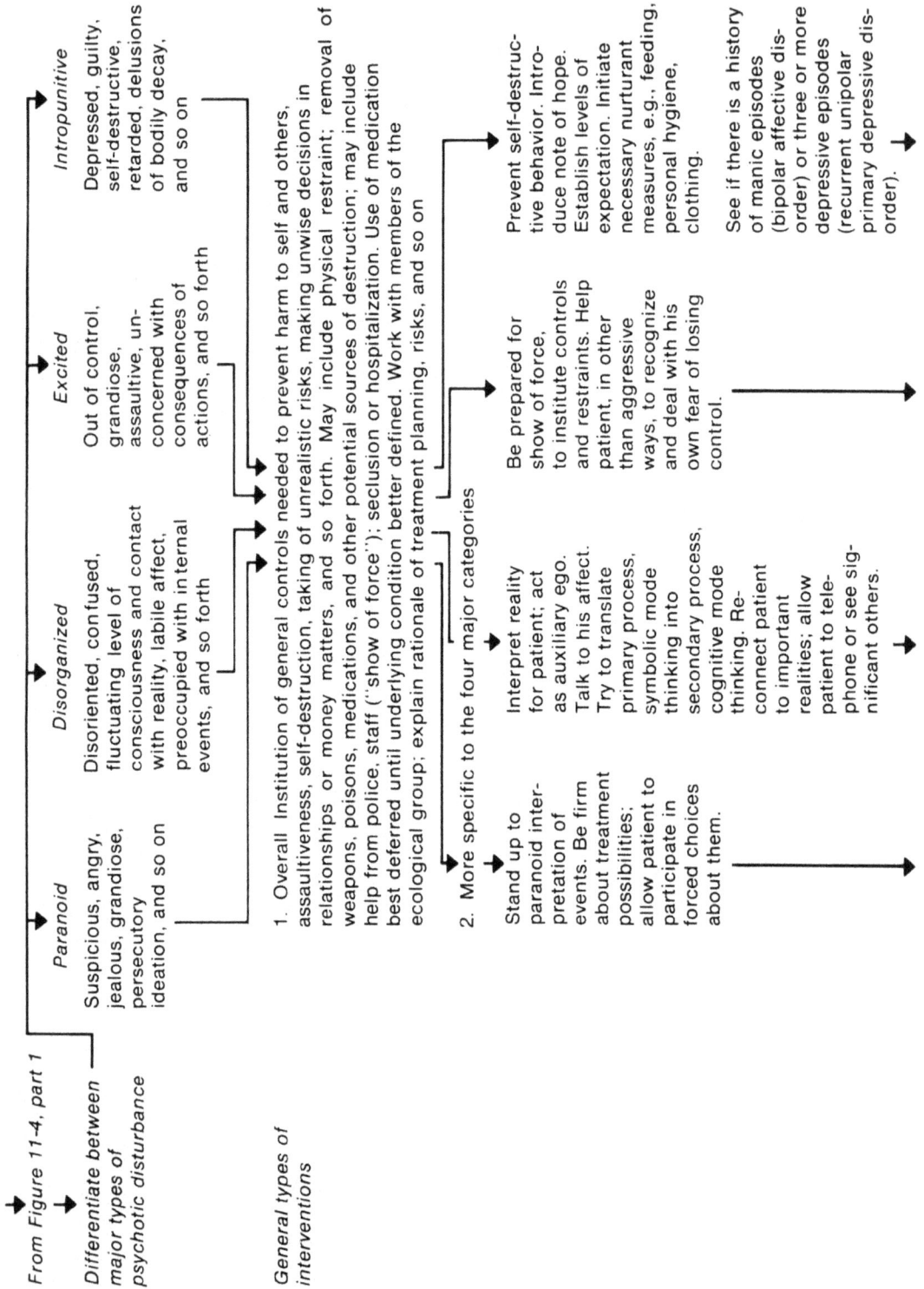

From Figure 11-4, part 1

Differentiate between major types of psychotic disturbance

Paranoid	*Disorganized*	*Excited*	*Intropunitive*
Suspicious, angry, jealous, grandiose, persecutory ideation, and so on	Disoriented, confused, fluctuating level of consciousness and contact with reality, labile affect, preoccupied with internal events, and so forth	Out of control, grandiose, assaultive, unconcerned with consequences of actions, and so forth	Depressed, guilty, self-destructive, retarded, delusions of bodily decay, and so on

General types of interventions

1. Overall Institution of general controls needed to prevent harm to self and others, assaultiveness, self-destruction, taking of unrealistic risks, making unwise decisions in relationships or money matters, and so forth. May include physical restraint; removal of weapons, poisons, medications, and other potential sources of destruction; may include help from police, staff ("show of force"): seclusion or hospitalization. Use of medication best deferred until underlying condition better defined. Work with members of the ecological group; explain rationale of treatment planning, risks, and so on

2. More specific to the four major categories

Stand up to paranoid interpretation of events. Be firm about treatment possibilities; allow patient to participate in forced choices about them.	Interpret reality for patient; act as auxiliary ego. Talk to his affect. Try to translate primary process, symbolic mode thinking into secondary process, cognitive mode thinking. Reconnect patient to important realities; allow patient to telephone or see significant others.	Be prepared for show of force, to institute controls and restraints. Help patient, in other than aggressive ways, to recognize and deal with his own fear of losing control.	Prevent self-destructive behavior. Introduce note of hope. Establish levels of expectation. Initiate necessary nurturant measures, e.g., feeding, personal hygiene, clothing.

See if there is a history of manic episodes (bipolar affective disorder) or three or more depressive episodes (recurrent unipolar primary depressive disorder). |

Specific interventions based on diagnosis (most commonly employed somatic treatments in parentheses)*	Paranoid	Disorganized	Excited	Intropunitive
	1. Paranoid stress reaction. Removal from stress or diminution of stress (antipsychotics).	1. The schizophrenias. Reality oriented, milieu, and supportive therapy. (Antipsychotics.)	1. Manic phase of manic-depressive illness (antipsychotics, lithium carbonate; sometimes ECT).	1. Psychotic depressive reaction (antidepressants, ECT if no response). 2. Primary depressive affective disorder. (a) First or second episode, unipolar type (antidepressants, ECT if no response).
	2. Involutional paranoid state (antidepressants, antipsychotics, ECT).	2. Organic brain syndromes, delirium. Correction of organic and psychosocial factors. (Sometimes antipsychotics in low doses; vitamins.)	2. Catatonic excitement in schizophrenia (antipsychotics; sometimes ECT).	(b) Third or more episode, unipolar type, "recurrent depression." (Lithium carbonate; ECT if no response). (c) Depressive phase of bipolar, manic-depressive illness. (Lithium carbonate; ECT if no response. Avoid antidepressants.)
	3. Paranoid schizophrenia (antipsychotics).	3. Secondary to drug use. Detoxification. (Sometimes antipsychotics, sedatives.)	3. Acute panic. Milieu and supportive therapy. (Antipsychotics.)	3. Involutional melancholia (antidepressants; ECT if no response).
	4. Paranoia secondary to drug use. Detoxification. (Some times antipsychotics.)	4. Secondary to other metabolic factors, e.g., brain tumor, carbon monoxide poisoning, endocrine dysfunction. Correction of underlying metabolic disorder.	4. Sociopathic personality in state of rage. Milieu and supportive therapy. (Minor tranquilizers.)	4. Schizoaffective disease, depressed type, first or second episode (antipsychotics, antidepressants). Third or more episode (antipsychotics, lithium carbonate; avoid antidepressants).
	5. Paranoia secondary to organic brain syndromes. Correction of organic and psychosocial factors. (Sometimes antipsychotics in low doses.)		5. Side effect of antipsychotics (change or reduce offending drug).	5. Secondary to drug use. Detoxification. (For persistent depression, antidepressants.)
	6. Paranoia in acute mania (antipsychotics, lithium carbonate).		6. Chronic schizophrenia in exacerbation (antipsychotics).	6. Secondary to organic illness. Treatment of organic illness; milieu and supportive therapy. (For persistent depression, antidepressants.)

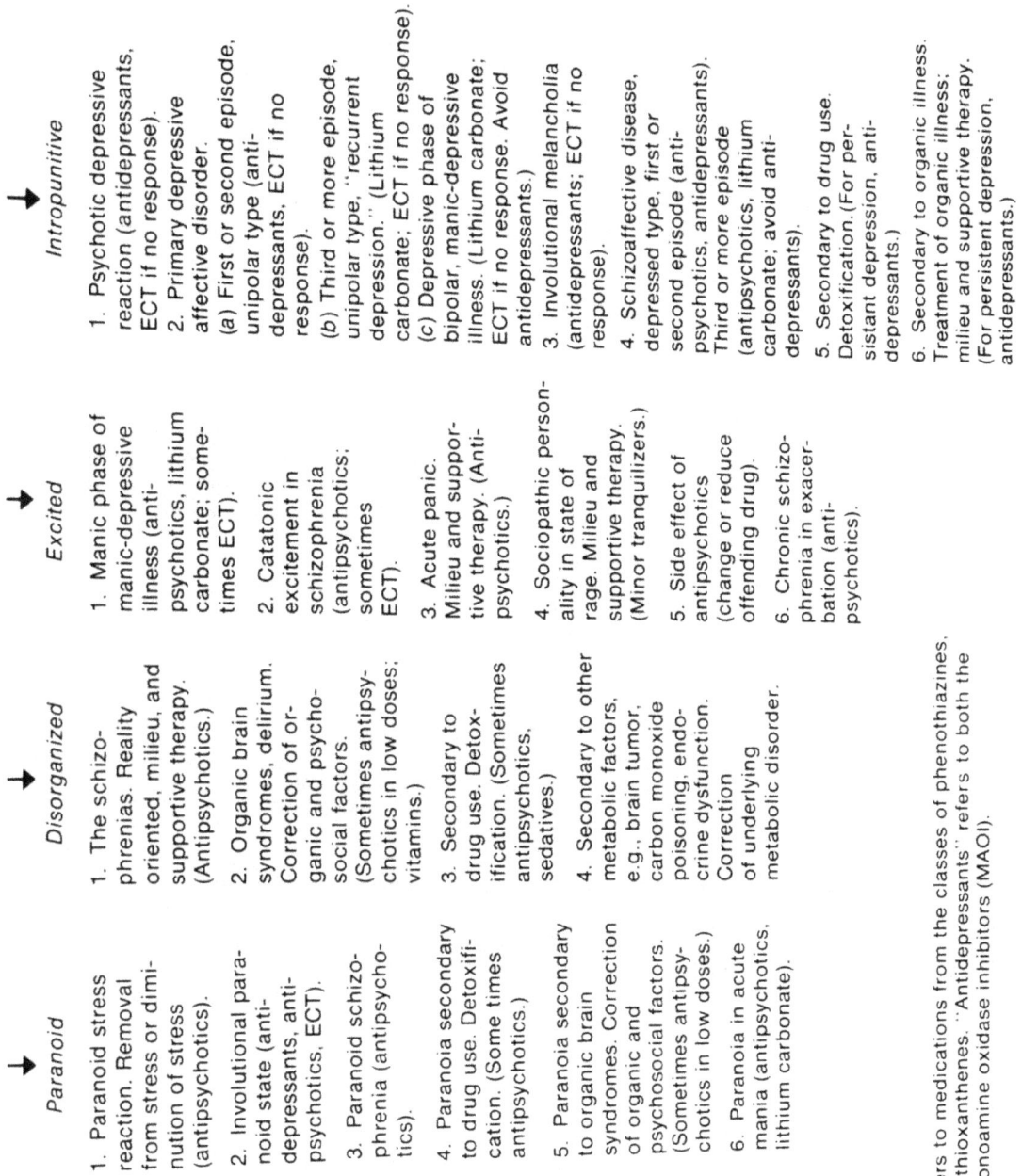

*"Antipsychotics" refers to medications from the classes of phenothiazines, butyrophenones, and thioxanthenes. "Antidepressants" refers to both the tricyclic group and monoamine oxidase inhibitors (MAOI).

Is patient in need of hospitalization? (Include
following in evaluation: information from old
chart, from family and friends; danger to self or
others because of delusional thoughts or hal-
lucinated commands; patient's degree of awareness
or insight into psychotic process and disability;
ask patient if he wants or *needs* to be hospitalized—
he may know best).

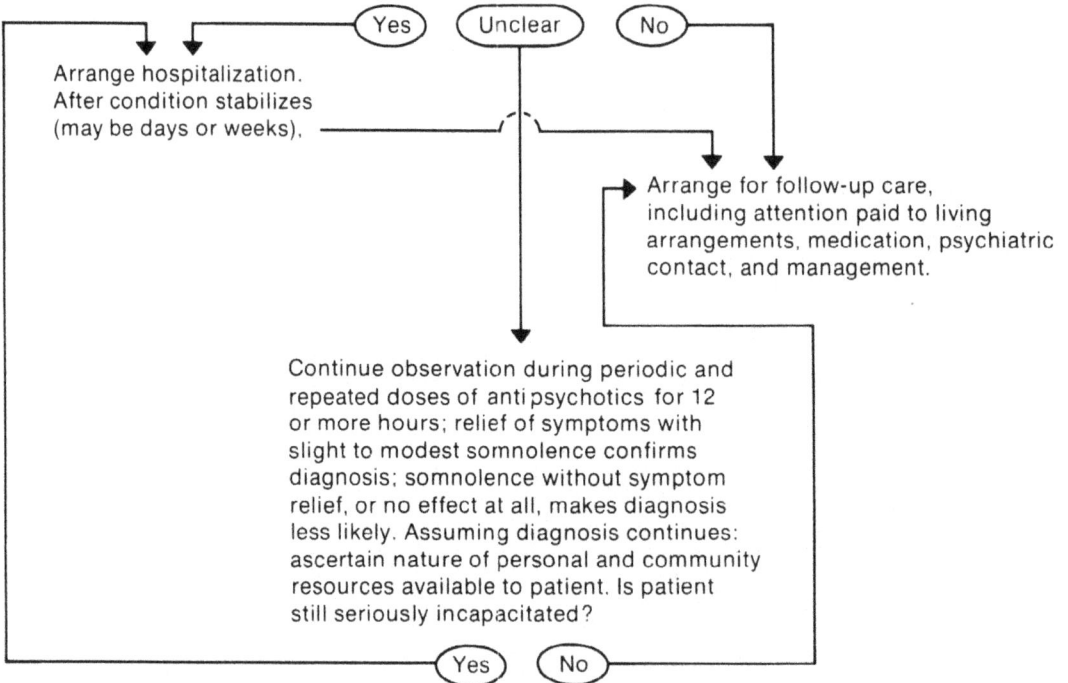

Figure 11-5 The schizophrenias.

Does patient have alcohol-related problem?

No   Yes

Complete usual psychiatric evaluation.

Does he show signs of deficits of reality testing, e.g., Wernicke-Korsakoff syndrome, pathological drunkenness, impending DT's, alcoholic hallucinosis?

Does he show signs of serious medical complications, e.g., gastritis and gastrointestinal bleeding, cirrhosis, and so on?

Yes   No

Arrange for emergency treatment of psychiatric-medical complications, including detoxification and withdrawal if necessary; then:

Is the patient acutely intoxicated?

No   Yes

Arrange for detoxification, including intramuscular injection of thiamine and chlordiazepoxide or hydroxyzine.

Then:

Is there strong suggestion of depression, suicidal, or homicidal emotion released by alcohol now or recently?

Yes   No

Arrange for follow-up psychiatric treatment and/or hospitalization.

Are there other evidences of alcoholism or alcohol problems?

Yes   No

Are there resources (family, friends, police, and so forth) to take patient home?

No   Yes

Help find place to sober up, sleep it off; enlist agency help for the resourceless person.

Send patient home.

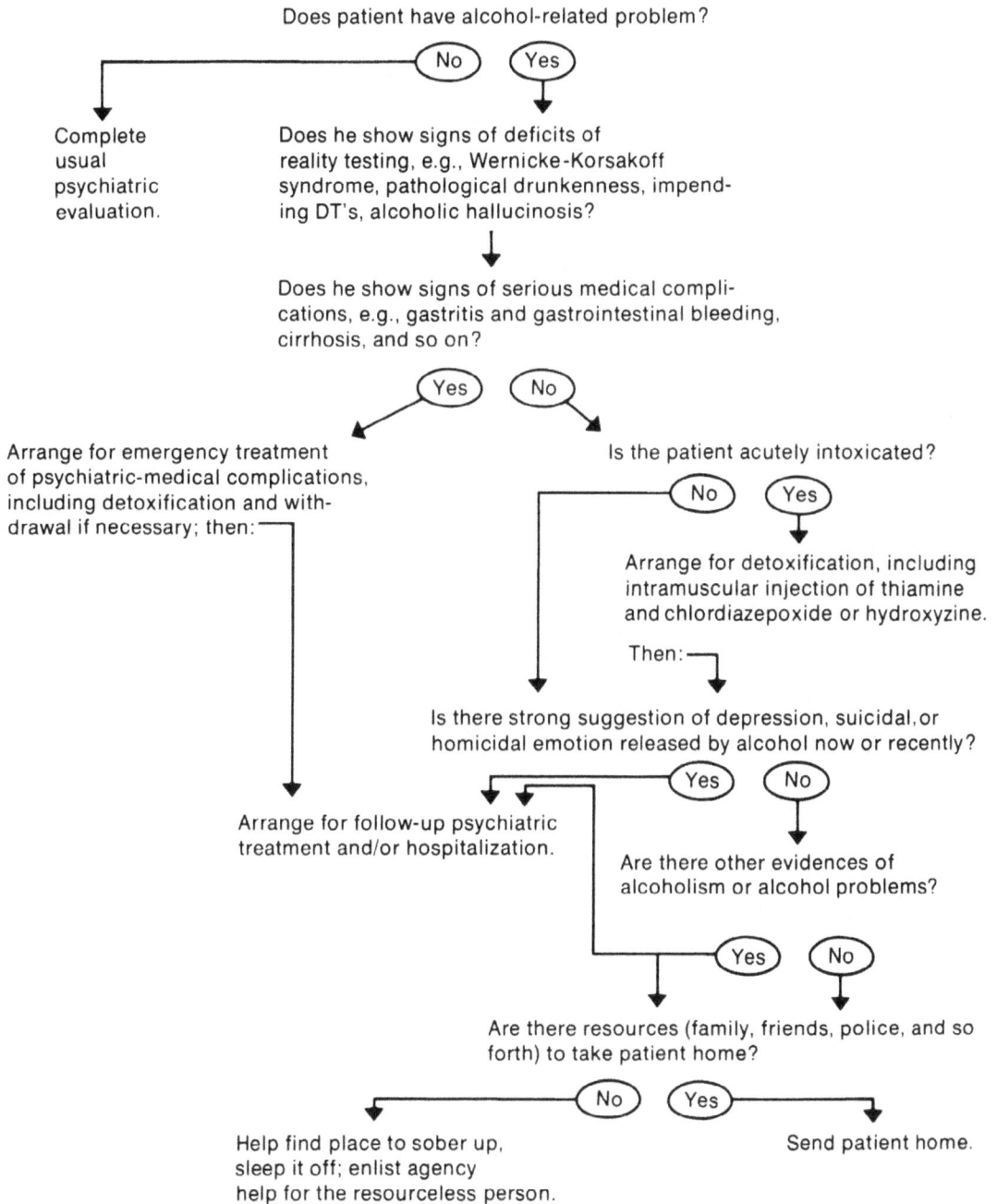

Figure 11-6 Alcohol and its complications.

Can ingredients of drugs be determined with relative certainty from patient or collaterals, including high reliability that supplier has given pure substance of named compound(s)?

No:

Unclarity exists about nature, quantity, or purity of drugs taken.

Further evaluation

1. Is local toxic drug screening panel available? If so, employ to clarify or rule out substances taken.
2. Is hot line to local drug treatment center available? If so, consult with their personnel as needed.
3. Arrange constant psychiatric observation and management; help "talk patient down" from bad trip. Talking down best done in comfortable ambience, often as well or better by family or friends as by medical personnel.
4. Be *exceedingly cautious* in use of phenothiazines, whose anticholinergic effects may act synergistically with street drug to produce "anticholinergic crisis."
5. Use diazepam, paraldehyde, and related drugs for severe anxiety and agitation.

Yes:

Arrange constant psychiatric observation and management; help "talk patient down" from bad trip. Talking down best done in comfortable ambience, often done as well or better by family and friends as by medical personnel. The following drugs may safely be treated with given antidote or antagonist:

Toxin	Antidote
1. Hallucinogen (LSD; mescaline).	1. Phenothiazines.
2. Anticholinergics, e.g., belladonna, scopolamine, related compounds. Diagnosed by "Mad as a hatter; dry as a bone; red as a lobster; blind as a stone."	2. Mild to moderate states: treat with diazepam, paraldehyde. Serious or life-threatening states: treat with physostigmine, IM, under close supervision. *Phenothiazines are contraindicated.*
3. Amphetamines; cocaine.	3. Diazepam for moderate states; phenothiazines for severe ones.
4. Opiates.	4. See Fig. 11-8 (opiates).
5. Marihuana.	5. Diazepam, paraldehyde. *Phenothiazines are contraindicated.*
6. Methaqualone (Quaalude)®; glutethimide (Doriden)®.	6. None; nondialyzable drugs. May look alert in emergency room, go into coma later. If in doubt, medical hospitalization for close observation, supportive treatment.

Has patient recovered well after 12 to 24 hours?

Yes:

Evaluate need for further psychiatric treatment for underlying problems; make appropriate recommendations.

No:

Consider possibility patient has taken long-acting hallucinogen, for example, DMT (dimethyltryptamine), STP and so on. Also consider possibility of underlying schizophrenia or other functional psychosis masked by drug intoxication; pursue treatment of psychosis.

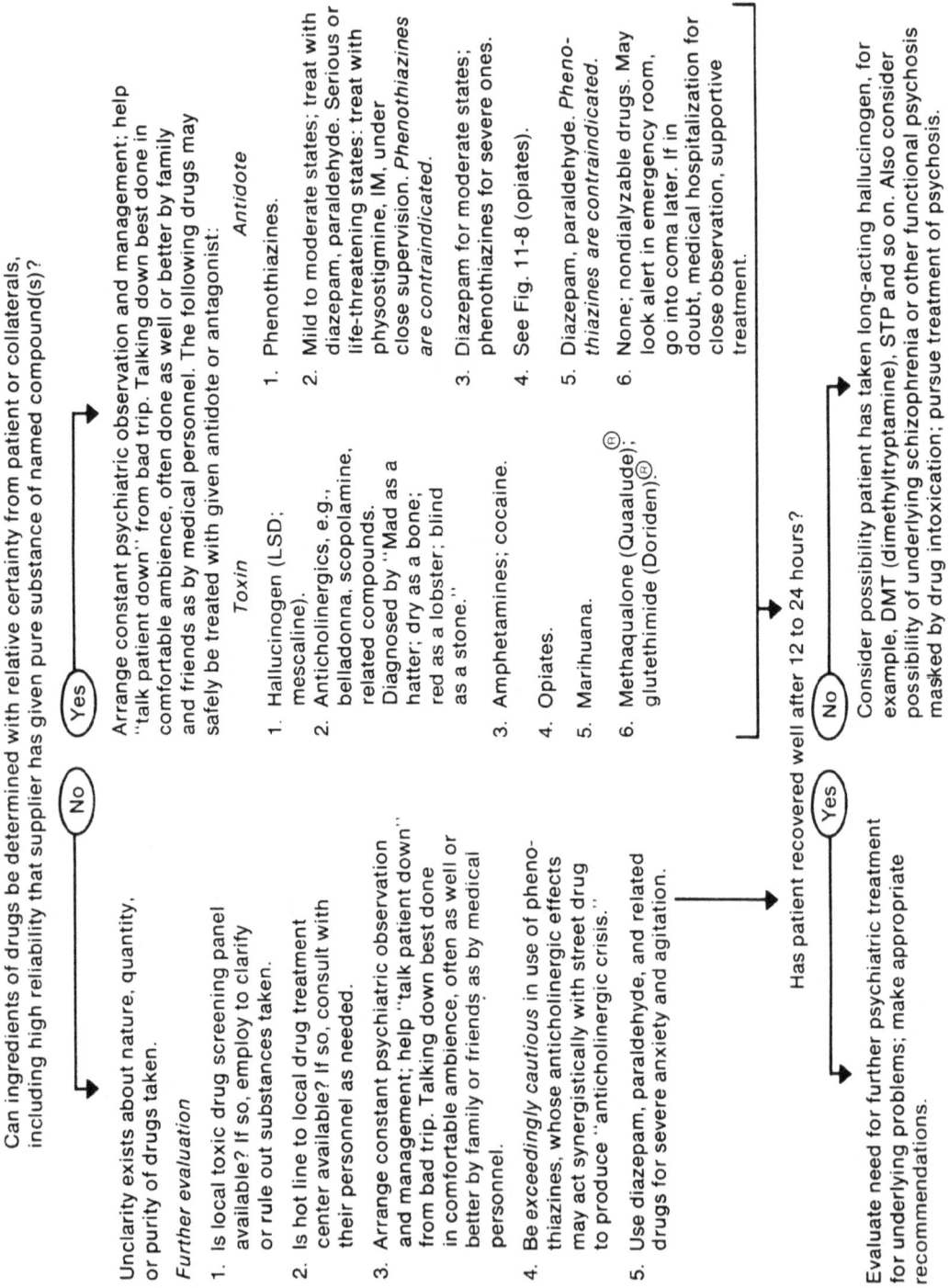

Figure 11-7 Street drugs and "bad trips."

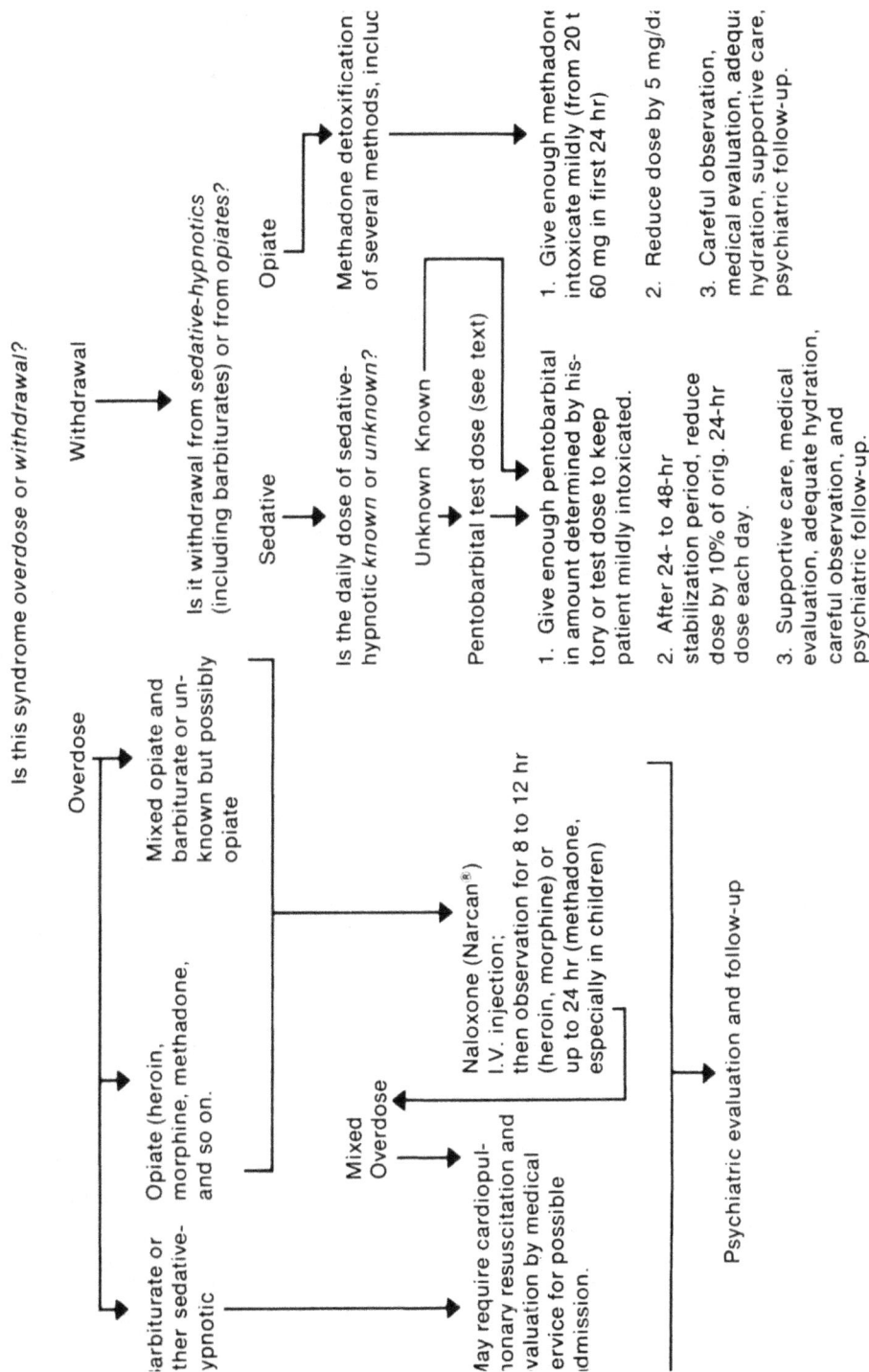

Figure 11-8 Opiate and sedative addictions.

DISPOSITION RESOURCES AND PRACTICES

Many communities have available a broad spectrum of disposition resources. What kinds they are, what they do and do not do, and who they do or do not accept for treatment are factors that will affect the practices of the emergency therapist. They range from facilities with locked rooms ("seclusion rooms") and high staff/patient ratios that can accept extremely disturbed, violently homicidal drunk paranoid schizophrenic patients to outpatient clinics or drop-in centers that are not equipped to deal with the out-of-control patient. In between these extremes are voluntary inpatient units, day and night care programs, emergency rooms, halfway houses, centers for the treatment of special problems such as opiate addiction, alcohol abuse, and street drugs, general outpatient clinics, and private practitioners and groups. These facilities are in marked contrast to those of two generations ago when the poor and middle-class had a choice only between a state or a county hospital in which all the wards were locked, or a public outpatient clinic with a long waiting list. The wealthy also had private sanitoriums, but with a limited range of treatments.

Not all patients are eligible for treatment at all facilities. Many county-operated facilities will not accept patients from outside the county; VA hospitals usually require that the individual have some connection with the military before they will offer treatment to him. Some insurance plans cover treatment for psychiatric problems; many do not. Some families have the money to pay for private treatment (especially short-term); many do not.

A Directory of Disposition Resources

The nature of available facilities and conditions of eligibility that must be met to enter them vary widely from one community to the next. The following directory of disposition resources is a general one that should be adaptable to the needs of a given area. The heading of Table 11-2 lists the kinds of treatment facilities that might be available in any given community; the kinds of patient eligibility that might be considered are listed along the side. (The emergency therapist can obtain some of this information from the patient or collaterals as he conducts his evaluation.) From these variables a grid is constructed and numbered; each number can be an index to a directory, available to the emergency therapist to suggest to him *all* the resources available to a given patient, not just the resources the therapist is already familiar with. Table 11-3 shows a sample excerpt from such a catalog.

Table 11-2 is reasonably comprehensive, but those who wish may refine it further. Under Partial Care Programs, one may want to insert those that deal with special populations, such as drug-using adolescents; under Special Problem Programs one may want to insert those that deal with patients from certain ethnic or socioeconomic groups, and so on. Thus, Tables 11-2 and 11-3 are to be used as models from which an emergency service can construct a catalog or directory to be used by all of its members. Such a catalog will need constant revision as new community services begin and old ones shut down.

Using a Resource Directory

Table 11-3 gives only a few of the 220 possibilities that were presented in Table 11-2. The following hypothetical situations are examples of how Tables 11-2 and 11-3 might be used. An enlisted Army man who lives in this county got drunk and belligerent and threatened to kill his wife. She called the police, who brought him into the emergency room. The emergency therapist ascertained that no medical complications were present and determined that he needed involuntary psychiatric hospitalization. Of all the categories under involuntary hospitalization in Table 11-2 (index numbers 1, 21, 41, . . ., 201), an army resource looked in principle to be the best for the patient. The therapist consulted his directory (Table 11-3), obtained the information about

TABLE 11-2: Available Facilities and Patient Eligibility

Patient Eligibility	Total Care Programs			Partial Care Programs			Special Problem Programs							Outpatient Clinics					Individual and Group Practice	
	Involuntary hospitalization	Voluntary hospitalization	Convalescent hospital and nursing home	Day treatment	Night treatment	Halfway house	Alcohol	Opiates	Other drugs	Suicide	Sexual	Geriatric	Retardation	General	Child	Crisis	Family service	Medical	Individual therapy	Couple group therapy
Federal programs																				
Military	1	2	3	4	5	6	7	8	9	10	11	12	13	14	15	16	17	18	19	20
Veterans	21	22	23	24	25	26	27	28	29	30	31	32	33	34	35	36	37	38	39	40
Public Health Service	41	42	43	44	45	46	47	48	49	50	51	52	53	54	55	56	57	58	59	60
State	61	62	63	64	65	66	67	68	69	70	71	72	73	74	75	76	77	78	79	80
This county	81	82	83	84	85	86	87	88	89	90	91	92	93	94	95	96	97	98	99	100
Neighboring county	101	102	103	104	105	106	107	108	109	110	111	112	113	114	115	116	117	118	119	120
This city	121	122	123	124	125	126	127	128	129	130	131	132	133	134	135	136	137	138	139	140
All patients above a certain income (including insurance)	141	142	143	144	145	146	147	148	149	150	151	152	153	154	155	156	157	158	159	160
All patients below a certain income	161	162	163	164	165	166	167	168	169	170	171	172	173	174	175	176	177	178	179	180
All patients without restriction	181	182	183	184	185	186	187	188	189	190	191	192	193	194	195	196	197	198	199	200
Miscellaneous other	201	202	203	204	205	206	207	208	209	210	211	212	213	214	215	216	217	218	219	220

TABLE 11-3: Some Sample Entries in a Mental Health Resources Directory

Index No.	Variable Interaction
1	*(Involuntary hospitalization)* X *(Military eligibility)* George Patton Army Hospital, 100 Main St., Greenville, 794-6000, Ext. 538, ask for medical officer of the day or report to infirmary, building 7. Limited to persons on active duty, U.S. Army, and immediate dependents.
21	*(Involuntary hospitalization)* X *(VA Hospital)* None within 50 miles
41	*(Involuntary hospitalization)* X *(U.S. Public Health Service)* None within 50 miles
61	*(Involuntary hospitalization)* X *(State Hospital)* Gardenview State Hospital, 7465 Bridge St., Gardenview, 846-8035, phasing out acute treatment facilities for mentally ill; units for the mentally retarded accepting admissions; call medical officer of the day.
81	*(Involuntary hospitalization)* X *(This county)* Morgan County General Hospital, 4739 Polk St., Hillsdale, 750-7744; 24-bed locked psychiatric unit; preference given to welfare, MediCare patients; beds often filled; admission determined at emergency room.
	* * * * * * * * * * * * * * * * *
86	*(Halfway house)* X *(This county)* Greenacres House, 3215 Parkview Avenue, Burlington, 893-2649, ask for supervising social worker. All residents of this county 21 years and older eligible regardless of income; fee on sliding scale; psychotic problems are their main interest. Holden Caulfield House, 5482 Oak Street, Greenville, 673-8573, ask for

youth counselor in residence. Accepts both sexes, ages 14 to 18, individual and group counseling, especially for those with drug problems and those who have left home without parental consent. No fees charged; contributions accepted.

---

the George Patton Army Hospital, and completed the referral.

A 17-year-old boy who lives in this county engaged in a fierce argument with his parents and went out with friends and took street drugs (a repetition of a previous pattern). He was not intoxicated when he went into the emergency room and wanted to "rap" with someone about where he might go. (He was determined not to go home.) The therapist saw that he would need a place to live away from home at least temporarily and decided on a halfway house as being the most appropriate resource. After consulting index number 86 of the directory (halfway house, this county), the therapist decided that of the two listings Holden Caulfield House seemed the better choice for this patient, who accepted the referral.

Centers with access to a computer can use it for such a directory in two ways. First, the information needed to compile the directory can be stored in the computer; for instance, the names, addresses and special features of the various treatment facilities as well as the varying kinds of patient eligibility. Second, the information can be retrieved easily from the computer. When the therapist referred the 17-year-old boy, he had only to ask the computer for the information stored in cell 86 to find out what resources were available in the community.

Actual on-call duty is the final test of an emergency therapist's executive skill. How might a therapist apply the information and the logic set forth in this and preceding chapters in a busy emergency room? The following hypothetical situation, the test of mettle we referred to previously, will give the reader a chance to apply his working knowledge of emergency psychiatry.

PART 2: EMERGENCY ROOM EXERCISE

We shall present an emergency room situation, describe the personnel and facilities available to the emergency therapist, and give a number of vignettes of the patients who are to be seen. The reader should: (1) decide in which order the patients should be seen; (2) make initial diagnostic and treatment decisions, including the use of medication and hospitalization; and (3) decide on the most efficacious use of personnel and facilities available. After noting his answers, he may then read the solutions to the problems. The reader's solutions will not be exactly like the ones given here; each person will have his own way of conceptualizing the problems. It is hoped, however, that the basic principles underlying the solutions will correspond with those in the preceding chapters.

SITUATION

It is 5 P.M. You are taking over as the on-duty (O.D.) therapist in the emergency room of a county general hospital. You can admit patients to the hospital's fifteen-bed open-ward, therapeutic community; currently it has one bed open. When its beds are full or the patient needs referral to another facility, a state psychiatric hospital (with a locked ward) is available ten miles away. You have the authority to authorize an ambulance or cab to transport patients to their residences or to other medical facilities. This emergency room has a locked room. Personnel include a surgical intern, a nurse, an orderly, and a clerk. A medical resident is on call for consultation.

The therapist who has been covering the emergency room is on the telephone with a patient who says she wants to kill herself, but who will not give her name or telephone number. He continues to listen to her and writes you a note stating that it is important that he leave soon. You signal that you will respond shortly.

You check in with the nurse. She gives you a message that the nurse on the psychiatric unit has just called to ask you to see a 40-year-old woman who has fainted. She is being treated with chlorpromazine for schizophrenia. She was unconscious for less than thirty seconds and is now lying awake in her bed. Her pulse rate is regular at 110 per minute and her blood pressure is 90/60. There is also a patient on the unit who wants to talk to a doctor about his medication.

The nurse lists the patients waiting for you. A 22-year-old bearded man is sitting with two friends who are unsuccessfully trying to talk him down. The patient appears extremely anxious and is screaming that his mind is dissolving. Friends say that he took an unknown pink tablet that had been given to him by a stranger on the street.

An "ingestion" was brought in by ambulance five minutes ago. The patient is a 35-year-old housewife who the husband says took fifty capsules of secobarbital about one hour ago. She is presently unconscious with normal vital signs.

An adolescent girl, recently discharged from the county hospital psychiatric unit after having been treated with phenothiazines for schizophrenia, is holding her hands over her face. Her parents are with her. She is waiting to go home. She had already been seen by the previous O.D. for increasing nervousness and feeling that her "tongue was getting larger." The O.D. had examined her and found questionable swelling of the tongue, but no other signs of edema or spasm of the tissues of the neck and throat. His impression was that she was having an anxiety reaction, and he asked her to stay for further observation. The nurse points her out to you because she seems to be getting worse as she waits to go home. At that moment she shows no psychotic symptoms.

The police arrive with a violent man in handcuffs. The man's wife called the police after her husband, who had been drinking heavily, assaulted her. Three officers are required to contain him. The patient was discharged from the service with a diagnosis of mental illness and has a history of several previous hospitalizations for alcoholism.

A man and his wife are sitting with their 18-year-old son who has recently started hallucinating and has developed the idea that someone is out to get him. He has not left the house for two weeks.

You must make decisions about the following patients:

1. The anonymous, female telephone caller who is threatening suicide

2. The 40-year-old woman on the ward, diagnosed as schizophrenic, who fainted and is now conscious

3. The patient on the psychiatric unit who wants to talk to a doctor about his medication

4. The 22-year-old man who thinks his mind is dissolving

5. The 35-year-old housewife who ingested fifty secobarbital capsules an hour ago

6. The adolescent girl who is anxious and thinks her tongue is enlarging

7. The police-escorted violent man in handcuffs who had been drinking

8. The 18-year-old son who is hallucinating and thinks someone is out to get him

THE SOLUTIONS

We think the patients should be seen in the order shown for the following reasons. First, the woman who ingested secobarbital (patient 5) is an acute medical emergency. You ask the clerk to call the nurse on the psychiatric unit and tell her that an acute emergency has come in, that the woman who fainted should be kept in bed, and that you will be up as soon as you have a chance. You write a note to the O.D. going off duty to keep the suicidal patient on the telephone while you tend to an emergency. You ask the clerk to call the surgical intern to examine the comatose woman immediately, and you ask the nurse to record her vital signs and prepare for gastric lavage until the intern arrives; you call the medical resident and ask him to supervise the intern's work. You explain to the woman's husband that you are the emergency therapist, that his wife will receive emergency medical treatment first, that you would like him to wait until after you have seen some other patients so that you can speak with him about beginning psychotherapeutic treatment.

Second, you must deal with the suicidal woman on the telephone (patient 1) because her life or physical well-being is at stake. You take the phone from the O.D., talk with the patient, and ask for her name and telephone number. You explain that you cannot be of further service to her until you have this information. She continues to withhold it. You explain that you have to attend to other emergencies, and that you will refer her call back to the clerk so that the necessary registration can take place. This firm stand causes her reluctantly to give the information, including her address, and to say with some conviction that she will drive in and talk with you in person. You hang up and give the information to the clerk and ask her to inform you if the patient has not arrived in fifteen minutes so that you can call the police to investigate.

Third, you talk with the bearded man who thinks his mind is dissolving (patient 4) and to his friends because he is acutely agitated. You confirm that he has taken an unidentified street drug and explain that there is every reason to believe his current panic will pass with their support and with an injection of a medication that counteracts anxiety. You ask the nurse to prepare an intramuscular injection of 15 mg of diazepam (Valium®). As she gives it, you explain to the patient that this will reduce his terror. (You do *not* administer a phenothiazine, thereby precluding a possible autonomic crisis.) You explain to the patient and his friends that you will check back with them at intervals and that you will repeat the injection every hour as needed. When the patient is finally calm, you will arrange for follow-up care.

Fourth, you go to the police and the violent man who has been drinking (patient 7). The police have had him under control and he has not appeared to be in a medically dangerous condition. You confirm the smell of alcohol on his breath and ask the nurse to prepare an intramuscular injection of 100 mg of hydroxyzine (Vistaril®) and 100 mg of thiamine. Although the police may be impatient, you point out to them that the patient is not dangerous as long as they hold him. You ask them to take him to the locked room, have them remove his shoes, belt, valuables, and possible concealed weapons for safekeeping, make sure there is a mat in the room for the patient to sleep on, and ask the police to help hold him down for the injection. You explain to the patient why you are giving the injection and why you will be keeping him in the locked room until he regains control. The police leave. The nurse, with the orderly's help, should obtain vital signs as soon as feasible. You are prepared to check on the patient every hour and to repeat the injection in four hours if necessary.

Fifth, you turn to the adolescent girl who thinks her tongue is swelling (patient 6). She has been sitting quietly and has not appeared to be in serious distress. Her tongue *is* swelling, probably in reaction to phenothiazines. The medical resident confirms your impression and takes over her management, starting with an intramuscular injection of 50 mg of diphenhydramine (Benadryl®). He makes sure an airway is available in case there is a spasm of the tongue and muscles of the throat. She will remain for observation until the swelling has definitely subsided.

Sixth, the woman who threatened suicide on the phone (patient 1) has come in, and you interview her briefly. She has been drinking a little but she is not drunk. She tearfully describes how her boyfriend broke up with her earlier that day. After twenty minutes she seems to have somewhat recovered her composure. You explain that you want to talk with her at greater length, that there are other patients who need to be seen, and ask if she will wait until you can devote more time to her. She agrees to this, and you escort her to the waiting room. You introduce her to the clerk and ask the clerk to call you if the patient wants to leave before you have had a chance to talk with her.

Seventh, you interview the boy who has been hallucinating (patient 8) and, separately, his parents. This patient had not been in acute distress and could safely be allowed to sit with his parents while you attended to more urgent matters. You try to talk to his affect, to enter into his experiential world. You conclude he is in the midst of an acute schizophrenic episode, an impression strengthened by the parents' report of his change in behavior over the last several weeks. You explain to everyone that he is having trouble with his thinking and that he needs to enter the hospital for further evaluation and treatment. They agree, and you arrange for his admission to the psychiatric unit. Because the other patients you have to evaluate are on the ward, you accompany the patient and his parents there, introduce them to the staff, and ensure that his case will be taken over by the ward therapist in the morning. You write orders for 100 mg of chlorpromazine orally, or half of that intramuscularly, if he becomes agitated, cannot go to sleep, or seems to want to slip away. If he remains calm and can sleep, medication can be deferred.

Eighth, you see the woman on the ward who fainted (patient 2), but who now is feeling all right. You deferred her because you surmised that she probably suffered from orthostatic hypotension caused by chlorpromazine. You explain to her the necessity of shifting positions slowly, that hers is a common reaction to this kind of medication and usually goes away, and answer in simple terms any questions she has without burdening her with gratuitous technical information. If there are any suggestions of lingering aftereffects of the fall, e.g., cranial injury, you ask the medical resident to examine her. You ask the nurse to hold the next dose of chlorpromazine until the patient's standing blood pressure is up to 100/60.

Ninth, you talk to the patient on the ward about his medication (patient 3). If he wants to talk about medication change or a physical complaint unrelated to his psychiatric medications, make certain he is not asking for immediate psychological help in a veiled way. Then suggest he take the matter up with his usual doctor. If no serious immediate problem, such as a concealed suicidal or homicidal impulse, is hidden behind the seemingly trivial complaint, make sure his doctor will learn about his medical concerns by writing a note in the chart. If a problem with impulse control does emerge, help the patient deal with it.

Now you have seen all the patients. You return to the emergency room to find that the woman who ingested the secobarbital has had her stomach pumped and is under observation in the intensive care unit. The young man who thought his mind was dissolving has had his second injection and is distinctly calmer but not yet completely lucid. You will return to him later. The girl with the swollen tongue responded to medication, and the medical resident sent her home with her parents.

The alcoholic man in the locked room is both tremulous and sleepy. You order the next injection for four hours after the first one, that he be allowed to sleep there overnight, and that he be given periodic observation of his vital signs. You leave orders for the next day's O.D. to continue to observe for and treat signs of acute alcohol withdrawal, to evaluate the meaning of the drinking (whether symptomatic or addictive) and his potential for violence, and to engage the patient in follow-up treatment for his drinking (using an initial hospitalization if desirable).

You return to the woman who had broken up with her boyfriend and threatened suicide on the telephone. After a half-hour she feels better and gives you the name of some friends she might spend the night with. You call them and explain that the patient has been very upset about losing her friend and felt like hurting herself. The friends are happy to have her stay with them until she feels more in control. You put her on the telephone to work out the plans for her friends to pick her up. She is worried about sleep that night. You give her two flureazepam (Dalmane®) capsules and

arrange for a follow-up visit in the clinic the next day. She returns to the waiting room to wait for her friends.

The young man's panic has passed. He no longer fears his mind is dissolving, and he is lucid but exhausted from his ordeal. His friends are willing to have him stay with them that night. They will make sure he comes in for a follow-up visit in the clinic the next day. You give them a few diazepam tablets to give the patient in case he has difficulty falling asleep.

You interview the husband of the woman who ingested the secobarbital. You check with the intensive care unit, and they give a guardedly optimistic report on her outlook. You tell the husband, and he begins to describe a marital rift of several weeks' duration that was precipitated by his wife's learning of his involvement with another woman. Today the wife had inadvertently seen the two of them together in a shopping center, a fact she revealed in the note lying next to her in the bedroom where he had found her. Although the husband feels embarrassed and guilty about his role, he is not suicidal. He readily accepts the suggestion that he become involved in therapy as his wife recovers. He can afford private care. You give him the names of two therapists who do marital couple work and find out where you can reach him the next day around noon to find out how he is doing with the referrals. There is nothing more to be done for the time being, and he departs.

Your tour of duty is off to a busy start. You complete your paperwork and relax with a magazine until the next patient arrives.

REFERENCES

1. Salamon, I.: "Management of Psychiatric Emergencies," *N.Y. State J. Med.*, **73**: 1066–1067, 1973.

SECTION 2 The Outpatient Clinic

JOHN E. BEEBE III, M.D.
C. PETER ROSENBAUM, M.D.

Outpatient Therapy: An Overview

PART 1: TRANSFERENCE REVISITED

PRESENTING COMPLAINTS

As we saw in Section 1 of this book, crises often force patients to seek psychiatric help, but many enter the clinic under different circumstances. Patients come with a wide variety of presenting complaints and for many reasons. Some come because they are bothered by psychological symptoms such as anxiety and depression; they may or may not have been able to connect their symptoms with interpersonal or intrapsychic events. Some patients come, understandably anxious and depressed, because of an upheaval in their lives, e.g., the breaking up of a marriage, the end of a love affair, the loss of a job and so on. Others come because they recognize certain recurrent self-defeating or neurotic patterns in themselves that they want to change.

Certain patients may have been referred by an internist who found the patient's physical symptoms to be functional and strongly suspected an emotional cause. Some patients who have broken the law have had psychotherapy made a condition of probation (compulsive stealing and certain forms of public sexual behavior are two frequent kinds of offenses).

Section 2 deals with patients who can be treated in the clinic. This chapter describes many of the theoretical issues on which treatment decisions are based. Chapter 13 discusses the rationale for specific decisions about treatment.

PSYCHODYNAMICS

We shall begin with an overview of psychotherapy and a detailed discussion of transference, and shall then proceed to examine the kinds of approaches a modern outpatient clinic offers the patients who come to it for help. Much of this section will deal with what to the psychoanalytically educated mind has always been "psychiatry." We shall retain from the analytic tradition its belief that formulation, an understanding of the psychodynamics of the individual patient, is indispensable to any decision about treatment, but we prefer to formulate dynamics from a range of theoretical models, not just from psychoanalysis. Excellent sources of information about psychodynamics and psychopathology are White,[1] Ellenberger,[2] Hillman,[3] and Whyte.[4]

Psychodynamics broadly refers to an understanding of the interactions of conscious, unconscious, and reality; of past, present, and future.* Without clearly understanding the inner workings of the situation at hand, the therapist is really powerless to make a reasoned intervention. Still too much of psychotherapy is irrational therapy, with the disadvantage that in addition to very lucky hits there are a number of quite unlucky misses. Therapists must understand psychodynamics. Until the therapist clearly understands what the patient's behavior is accomplishing for him and what its probable antecedent causes are, he is in a very poor position to make definitive interventions.

The dynamic formulation is that part of the psychiatric examination that attempts to explain how the present situation came into being and what forces are causing it to continue to persist. It is an indispensable part of the treatment process (it is described more fully in Chapter 14).

The decision to enter therapy may be a momentous one for the patient. Very primitive emotions of hope and fear are usually operating. There is also considerable lack of clarity; patients frequently do not know, cannot say, why they seek psychiatric help. The therapist needs to develop a sensitive friendliness to the state of confusion that so frequently accompanies the entry into psychotherapy. The novelist Doris Lessing[7] describes in *The Four-Gated City* how hard it can be even for an intelligent patient if this initial feeling of confusion goes unrecognized:

> She went to her doctor, who sent her to a psychotherapist. This was a woman. The relationship lasted for a couple of confused

---

*The term *psychodynamics* seems to have originated with Jeremy Bentham,[5] who stated in 1817, "Psychological *dynamics* (by this name may be called the science, which has for its *subject* these same springs of action, considered as such) has for its basis psychological *pathology*." As Hillman[6] notes, Bentham characterized psychopathology as "the unseemly parts of the mind." Hillman points out that this nineteenth-century pathological bias is still with us when we try to formulate the "springs" of our patients' actions in the language of psychopathology.

months. The central fact here was glaringly obvious, like the sun in the tropics: both women were stupid about people and their relationships with each other. Both were perfectionists, and managing and dogmatic by nature. Mrs. Johns . . . knew all about Phoebe from her first interview with her. Phoebe believed in self-control, doing one's duty, and behaving well even when others did not – she could not see what was wrong with this.

The thing is, no one ever gets to that point of moral confusion where one finds oneself sitting before a human being privileged to pronounce on one's state of being without having wondered and suffered and doubted. Phoebe knew well enough that she was a sadly rigid soul. But here she was, seated opposite another! Who was Mrs. Johns to pronounce on her, Phoebe? Phoebe kept wishing that Mrs. Johns would come to the point: there must be one, surely? For it was implicit in her manner that truths were there to be seen, but every time a truth or the intimation of one emerged, Phoebe thought it was suspect.

The sort of impasse found in Lessing's example is preventable. The aim of this chapter is to give the therapist an idea about how he can get off to a different kind of start. It seems to us that good therapeutic sense begins with an understanding of transference.

TRANSFERENCE – THE KEY CONCEPT

Transference as An Intrapsychic Phenomenon

It is to Sigmund Freud, of course, that we owe the first formulation of the idea of transference. For Freud, transference referred to the *unconscious* attribution to a person or institution of qualities this "object" may or may not possess, these attributions reflecting repressed attitudes, beliefs, and feelings from childhood. As Ralph Greenson[8] says,

> Transference is the experiencing of feelings,

drives, attitudes, fantasies and defenses toward a person in the present which do not befit that person but are a repetition of reactions originating in regard to significant persons of early childhood, unconsciously displaced onto figures in the present. The two outstanding characteristics of a transference reaction are: it is a repetition and it is inappropriate.

Traditional psychoanalysis directs that the therapist often make himself a blank screen so that the patient's transference projections can be seen quite clearly. This means in practice that the therapist is mostly silent and non-self-disclosing to create a situation in which the patient's perception becomes colored as much as possible by his own intrapsychic habitual modes of perceiving. What emerges is a definite neurosis in which the person of the therapist is distorted in accordance with the patient's internal dynamics. The elucidation of this "transference neurosis" is felt to be indispensable to successful treatment, for it is thought that here, in relatively pure culture, the analyst can see what typically contaminates the patient's experience.

Psychoanalysis structures the situation rather as if the patient were a slide projector, and the therapist, in addition to being a blank screen, gives the patient no slide but turns on the projector. Often an unsuspected slide stuck in the projector shows upon the screen, the very picture of an unresolved infantile conflict. The hope is that such major, distorting carryovers from the past can be worked through in psychotherapy so that the patient-projector is able to approach the world sending out a mostly clear beam, capable of projecting whatever current slide is in his projector without distortion. Psychoanalysis, then, is an attempt to modify the patient's perception of the world by freeing him from the contaminating influence of past perceptions, and the famous inactivity of the traditional analyst is felt to be essential if the contaminating past is to be identified.

The model of perception on which psychoanalysis is implicitly based has been attacked by nearly every other major school of psychology, and the inactivity of the psychoanalyst abundantly caricatured, but the *experience* of transference in the psychoanalytic situation remains one of the fundamental discoveries of our era. In a famous conversation, Freud once asked Jung what he thought about transference, and Jung replied, "It is the alpha and omega in treatment." Freud then answered, "You have understood."

Indeed, it would scarcely be possible to understand psychotherapy without appreciating the central position of transference phenomena. Furthermore, it would seem that all emotional interaction contains much of what we experience in individual psychotherapy as transference. Choices of jobs, husbands, wives, friends, penchants for behaving in certain ways, ways of experiencing others in the environment, all these involve projections based on the past, a special sort of experiential conditioning. Thus it is no accident that as a patient first enters the psychotherapist's office, he brings with him his own highly charged, individual atmosphere of feeling and perception that immediately expresses itself in the ways he reacts to the therapist and the office, and which elicit, in turn, feelings and emotions in the therapist that partly existed before the appearance of the patient.

Transference as An Interpersonal Phenomenon

When we consider that transference also involves the therapist's experience, the slide projector model is inadequate. It becomes necessary to deal with transference in its interpersonal aspects. This next step from Freud has been hard to take. Freud's original model, for all its limitations, has fascinated the modern mind, which continues to wonder at its own capacity for self-deception and projection. Therefore, attempts to expand it to include the interpersonal seem never quite satisfactory, seem always to dilute Freud. Every five or ten years another theorist still feels the need to comment on the dimension that Freud left out, only to discover that his is received as the weaker formulation.

Interpersonal theorists' formulations are considerably more complicated than Freud's in explaining countertransference, the therapist's (largely) unconscious reactions. For the interpersonalists, it is as if the patient and therapist meet together at both a conscious and a transference level — unconscious shaking hands with unconscious — so that the emotional atmosphere of one encounters the emotional atmosphere of the other, creating together a new experiential world in which both persons participate. Consciousness allows the therapist and patient to collaborate, together studying their mutual effects on each other.

Interpersonal theorists are usually less pessimistic about the unconscious than Freud; unconscious transference effects are often viewed as positive, not merely distortions, as Kaiser[9] describes so well in his *Effective Psychotherapy*. Traditional psychoanalysts have commented on the difficulties in studying the patient at all, once the therapist enters into active intervention. In interactive therapy, the therapist brings his own relationship-ego to the transference atmosphere created by the interaction of the patient's and his own dynamics, and he makes verbal use of this ability to watch from within to help the patient become more aware of the transaction in which they are both involved. Sullivan calls this method "participant-observation."

Transference as Recapitulation of Past Coping

Thus far we have discussed transference as a *process*, first as an individual phenomenon, then as an interpersonal one. Now we look at its *content*. Content is not as popular now as it once was, but content remains the ground of experiencing; content is the ultimate information about the self which can be learned in psychotherapy. Content information becomes relevant whenever psychotherapy is conceived, not merely as an unconscious transition from a less adaptive to a more adaptive state of being, but also as an educative experience

in which conscious understanding of how the individual has changed takes part. Patients want and deserve such understanding.

Transference is first of all a recapitulation of past coping strategies in the stress of a new situation. The following example is a stereotyped situation with which many therapists will be familiar.

> *Example 12-1.* A drunken, chronic alcoholic man comes into the emergency room. He is hungry, tremulous, and boisterous. He is received by the night shift receptionist who requested night duty when she became estranged from her own alcoholic husband. She calls the emergency therapist, who has a problem drinker brother-in-law and who, moreover, has been awakened at 2 A.M. four times previously this week because of drinking patients. The alcoholic patient himself despairs of receiving much good treatment for his current dilemma (and privately, in his more sober moments, he considers himself a hopeless failure, unworthy of decent care by anyone), and both the secretary and the intern find themselves quite angry at this intruder. The secretary says on the telephone to the therapist, "We have another one for you," and the therapist says back to the secretary, "Oh God! Well, I'll be down."

The interaction begins on a note that promises a highly stereotyped pattern of rejection. The patient, for his part, can be viewed as a help-rejecting complainer. The doctor is more likely than not to behave as a help-pretending rejector. And yet this is the first meeting of a new patient with a new doctor. Each brings to a situation *which is in fact new for both* old ways of operating. If both continue to behave in accordance with unconscious stereotypes, the transition will reinforce both in their belief that alcoholism is a frustrating, hopeless condition that can only be managed by grudging, temporary, ineffective support. This is, in fact, how both have coped with alcoholism in the past, and each time a new experience is forced into the old unconscious transference mold, the stereotyped solution becomes more fixed, seemingly all the more supported by evidence.

The content of both transference and countertransference starts before the patient walks in the door. The actual encounter can be said to "constellate" this content so that an unconscious decision about how treatment will proceed is reached by both participants with remarkable speed. Unless one or the other makes a conscious effort, there will be no exploration of the implicit contract, and the therapy will proceed unconsciously, and almost always in a neurotically stereotyped fashion.

The therapist has to be aware of this stereotype if he is to overcome it. Much of the early work of therapy is trying to make conscious the initial pull into an unconscious contract. Supervision often identifies a therapist's unwitting participation in the patient's pathologic approach to problem solving. Every supervisor is aware that the pretty, girlish patient who treats her therapist as if he were a father often elicits from the inexperienced therapist a certain paternal pomposity, and that the work of therapy can proceed only when one or the other takes the risk of exploding the tight bind this very common transference places on their interaction. Although it can sometimes be adaptive for a woman to behave like a pleasing little girl with men, and for a professional man to carry paternal authority, overemphasis on these styles in a recapitulation of past coping behavior precludes any new learning about the interaction of an adult man and woman.

Transference as Anticipation of Future Coping

Undue emphasis upon the regressive and maladaptive elements of transference distortions is one of the gravest drawbacks of the original psychoanalytic formulations of transference. Henri Ellenberger[10] has shown that the roots of this bias lie in the psychologies of self-deception, which were extremely popular during the late nineteenth century. Jung recognized early that transference distorts as well in a progressive direction, projecting onto the therapeutic relationship and the therapist the possibility of new development. Although at the outset of therapy the projection may be unrealistically positive, it may also contain a picture of the self the patient is able to become as a result of therapy. Similarly, the therapist can find himself responding to the patient in a new, fresh way at the outset of treatment, as if he were finding in himself a new way of relating to such persons. This anticipation of a possible new kind of coping lends hope and excitement to the process of therapy.

The beginning of therapy often is slanted toward either past experience of repetitive failure or the hope of future success in interpersonal relationships. Either transference reaction can become too extreme. Hope can be a subtle trap for both the patient and the therapist; it can substitute for the necessary acceptance of frustration which is essential to realistic functioning. Pessimism can slowly poison therapeutic life.

In general, it is wise for the therapist to pay attention to the content of initial dreams, fantasies about therapy, and comments about therapy, in himself as well as in the patient. This initial transference, often very strong, frequently tells how therapy is likely to proceed. Optimistic fantasy can give confidence; pessimistic fantasy should give pause. Is this a case in which therapy could do harm?

Particular emphasis should be given to accidents occurring outside therapy in early weeks, or to dreams portending disaster, danger, and the like. These often have predictive significance as to the impact of therapy.

The Real Relationship – A Base Line

It is necessary to have a base line upon which to gauge transference. This base line is the real relationship between the patient and therapist. The "real relationship" is perhaps a misnomer; more precisely, it is the conscious relationship between the patient and therapist. This involves events such as the therapist's behavior, his office and dress, his punctuality, all of which should be uniform enough to give the patient a certain experience of regularity and to give the therapist a certain sense of self-continuity. Most therapists will now concede it is both impossible and undesirable to maintain a totally blank screen for patients, but it is nevertheless possible to provide a certain base line against which the intrusion of emotional distortion can be measured.

The therapist's attempt to establish a base line shoul l not be extremely rigid and punctilious. The base line should not be a straitjacket; it should be a comfortable, working rapport that enables both the therapist and patient to experience major variation as the effect of strong emotion, which can then be examined.

At a deep level, of course, even the comfortable, working relationship is a transference fiction, a still largely unconscious arrangement predicated in large part by interpersonal attraction and need. Whitehorn and Betz[11] have suggested that successful psychotherapy depends upon a kind of unconscious fit between the therapist and patient, in which the therapist's need to work with a particular kind of person may be as important as the patient's need to work with a particular kind of therapist. Although it is impossible to avoid unconscious relating, it can be examined to ensure that the fit furthers rather than hinders therapy.

In exploring transference, therapists usually do not initially interpret the base line of general mutual liking and respect. Transference interpretations are confined to intrusions of excessive positive or negative affect that interfere with the working relationship. Generally, it is not a good idea to tamper too much with the base line if meaningful work is to be done on other areas of the patient's life. There is no theoretical end to the process of making unconscious transactions conscious, but there must be a practical abstention from too much examination of a transaction between the patient and therapist. Otherwise no other content can be discussed. Also, what is working well at an unconscious level does not *need* to be explored; we take apart the watch that *does not* tick.

Toward the end of therapy, most therapists like to get some discussion of the real relationship that has been the vehicle for therapy all along. At the beginning of therapy, such discussion merely makes the process more difficult for the patient and deprives him of the interpersonal security and unselfconsciousness that permit him to discuss openly and fully disturbances in all areas of his life.

Institutional Transference

Transference does not occur only between individuals. Important transferences are also made to institutions, including the institution of the healer's role. When patients perceive therapists as agents of societal authority more than as interested persons, therapy is comparable to going to confession and not noticing the priest. Often, the therapist is initially made to feel anonymous. Therapists who dislike this anonymity sometimes forget that their role, or the institution in which they serve, is providing an important base of their effectiveness to some patients.

Therapists and patients working in an institutional setting accord a mutual transference to that institution, and the support it gives to both should not be underestimated. Therapists who go into private practice often report what an astonishing experience it is to be without the symbolic support of an institution's walls. As one therapist reported, it was as if suddenly she were out in a boat on an open sea, alone with each patient, and her right arm grew sore from bailing out water whenever an unconscious leak occurred.

Many therapies make practical use of the institutional aspects of the transference. Chapter 18 ("Supportive Psychotherapy") illustrates this kind of treatment.

STAGES OF THE TRANSFERENCE IN ALL PSYCHOTHERAPIES

In any psychotherapeutic treatment, the transference relationship evolves with time. As therapy progresses, or if it progresses, it is possible to observe certain typical sequential stages of the transference. It is quite possible for therapy to get stuck at any of the stages. Each stage, moreover, depends upon successful evolution of the previous stage. Finally, these stages seem to be common to all psychotherapies.

In our view four distinct stages are discernible: contact, confrontation, initiation, and individuation.* Our descriptions of the stages are designed to give the therapist a sense of where he is with a given patient at a given time so he knows what he can and cannot expect of the therapy at that point. This model is intended to replace the more traditional view of psychotherapy as a three-stage process involving beginning, middle, and end of treatment.[14] These four stages are most likely to be seen in long-term, uncovering psychotherapy. In the reality-oriented therapies, perhaps only one or two of the stages will be apparent; for example, in supportive work with schizophrenic patients, the stages of contact and confrontation may predominate, and in behavior modification the stages of confrontation and initiation are the main ones.

Contact

In the first stage of therapy, the therapist and patient must make psychological contact with each other. Rogers[15] postulates psychological contact as the condition in which the client feels psychologically received by the therapist, that certain qualities in the therapist — genuineness, accurate empathic understanding, nonpossessive warmth — are requisite to successful psychother-

apy, and that the client must be able to perceive these qualities in the therapist. Much has been said in praise and criticism of Rogers' ideas of the "necessary and sufficient" ingredients of the successful therapist's personality. Less well known is his conception of neurosis as a condition in which a person becomes separated from his experiencing in infancy by the need to satisfy certain "conditions of worth" that he perceives as coming from his parents. It is Rogers' deliberate aim to remove from the therapeutic situation all such conditions of worth so that this living against (or at some remove from) felt experiencing can come to an end in an atmosphere of "unconditional positive regard."

Harry Stack Sullivan has called the ways in which neurotics avoid their natural experiencing in order to satisfy fantasied environmental demands as "security operations."[16] Franz Alexander and Thomas French[17] have talked about psychotherapy as a "corrective emotional experience," and they stress too that the therapist needs to supply an atmosphere in which constructive change is made possible.

Contact occurs between the therapist's listening or treating consciousness and the patient's preconscious experiencing. This contact is described in Freudian circles as the "working alliance." This alliance is the basis of all later therapeutic work. Unconscious factors play a part in the making of a working alliance. For example, it is often sufficient that the patient like the therapist and that the therapist like the patient for the first stage of transference to come into being and for the entire therapeutic process to be set in motion. Rogers once said in response to a beginning therapist's question that it could even be of help if the therapist felt sexually attracted to the patient. The opposite, an attraction based on power needs in the therapist, can also be effective in certain situations. Many authoritarian patients like authoritarian therapists. Some therapists intuitively relate better to men, others to women. Some therapists are able to relate well to older people but have difficulty with younger people. We are still very

---

*The four-stage conception is derived from the comparative study of healing systems as found in Jerome Frank's *Persuasion and Healing*[12] and C. G. Jung's *The Integration of Personality.*[13]

much in the process of learning why it is that people are able to make psychological contact with each other in some circumstances and not in others.

Often psychological contact is *implicit.* A great deal has occurred psychologically before a patient can approach a therapist and say, "I have such-and-such a symptom that I would like to overcome." To be able to make such a request, the patient must be able to accept the therapist's approach and to trust him with the responsibility of dealing with his problem. If the patient has not made psychological contact with the therapist, he simply cannot submit to treatment.

Sometimes, psychological contact is *faked.* Then we see patients who seem to be in treatment, who make verbal assurances that they are participating meaningfully in the process, but whose actual therapeutic progress is nil or marked by missed appointments, unpaid bills, dramatic evasions, and so on. The therapist needs to realize that such patients, despite their protestations to the contrary, have not made contact and thus have not really entered therapy.

Many patients find it difficult or impossible to make contact with anyone. For them, the most important part of therapy is the process of making contact. This sensitivity is particularly true of schizophrenic patients, schizoid personalities, and certain adolescents. Equally, there are some patients who can make contact *only* with their therapists and resist any movement that might lead them out of the state of symbiotic fusion with a helping person. In this group belong the "therapy addicts," including unhappy women with somatic complaints who go through long and moderately satisfying periods under the care of fatherly internists. They do not proceed beyond the stage of psychological contact in their transference relationships to their physicians, nor do they want to. They are paying for very real gratification. Erotic transferences, as Freud[18] pointed out, are a way of clinging to the therapist as a defense against further movement. In some circumstances, they must be interpreted as such.

Confrontation

For most patients, the state of being psychologically received by the therapist is not sufficient to satisfy the pressure to health. The appetite for healing asks not just a feeling of being valued or needed, but also mastery of the difficulties of living. At the stage of confrontation, patient and therapist begin to grapple with the *content* of what is wrong. The stage of confrontation has been reached when the therapist is able to make a direct comment about the patient's life without loss of rapport. At this point, the patient starts commenting on himself with an emphasis on his pathology. He begins actively to point out areas in which he feels he needs to do work.

Probably the stage of confrontation cannot proceed naturally until the stage of contact has been adequately experienced. This point is often unappreciated in the modern lust to confront. At present, confrontation is an extremely popular therapeutic technique; there are confrontation groups and confrontation wards. An almost Messianic quality is discernible in some who use confrontation; they talk as if they were rescuing psychiatry from overinvestment in gentle, passive listening. Such evangelism ignores the fact that confrontation has always been a part of psychotherapy, and although the new emphasis on confrontation is a good corrective to therapy that stresses only the contact stage of transference, meaningful confrontation grows of itself out of the condition of psychological contact in patients who are ready to go further. It is often wiser not to push. We are learning, indeed, that not everyone can handle confrontation. Harold Searles[19] pointed out that one of the several ways of driving another person crazy is to continually point to areas of himself of which he is unaware. Yalom and Lieberman's[20] report of encounter group casualties, persons who developed serious neurotic depressive or anxiety states or psychotic breaks in the course of T group or encounter group experiences, is good testimony to this.

The most common disadvantage of confronting

someone with whom the other person is not in contact is that the confrontation is not heard. Almost every experienced therapist has had his patients tell him that in therapy they learn things about themselves that friends and family members have been telling them for years. The difference is that the therapist's word is trusted and believed. If he confronts too early, it may not be.

It is common to hear experienced therapists who have worked for some time with a difficult patient say, "Well, he's finally *in treatment*," meaning the patient is engaged and the working alliance is operating after a frustratingly slow start. This development corresponds to having arrived squarely at the stage of confrontation.

Like contact, confrontation can become an addiction. Some patients are quite willing to come to therapy for years, repeatedly telling their therapists and themselves what is wrong with them. This kind of patient frequently elicits highly critical comments from the naïve therapist, who assumes that by joining the patient's attack on his pathology he is somehow assisting him to achieve self-understanding. In fact, the therapist may only be satisfying the patient's masochistic need to recreate a childhood situation in which he was repeatedly verbally abused. Along with patients who can only be confronted, we have to mention therapists who can only confront. Sometimes therapists have to balance the urge to confront angrily with the need to confront therapeutically.

A kind of stalemate comes toward the end of the period of confrontation. It seems as if the problem, although named, can never be solved. Both the patient and therapist are likely to feel intense frustration during this period. To avoid getting stuck at the stage of confrontation, it is frequently better to admit the perplexing, defeating feel of the situation than to attempt fresh confrontation, as if to whip the unconscious into coming up with some answer. When the therapist finds himself in the bind of repeatedly confronting the same situation, it is better for him to recognize the impasse than to turn the therapy into a weekly brutal, sadomasochistic ritual. Impasse is natural, and necessary to being convinced of the need for a new solution, which appears in the stage of initiation.

Initiation

The word initiation is used to discuss the next stage of psychotherapy because it suggests the idea of a kind of rite of passage into the stage of health. Such a rite of passage, very similar to those rites by which traditional cultures mark the move from the stage of childhood to that of adulthood, is both a natural stage in the psychology of the patient as he moves from one state of being to another, and a period of active treatment on the part of the therapist, who functions very like a shaman according to his own special skills. This is the point in psychotherapy when both the therapist and patient feel that something must be done, that something has to happen.

Here is where the schools of psychotherapy differ in all their glorious variety, just as initiation rites vary from tribe to tribe. Each school has its own idea as to the right content of the rite of passage from the "sick", undesired state to the "healthy", desired state. For psychoanalysis, initiation is "working through." For behavior therapy it is some form of new learning, conditioning, or desensitization. In Jungian therapy, it is frequently dream analysis. In client-centered therapy, it is the unfolding of the experiential process in response to accurate reflections of feeling.

At this discrete psychological stage of treatment, the patient and therapist feel that they are actively tackling the problem, that the neurotic walls are tumbling down, and that meaningful therapeutic change is occurring. This is the period during which the patient and therapist feel most intensely that therapy is working. This is also the stage during which the patient becomes most evangelical about therapy, telling family and friends how helpful it is and encouraging them to undergo the exact same initiation he is experiencing.

However, not every patient can be initiated in the same way, nor can every therapist initiate in every way. Even though it is helpful for the therapist to try to develop as large a repertoire as possible, the fact remains that each therapist becomes comfortable with some ways of guiding patients at this stage and not with others. So it is that a patient who has passed successfully through the stages of contact and confrontation and can now see what is wrong may not always be able to work on what is wrong with the same therapist. It is not inappropriate to refer a patient at the stage when he is ready for a meaningful initiation that can be conducted better by another therapist. Sometimes patients leave therapy at the point that they know what is wrong and go into a life experience that can, far more satisfactorily than therapy, provide the necessary initiation.

As with the stages of contact and confrontation, the stage of initiation also has its addicts. Among these are some therapists who become unconscionable dogmatists, expounding the joys of their own method of initiation in an inflated fashion, as if theirs were the only way to help people develop. Many initiation addicts are patients who, although they have been successfully helped by therapy through the stage of initiation, seem destined to repeat that initiation ad nauseam, bringing its once rich content into every situation, however inappropriate. Anyone finding himself in the bind of becoming too sold on the glories of what he has already experienced ought to acknowledge that he has begun to repeat himself and to wonder why this is so. For therapy can proceed beyond the stage of initiation.

Individuation

This in Jung's[21] sense is that process by which the personality becomes integrated according to its own plan, now not dependent upon models derived from the infantile, the environmental, or the therapeutic situation, but somehow differentiated into "that self which one truly is." When therapy enters this stage, the developmental process becomes conscious, and the patient actively seeks to futher his own maturation. The inappro-

priate and repetitious transference distortions from the past are no longer dominant, although some always persist: the "completely analyzed person" is a myth, but successfully treated, more independent people are many.

In the transference, this stage is heralded by a new kind of resistance, a resistance that the wise therapist will recognize as healthy. It is a resistance to the therapist's way of conceptualizing and initiating, a withdrawal from the earlier processes of contact, confrontation, and initiation that have made this stage possible, into a more actually self-defined condition. Now the Messianic inflated praise of therapy and therapist begins to fold its tent, and the patient starts taking his own life firmly in hand, withdrawing previous projections from the therapist. We believe this stage can only take place in the company of a therapist who is himself individuated enough not to need his patient to immortalize his own style. This is the stage at which the patient makes therapy his own once and for all. The therapist at this stage, according to Joseph Henderson,[22] becomes now a "symbolic friend," who helps the patient out of his general understanding of psychology wherever he can, but is in every other respect very much at the level of a peer in the patient's life. There is much less active "treating" of the patient at this stage, but the therapist stays available to further the patient's own process at any point that his information and experience might contribute.

A Jungian therapist, for instance, might be useful to a patient when a particularly puzzling dream can be elucidated by the comparative symbolism at the Jungian analyst's disposal. A behavior therapist might be able to suggest some new form of desensitizing procedure for a particular kind of maladaptive behavior that the less anxious patient might wish to work on.

As with every other stage, even individuation has its addicts: those who will not depend especially upon any particular therapeutic style or therapist but are perhaps too sold on their individual approaches to life to be comfortable in relating to others. Meaningful psychotherapy, like successful personal growth, never ends; but to the degree that therapy is successful there should be a kind of dissolving of the entire transference into some kind of living in the world so that the outlines of the now strong enough individual become less important than the experienced flexible adaptation to living. Descriptions of self-actualization are generally impossible, for the simple reason that self-actualization is a process, not a pose. Such people, innately themselves, tend to be immediate and real; and, at the risk of being flippant, it might be said that the "well-analyzed" person may in his relation to therapy be compared to the perfect haircut which conjures up no image of barber chairs either before or after.

Although formal therapy may end after a few years, informal therapy may be a lifetime process. The former patient, now accustomed to thinking about his life in psychological terms, continues to do so, especially at times of personal distress or puzzlement. He notices that he feels depressed or anxious and wonders why. Often, on introspection or thinking about his dreams, he can figure out why, and then either accept the upsetting situation more comfortably or figure out adaptive ways of dealing with it. If the distress continues, he may wish to reenter therapy to do some "postgraduate" work.

HANDLING OF THE TRANSFERENCE IN VARIOUS THERAPIES

Psychoanalysis

In this form of therapy the therapist does very little reaching out to produce contact. Rather he selects as his patient someone with a relatively strong ego who is capable of enduring a relatively low level of actual gratification in the therapeutic situation, but who accepts the basic premise that the therapist is working in his own best interest by refraining from much engagement with him. The patient's healthy ego then maintains the contact at an implicit level, while a kind of explicit frustration is undergone.

Confrontation takes place in the early weeks and months of therapy as the patient comes to see how he reacts to the therapist and to significant others in his life in neurotic and overdetermined ways that hamper his full effectiveness. As treatment proceeds, new, different, or more profound levels of conflict may be identified – the peeling of the layers of the onion – so that confrontation in one form or another extends deep into the treatment as new areas first of resistance and then of comprehension make their appearance.

As awareness of intrapsychic phenomena increases, the patient's perception of the therapy and of his interpersonal relations becomes based more on current reality and less on previous transference distortions. To the extent that insight leads to behavior change (and it often does, despite criticisms to the contrary), the patient is in the stage of initiation. Even "purely intellectual insight" (as contrasted with emotional or affective insight) can lead to behavior change. Freud[23] said, in another context, "The voice of the intellect is a soft one, but it does not rest until it has gained a hearing. Ultimately, after endlessly repeated rebuffs, it succeeds."

The combination of confrontation and initiation, the repeated assessment of neurotic perceptions and emotional responses to situations, the chipping away at the core of the neurosis, is what psychoanalysts have termed the "working through," and when it is complete the patient is into the stage of individuation.

Analytical Psychology

Jungian analysis takes a markedly different view of the transference situation. It is accepted that the therapist's own actual personality is required to "constellate" from the patient's unconscious that "archetype" that will guide him through the therapy. Thus, a patient who has suffered paternal deprivation may, in contact with a male therapist, begin to experience the father archetype that is needed to guide him in the maturation of his personality. For this reason, Jungians frequently spend much time deciding whether the patient will see a male or female, or an older or younger, therapist, and make a considerable effort to match the therapist and patient to each other according to personalities. (Often a patient will change therapists to experience another healing arche-type.)

The stage of confrontation in Jungian analysis is viewed as the experience of the "shadow," or unacceptable identity, and considerable effort is made to help the patient achieve a conscious relationship to this. The stage of initiation involves the experience of positive features of the shadow which carry the seeds of new growth. These usually involve contrasexual aspects of the per-son's psychology, the discovery of the "anima" in a man and "animus" in a woman. A considerable amount of education is done by the therapist with the patient to help him see the value in unaccepted or unrecognized parts of himself, which formerly were encountered only in projection onto others. The stage of individuation in Jungian analysis comes when the once unowned, dissociated, and projected parts of the self are now owned as related to the conscious personality in a relation-ship of polar opposition. For the Jungian, finding the opposite to his own point of view and holding onto it as his necessary complement is the essence of wholeness. At this stage, few projections oper-ate to divide the personality, and the therapist no longer carries the image of the patient's needed strength. As in Freudian analysis, the projection onto him of the guiding light of therapy is withdrawn.

Interpersonal Therapy

Sullivan conceptualizes the transference relation-ship as an interpersonal field in which the patient creates "parataxic distortion" of the relationship based on his early experience. The patient system-atically distorts aspects of the relationship pri-marily by the mechanisms of selective inattention, sublimation, and obsessionalism. The therapist deals with these parataxic distortions not only by direct confrontation, but also by making use of his own experience of the interpersonal situation. The therapist becomes an expert commentator upon the interpersonal field as he knows it from "participant observation." In this interpersonal field, the therapist is well aware that he, too, makes parataxic distortions by selective inatten-tion. By his own courageous willingness to discuss his experience of the patient in the hour, however, he renders these distortions accessible to feedback from the patient. The therapist's acceptance of correction is a model for the patient to receive feedback from the therapist in turn when he is distorting the emotional field. The therapy then becomes a kind of intense collaboration in which the major therapeutic initiation consists of work-ing through parataxic distortions until a relatively distortion-free interpersonal atmosphere obtains.

Perhaps no one has described more fully the need for the therapist to freely offer up his own parataxic distortions to the scrutiny of the patient than Searles,[24] whose book *Collective Papers on Schizophrenia and Related Subjects* describes the handling of countertransference phenomena by means of self-analysis and self-disclosure in the service of ever-increasing clarification. It should be said that Searles' formulations are very akin to the concept of "participation mystique" in Jung's work and "projective identification" in the writ-ings of Melanie Klein. These theorists all attempt to formulate the intense interpersonal mutuality that is integral to the phenomenon of transference. What distinguishes members of these schools is their willingness to discuss openly the ways in which the patient makes the therapist feel, in order to free the patient from an unconscious identification with him.

Adlerian Therapy

Adlerian therapy consists primarily in the rigor-ous examination and confrontation by the thera-pist of the patient's lifestyle. To Adler is owed a great deal of the understanding of the psychology of the ego and its typical adaptive and maladaptive ways of dealing with society. Once the lifestyle is grasped in the stage of contact, the relationship with the patient is used primarily to make vigorous confrontation acceptable to the patient. Advice and exhortation are common in this form of therapy.

Bierer[25] states:

> For suggestion Adler substituted persuasion, and relied upon the dialectic [which], in the case of both Adler and Socrates, starts from the assumption of ignorance on the part of both parties and endeavours a joint pursuit of truth by means of questions and answers. . . . The task of the psychologist is to prove to the patient out of his own mouth that his method of thought is a wrong one.

Typical of Adler is the view that the position of the ego is a stance, and that the neurotic syndrome is an "arrangement" by which the patient satisfies his needs for power in the world. By taking this position toward the patient's system of emotional attitudes and behaviors, the Adlerian therapist assumes from the outset that the patient has choice in his manner of presenting himself and a responsibility to find a socially satisfactory means of expressing his own individual needs for power in relationship to others. Confrontation then becomes a form of initiation. The therapist takes a strong position vis-à-vis the patient's ego, which is assumed to be basically powerful, responsible, and capable of choice, including the choice of resisting the therapist.

Client-centered Therapy

Client-centered therapy has been distinguished since its origins in Otto Rank's "will therapy" [26,27] by its emphasis upon the here-and-now experiencing of the "client." (It is consistent with Rogers' entire point of view that the medical term "patient" has been dropped.) In classical client-centered therapy the therapist does not engage in much frank self-disclosure or direct confrontation with the client, but he does vitally attach himself to the client's experiencing of the here-and-now situation during the therapeutic hour, and the therapist's every response is aimed at an accurate "reflection of feeling," emphasizing always the "affective" aspects of the client's comments in an attempt to bring to the client a profound acceptance first by the therapist and then by himself of his own experiencing. This acceptance implies confrontation with the possibility of one's own affective life as well as passive contact with the therapist. Client-centered therapists feel that it is affect which drives the process of self-actualization, and it is sufficient for healing that a client come to experience his own affective track and to follow it wherever it leads him. The therapist is thus a maximum facilitator who is using the interpersonal relationship to promote an intrapsychic process.

In this respect client-centered therapy is very similar to both Freudian and Jungian analysis in the attempt to use interpersonal dialogue as a means of promoting intrapsychic communication. The pièce de resistance of client-centered therapy is the client's discovery of his own experiential process and his moving to "greater stages of process" as he takes more seriously the affective dimension of himself.

There is remarkably little emphasis on content in client-centered therapy; thus specific dream motifs or supposedly pathogenic complexes have in themselves no interest for the traditional Rogerian. Instead, the self is considered purely as experiencing. Rogers feels that in this kind of therapy no transference neurosis develops because immediate gratification in reality is provided by the therapist's attention to the client's experiencing. The decisions about what to confront are made entirely by the client, as his own experiencing leads him into areas in which he is not happy about himself.

In a sense, individuation is assumed from the beginning of client-centered therapy, and it is indeed disarmingly individuating to the patient to have his every statement returned to him with an affective resonance by an experienced client-centered therapist. This style Rogers has always employed in responding to his critics: he simply takes the felt meaning of what they are saying to him with unconditional positive regard. More than one critic has gone away from Rogers saying, "Well he finally understood what so many others have tried unsuccessfully to tell him," without realizing that he is the beneficiary of Rogers' remarkable technique.[28]

Behavior Therapy

In this form of therapy the initiation stage of treatment is the most important. However, before a successful desensitizing or avoidance-conditioning procedure can be applied, preparations resembling the stages of contact and confrontation must be undertaken. (These preparations are described in Chapter 21.) Equally, many analysts who work with severely neurotic and borderline patients feel about behavior therapy that by the time the patients are quite clear about what is wrong with them and are willing to go to a behavior therapist, most of the work that consumes them with the patients they see has already been done. To formulate a goal clearly is not easy for many patients in therapy, and many patients who present themselves to therapy do not come to have a specific symptom removed.

Although other schools of therapy have much to offer with understanding of the stages of contact and confrontation, many of their therapists are surprisingly lacking when it comes to the specific initiatory procedures necessary to help the patient over the specific difficulties that finally emerge. It is to the credit of behavior therapists that they have brought us a whole new emphasis on specific means of helping those with specified problems.

Behavior therapy is a narrowing of the great stream of directive therapy that received so much attention before World War I, primarily as the result of Pierre Janet's major influence. Janet, as Ellenberger[29] has shown, was a master of the practical. His understanding of the destructive and constructive use of psychological energy, and his practical suggestions for avoiding wastes of nervous force and achieving greater degrees of psychological organization (or "tension") remain a landmark of practical psychotherapeutics. The triumph of Viennese psychoanalysis over French psychological analysis led to two generations of neglect of the role of directive techniques in dynamic psychiatry. In the past decade directive psychotherapy has staged a remarkable comeback, coinciding with a general decline of faith in psychoanalysis as the sole or preeminent mode of treatment.

What is characteristic of suggestive, hypnotic, prescriptive, and behavioral techniques is that the transference relationship is assumed and manipulated rather than discussed. Nevertheless, the stages of contact and confrontation have been reached. A very specific behavioral analysis of the problem, and sometimes a dynamic formulation of it, has usually been attempted. Based on the analysis, specific procedures are recommended. So long as direction is not undertaken in a way that suggests that the therapist is able or about to take control of every part of the patient's life, the specific initiatory procedures employed by even these very directive therapists need not interfere with the patient's later individuation into someone who can learn to control his own behavior according to the techniques he has now learned from the therapist.

Comment

A final way to review the schools involves a sense of the human life cycle.[30] It has been remarked that, "If you need therapy when you are an adolescent, see an Adlerian; during young adulthood, a Freudian; and in maturity, a Jungian." Adolescents are concerned with power, autonomy, and sexuality, of establishing an arrangement with the world, and Adlerians deal with these issues. Young adults have already come to some kind of arrangement with the world, but often find the arrangement unsatisfactory and need to explore the neurotic limitations they unconsciously impose on the arrangement. Patients in their middle years have grown largely past a vital interest in struggling with their arrangement and more often seek inner ways of making their lives more rewarding and fruitful. And of course, the concerns of adolescence, young adulthood, and maturity intertwine in the emotional life of every adult, so that many therapists will find themselves working now like Adler, now Freud, now Jung, and now Sullivan, by whatever names they call themselves. And at every stage of life, the need for specific behavioral remedies for long-standing behavioral impasses will emerge. Sometimes the therapist will show the way; often, the patient will come up with a surprisingly complex behavioral program for himself, just as he had earlier surprised the therapist by his ability to befriend himself, interpret his pathology, and accept his limitations.

REFERENCES

1. White, Robert W.: *The Abnormal Personality*, 3d ed., Ronald, New York, 1963.

2. Ellenberger, Henri: *The Discovery of the Unconscious*, Basic Books, New York, 1970.

3. Hillman, James: "The Language of Psychology and the Speech of the Soul," *Eranos Jahrbuch 1968*, Rhein-Verlag, Zurich, 1970, pp. 299–356.

4. Whyte, L. L.: *The Unconscious before Freud*, Basic Books, New York, 1960.

5. Bentham, Jeremy: "A Table of the Springs of Action," in John Bulmer (ed.), *The Works of Jeremy Bentham, Vol. I*, William Keit, Edinburgh, 1843, p. 205.

6. Hillman: op. cit., p. 309.

7. Lessing, Doris: *The Four-Gated City*, Knopf, New York, 1969.

8. Greenson, Ralph R.: *The Technique and Practice of Psychoanalysis, Vol. 1*, International Universities Press, New York, 1967, pp. 154–158.

9. Kaiser, Hellmuth: in Louis B. Fierman (ed.), *Effective Psychotherapy*, Basic Books, New York, 1965.

10. Ellenberger: loc. cit.

11. Whitehorn, John C., and Barbara Betz: "A Study of Psychotherapeutic Relationships between Physicians and Schizophrenic Patients," *Am. J. Psychiat.*, 3:321–331, 1954.

12. Frank, Jerome: *Persuasion and Healing*, Schocken Books, New York, 1963.

13. Jung, C. G., *The Integration of Personality*, Stanley M. Dell (trans.), Farrar & Rinehart, New York, 1939.

14. Colby, Kenneth M.: *A Primer for Psychotherapists*, Ronald, New York, 1951.

15. Rogers, Carl R.: "A Theory of Therapy, Personality, and Interpersonal Relationships as Developed in a Client-centered Framework," in S. M. Koch (ed.), *Psychology: A Study of a Science*, McGraw-Hill, New York, 1959, vol. 3.

16. Sullivan, Harry S.: *The Psychiatric Interview*, Norton, New York, 1954.

17. Alexander, Franz, and Thomas French: *Psychoanalytic Therapy*, Ronald, New York, 1946.

18. Freud, Sigmund: "Further Recommendations on the Technique of Psychoanalysis, Observations on Transference-Love," in *Collected Papers*, Joan Riviere (trans.), Basic Books, New York, 1959, vol. 2, pp. 380–381.

19. Searles, Harold: *Collected Papers on Schizophrenia and Related Subjects*, International Universities Press, New York, 1965, pp. 254–283.

20. Yalom, I. D., and M. A. Lieberman: "A Study of Encounter Group Casualties," *Arch. Gen. Psychiat.*, 25:16–30, 1971.

21. Jung, C. G.: "Definitions," *The Collected Works of C. G. Jung*, H. G. Baynes (trans.), revised by R. F. C. Hull, Princeton, Princeton, N.J., 1971, Vol. 6, p. 448.

22. Henderson, Joseph: "Resolution of the Transference in the Light of C. G. Jung's Psychology," *Acta Psychotherap.*, 2(3):267–283, 1954.

23. Freud, Sigmund: *The Future of an Illusion*, W. D. Robson-Scott (trans.), International

Psycho-analytic Library, no. 15, Ernest Jones (ed.), Liveright, New York, 1949, p. 93.

24. Searles: op. cit., *passim.*

25. Bierer, Joshua: "Transference in the Light of Adlerian Theory and Its Developments," *Acta Psychotherap.*, 2: 250–266, 1954.

26. Rank, Otto: *Will Therapy and Truth and Reality*, Jessie Taft (trans.), Knopf, New York, 1945.

27. Rogers, Carl R.: *On Becoming a Person*, Houghton Mifflin, Boston, 1961, chap. 1.

28. Rogers, Carl R.: "A Dialogue between Therapists," in C. R. Rogers, E. T. Gendlin, D. J. Kiesler, and C. B. Truax (eds.), *The Therapeutic Relationship and Its Impact*, University of Wisconsin Press, Madison, 1967, p. 515.

29. Ellenberger: op. cit., pp. 337–386.

30. Erikson, Erik H.: *Childhood and Society*, Norton, New York, 1950.

Outpatient Therapy: An Overview

PART 2: APPROACHES TO THERAPY

Although transference phenomena in the various stages are present in all therapeutic relationships, not every school of therapy handles the transference in the same way. How, then, does the general practitioner of psychiatry begin treatment? Traditionally therapists have recognized two main approaches to therapy: the uncovering approach and the reality-oriented approach. Although the distinction reflects the era when psychoanalysis was viewed as the yardstick against which all the therapies were measured, it is still helpful for the therapist to recognize this broad division in the kinds of treatment when he is trying to decide what kind of therapy he wants to offer.

THE UNCOVERING APPROACH

This term is used whenever therapy seeks to make unconscious dynamics conscious, to uncover that which was out of awareness and bring it to awareness, and to educate the patient to his transference or "parataxic" distortions.

Nowadays it is extremely common to attack the "insight" goal, which is the main aim of the uncovering approach. Freida Fromm-Reichmann[1]

said, "Patients don't need an explanation, they need an experience." Carl Rogers[2] has questioned the value of dynamic formulations in therapy. Jay Haley[3] and Paul Watzlawick[4] feel both that (1) insight does not lead to change, and (2) insight can even be a dangerous goal, leading to that paradoxical situation in which the patient creates a hell for himself out of his pursuit of the heaven of complete self-understanding.

To answer these criticisms it is first necessary to give a careful definition of insight. We prefer the term "meaning," which implies an experiential as well as a logical and empirical approach to self-understanding.[5] The experience of meaning is very powerful indeed — leading to new experiencing. It is similar to the experience of trance or orgasm; it involves an altered state of consciousness with intense reliving and far-reaching self-consequences. Eugene Gendlin[6,7] suggests that it is upon the experience of meaning that the unfolding of experiential process depends. The purpose of an insight is not so much to change the behavior that the insight comprehends as to further the experiential process of the person who has been behaving. The worst consequence of a repetitive behavior can be its effect in trapping the patient's experiencing. The insight into the behavior may not change *that* behavior, although it often does; the insight does make it possible for the patient to experience himself in a new way and to select out of that new experiencing many new kinds of behavior.

Thus, the often quoted joke that ends with the patient saying, after several years of therapy begun when he complained of a particular symptom, "Yes, I still do that, but it doesn't bother me any more," is not so ridiculous as it seems. What is uncovered is not just the reason for that particular maladaptive or puzzling piece of behavior, but the whole experiential process which that behavior has implied. Frequently, it is the liberation of the experiential process rather than a change in behavior that satisfies the patient, providing him with the relief he was originally seeking.

> *Example 13-1.* A woman had undergone a stormy, five-year psychoanalysis during her 40s. One result was that she was able to move to the suburbs after her neurosis had kept her city-bound for many years. She took up gardening and described her situation in a letter to a relative who knew a good deal about psychotherapy, saying:
> "Very zany and spasmodic gardening. I find I just love ripping things out of the garden, but that does not get me the most beautiful garden in time. However, it keeps me happy. As soon as something has the temerity to push its way through the ground, I stand around palpitating until I can either cut it off or pull it out. I know what you're thinking, but I don't give a damn. Better I do it to my plants than my children. One thing analysis did for me: I got all through only to find I had the same problems I always had, but with a difference, sometimes I could do something about them, and most of the time they don't bother me very much, and that's enough for me, so I'll never find out why I enjoy ripping things out. Look at all the things I can plant for far less money. I think it's all well worth the time and money, don't you?"

Uncovering the experiential meaning of a pattern of behavior does frequently lead to change in that particular behavior. Otherwise, patients with very practical problems would be ill advised to seek help from an uncovering approach. What kinds of behaviors can be changed by an uncovering approach has yet to be completely determined. But the main advantage of uncovering therapy is its role in helping a process of maturation by freeing trapped experiencing.

THE REALITY-ORIENTED APPROACH

These approaches to therapy attempt to leave the patient's general level of experiencing pretty much alone and do not dwell too much upon the meaning of the patient's symptoms. We use the term *reality-oriented* to emphasize that the primary focus of treatment is on the two realities most easily accessible to the patient and therapist: "external, objective" reality (the patient's life situation as he perceives it and as it might be perceived by others); and "internal, subjective" reality (consciousness, awareness of how external reality impinges on the patient, how he thinks and feels about what is going on around him and inside him, including rumblings from the unconscious which may be only dimly perceived). The term *reality-oriented therapy* should not be confused with Glasser's *reality therapy*, [8] which is only one of many approaches that fall under this rubric. Crisis intervention, behavior therapy, symptom prescription and hypnosis, brief psychotherapy, supportive psychotherapy, and many other therapies have as a common and important feature the support of the patient's ego in its ability to make decisions and to modify those behaviors and their disruptive effects that interfere with harmonious living in the world. Some exponents of these approaches do not believe in the existence of a dynamic unconscious influencing consciousness and behavior. We believe that the unconscious is there in reality-oriented therapy too and that it has an important impact on treatment which must be appreciated.

In speaking of the patient's ego, both the "I," that center of consciousness the patient knows as himself, and the executive, that often unconscious part of himself that makes decisions, are meant. This definition of ego is about midway between the Freudian and the Jungian definitions, but it is empirically useful in doing reality-oriented work. This approach can be very aggressive and challenging to the patient, despite the rather nurturant connotations of the word "support," often used in this kind of therapy. Attack of a particularly self-defeating form of behavior can, paradoxically, be a form of support, if the patient receives the therapist's criticism as a concerned attempt to inject more health into his life. When this approach is used, it is frequently spoken of in therapeutic circles as "lending the patient one's ego."

In common usage, "supportive psychotherapy" is often used as a near synonym for reality-oriented therapy; by this usage, pharmacologic and behavioral approaches to symptoms are supportive techniques. (Supportive psychotherapy is described in Chapter 18.) Crisis intervention in brief psychotherapy that aims at getting the patient back to where he was, not "opening up" a new mode of adaptation to him, also is a reality-oriented approach.

COMPLEMENTARITY

In practice, the ideal therapist should be able to work in both an uncovering and a reality-oriented capacity as is needed. This ideal situation does not always obtain. Presently community mental health centers offer primarily reality-oriented therapy, and many private practitioners devote much of their professional energies to uncovering psychotherapy. Such stereotypes are not confined to professional categories. There are psychiatrists who offer primarily reality-oriented therapy and social workers who do mostly uncovering psychotherapy.

Certainly some therapists are more in touch with the needs of the ego to maintain its position and to improve its methods of coping with stress,

whereas other therapists are more comfortable with the unconscious and its need to express itself more completely and to open up new forms of experiencing. Disagreement between those who practice reality-oriented therapy and those who practice uncovering therapy has made it seem as if one or the other approach were the "real psychiatry." In fact, both approaches are needed, often with the same patient. It would be better to see them as opposite ends of a single continuum. More than one analyst has found himself giving valuable advice during a period of stress, and more than one community psychiatrist has allowed a situation to open up considerable anxiety and depression before it is able to be resolved adequately. It should be remembered that the emergency psychotherapy of grief, a cornerstone of crisis intervention theory, is essentially an uncovering approach.[9]

INDICATIONS FOR THE UNCOVERING COMPARED TO THE REALITY-ORIENTED PSYCHOTHERAPIES

Were there psychoanalysts enough and time, not every patient would benefit from uncovering psychotherapy. Many patients would not possess the strength and determination that the procedure requires, but they still could make excellent use of reality-oriented psychotherapy. Nor is attention to reality lacking in dynamic consequences. A therapist's appreciation of his patient's unconscious struggles need not be used in treatment only to uncover these conflicts; the therapist can also support reality actions that lessen or minimize these struggles.

Indications

The most common indications for uncovering and reality-oriented psychotherapies are shown in Table 13-1 and will now be expanded upon.

Motivation. The patient who is suitable for dynamic, uncovering psychotherapy is consciously

TABLE 13-1. Comparison of Indications in Uncovering
and Reality-oriented Psychotherapies

		Indication	
	Parameter	Uncovering	Reality-oriented
1.	Motivation	Personality change	Symptom relief; environmental change
2.	Mental health	Moderate to good	Very poor to very good
3.	Perception of symptoms	Ego dystonic	Ego dystonic or syntonic
4.	Ego strength; capacity to endure painful affects; formal diagnosis	Strong ego; capacity to endure painful affects; symptom or character neurosis	Weaker ego; lesser capacity to endure painful affects; personality disorder, sociopathy, psychosis, organic brain syndrome
5.	Quality of interpersonal relationships (including previous therapy)	Successful; useful	Unsuccessful; sparse
6.	Presenting circumstances	Stable life situation	Stress, crisis
7.	Age	20–40 years	Childhood to old age
8.	Psychological mindedness	Considerable ("Dostoyevsky")	Moderate to negligible ("Hemingway")
9.	Intelligence	Sensitive; bright	Wide range
10.	Value orientation	Future: desires self-improvement and personal growth	Present or past: desires current relief or return to tradition

motivated to change his basic personality or character structure through realistic effort. (The common magical expectation that contact with a psychiatrist will ipso facto produce change cannot be counted as a sign of realistic motivation.) The usual understanding between the patient and therapist is that psychotherapy will help him to mature.

Other patients may come because they are anxious, depressed, and distraught. They may also be caught in a turbulent environmental situation. Their motivation is for relief of distress and help in controlling and improving the environmental disruption. When these objectives have been accomplished, they may very well not be interested in further exploration. Such patients are most suitable for reality-oriented therapy.

Mental Health. Some patients who are experiencing distress may strike the interviewer as basically quite healthy, with strong egos and little evidence of severe unconscous conflicts. Such patients may be caught in a life crisis for which a reality-oriented approach is indicated. Other patients have few external difficulties but are experiencing much internal conflict. Their difficulties often yield to an uncovering approach, provided their egos are strong enough. Ego strength is a concept that will be discussed later.

For the majority of patients, there is some external difficulty, some internal conflict, ego strength in some areas, and ego weakness in others. It is necessary for the therapist to understand the interactions between external reality, conscious ego, and unconscious personality structure to make the decision about how much he should use the reality-oriented approach and how much he should use the uncovering approach.

We offer the examples of Allen, Ben, Colin, and Daniel to illustrate the range of possibilities. These examples are not to be taken as rigid indications of the kinds of patients who are "suitable (or unsuitable) for uncovering (or reality-oriented) psychotherapy," but rather as kinds of presenting pictures for which different approaches to therapy are indicated. In the course of therapy, as tensions wax or wane, the same patient may come to resemble any one of the four profiles, and the approach of the therapist must change to suit the patient's needs. (Such changes may come when a seemingly healthy patient faces a major health crisis, or when a formerly psychotic patient has found the courage to separate himself from a toxic relative.) The different dynamics in each profile will be represented in the form of a diagram.

Example 13-2, Allen. Allen, a college student home for Christmas vacation, saw his father die of cancer and became engaged to a girl he had gone with for several years. On returning to school, he started having trouble concentrating, felt "sad and blue," lost his appetite, and began waking up at 5 A.M. feeling unrested. He had never experienced such feelings before, and he sought psychiatric consultation.

In consultation Allen expressed considerable concern that his symptoms might represent signs of impending insanity. The consultant reviewed his past, found that he had had many successful and gratifying social and academic achievements, and that he came from a closely knit family. He thought the student's ego was strong, that there was no evidence of significant neurotic conflict, and that, aside from the presenting symptoms, the student seemed mentally healthy.

The consultant told him he was having an acute, reactive depression, that it probably was the result of his not having been able to express all his feelings about his father's death and of being away from his fiancée, that such

depressions usually responded to psychotherapy, and that the symptoms did not portend psychosis.

Allen was greatly relieved to hear this and left the session visibly less anxious than when he had come in. He started therapy later the same week. His therapist reported that after nine sessions the patient had expressed considerable affect about the loss of his father and the separation from his girl, that there was a complete remission of symptoms, and that treatment ended by mutual consent (see Figure 13-1).

In contrast, in the case of Ben, external reality was not so stressful, but unconscious neurotic conflict was troubling him. He was motivated to change, and he seemed generally to fulfill the indications for uncovering psychotherapy described in this section.

Example 13-3, Ben. Ben, a graduate student in physics, applied for treatment of acute anxiety about a serious marital quarrel. During the course of the first few sessions, some of the marital frictions were resolved with a concomitant decrease in anxiety, but it became apparent to the therapist that the student was far from utilizing his rather considerable intellectual potential. Evidence began to emerge that conflicts about authority prevented him from working effectively with his thesis sponsor, and sibling rivalries prevented useful interchanges with his fellow students. The therapist found the patient's general level of functioning to be good, as was his ego strength.

The therapist presented these ideas and the data from which they derived in the third session, concluding, "I think you have some serious neurotic conflicts about authority, rivalry with your fellow students, and achievement, all contributing to the slowness of your progress on your thesis, and I think you need long-term psychotherapy if you are to resolve some of these problems."

Ben was taken aback by such a direct statement, but on reflection saw that there was a

Primary conflict is between stressful reality and
healthy ego temporarily unable to cope with stress.
Intervention *brief*, aimed at resolution of stress and
coping;   long-term treatment not called for, e.g.,
student with reactive depression

Figure 13-1   Allen.

good deal of merit in what the therapist had
said and entered into what turned out to be a
quite profitable three-year period of intensive,
uncovering psychotherapy (see Figure 13-2).

Perception of Symptoms. The way the patient
perceives his symptoms is closely linked to his
motivation for treatment. If the patient dislikes his
symptoms and what they represent, that is, if they
are *ego dystonic*, he will be more motivated to give
them up in intensive psychotherapy, even at the
cost of experiencing anxiety and pain in the
process. On the other hand, if he is relatively
comfortable with them, that is, they are *ego syntonic*, he will be less motivated to change, particularly because change in intensive therapy means
more work for the ego. Ben was distressed by his
symptoms and was willing to suffer to give them
up.

Many patients who enact their conflicts sexually

not only enjoy the actions but also dread the
experience of anxiety not acting would release.
Only when social disapproval of the sexual
behavior, or realistic frustration of the means of
gratification, is strong will the patient want therapy, and then more often to grieve the loss of a
once-effective solution than to work through the
original basis for taking up that solution.

Example 13-4, Colin. Colin, a 54-year-old
cook who had lived homosexually his entire
adult life, had recently been left by his partner
of several years. In the weeks that followed he
started doing two uncharacteristic things: he
drank heavily, and he sought out new partners
in bars and public lavatories. The police picked
him up in a lavatory; he was arrested, jailed,
and lectured sternly by the judge and told to
seek psychiatric help as a condition of probation.

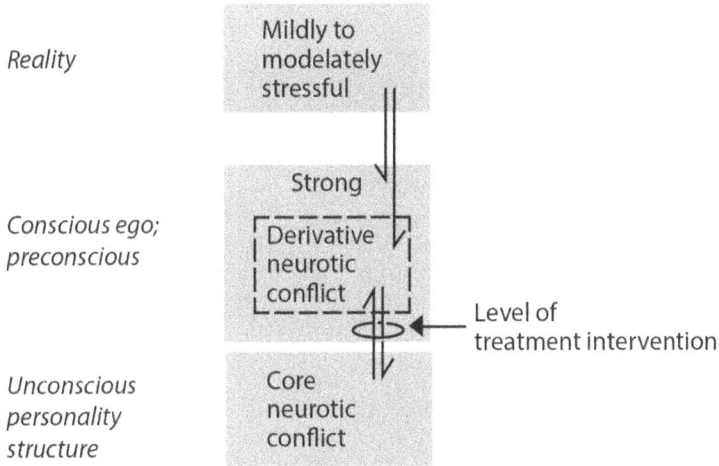

Current reality revivifies derivative conflict symptomatic
of core neurosis in patient amenable to uncovering therapy.
After initial stress resolution, *long-term* uncovering therapy
for core neurosis attempted, e.g., graduate student in physics.

Figure 13-2 Ben.

His father had brutalized Colin as a child and had favored Colin's sister. Colin's mother had ineffectually tried to protect him from his father's verbal and physical assaults. The arrest by the police and the judge's lecture stirred up Colin's fears of abuse at the hands of adult males (against which his homosexuality was presumably a reaction), and he was extremely anxious and depressed when he came for his first therapy session.

One of the first things Colin brought up was whether he was going to have to change his sexual orientation as part of therapy. After exploring the history a bit, the therapist said that it appeared to him that Colin's homosexuality had by and large worked well for him over the years, that if Colin wanted to work on it further in therapy they could, but that helping him find some relief from his current anxiety and depression seemed to be the first order of business. Colin was relieved to hear

this and did not bring up again the issue of wanting to change his sexual orientation.

Instead, therapy was aimed at finding the causes of the break with his partner, how his partner could be approached, how a new partner might be found in less self-destructive ways, and so forth. Such an approach served to make him less anxious, depressed, hopeless, and ashamed. After twelve sessions Colin felt added security about his way of life, had had some initial successes in establishing new relationships, was feeling much better, and treatment ended by mutual consent (see Figure 13-3).

The fact the symptoms are initially ego syntonic does not automatically mean a patient cannot profit from intensive psychotherapy. Sometimes one of the major tasks of the initial period of therapy is to raise anxiety in the patient's mind concerning the nature and implications of his symp-

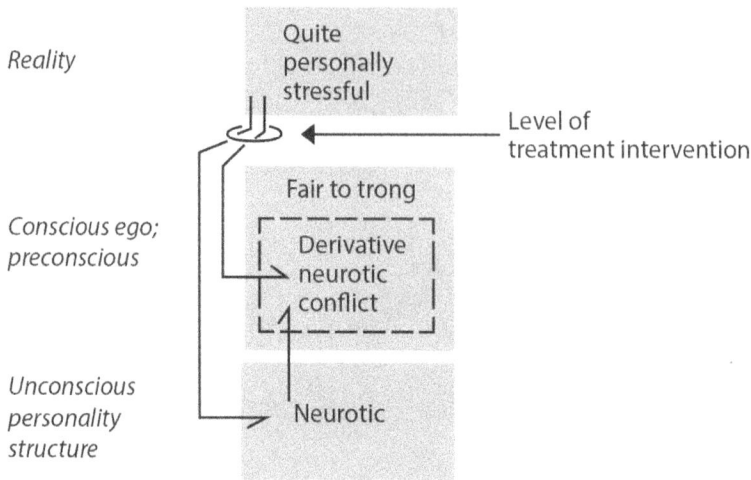

Current stress revivifies personal neurotic core conflict
in latter-day, derivative form. Patient not suitable for
uncovering therapy. Intervention *brief*, aimed at resolution
of derivative conflict; work with core neurosis not attempted,
e.g., the 54-year-old cook with conflicts over homosexuality.

Figure 13-3   Colin.

toms so that they cannot remain purely ego syntonic. In cases in which this kind of transformation seems to be a feasible goal of early intensive
therapy, the paradoxical phenomenon of trying to
make a patient feel worse about himself so that
ultimately he can feel better will occur.

Here, of course, the values of the therapist and
his judgment as to *where* to make the patient
anxious come into play. And just here, contro-
versies abound. It is well to remember that a
symptom is never an a priori item in psychiatry; it
is always a judgment involving the therapist.
the patient, and society in a complicated decision.
which is itself always open to change as part of the
therapeutic process.[10] In short, what is seen as
symptomatic at one point in therapy may not
seem so at another, depending on its meaning and
impact on the life of the individual and the
environment in which he lives.

**Ego Strength; Capacity to Endure Painful Affects;
Formal Diagnosis.** People vary in the way they
respond to anxiety and stress. Some tolerate it,
live with the anxiety, continue to function, and
seek to resolve the underlying sources of stress;
they can "muddle through," as the English did
during World War II. Such persons are said to have
a "strong ego." Others do not cope so well: they
may become paralyzed with anxiety and depression; they may discharge their feelings impulsively;
they may become psychotic. They are seen as
having a "weak ego," with the amount of weakness more or less in proportion to the amount of
incapacity or maladaptiveness of their response to
stress. Patients with compromised brain function,
such as the "syndrome of cerebral insufficiency"
(described in Chapters 30 and 31), also have a
reduced capacity to respond to stress.

Uncovering psychotherapy is itself a source of

stress because it asks that the patient be able to experience once again feelings and fantasies buried because they were painful to begin with. Therefore, uncovering psychotherapy is most appropriate for patients judged to have strong egos, those who would most likely be diagnosed as having a symptom or character neurosis. Reality-oriented therapy is most appropriate for patients whose egos are weaker, those who would most likely be diagnosed as having a personality disorder, a latent or overt psychosis, or an organic brain syndrome.[11,12]

With psychotic patients, the therapist will often have to direct his attentions to two levels of reality: he will have to help the patient with external reality and the problems of day-by-day living, and he will have to intercede against disturbing irruptions from the unconscious, as shown in the case of Daniel.

Example 13-5, Daniel. Daniel was a 22-year-old schizophrenic patient, first hospitalized when he was 18, who impulsively left his home in St. Louis, where he lived with his mother, older sister, and aunt, to fly to Los Angeles. He arrived there without warning at the home of his father, who had divorced his mother when Daniel was four. The father had remarried and started a second family. Daniel thought that if he left the women he had been living with, took up residence with his father, and also, for the first time, took his father's last name, he would somehow "become a man" (symbolically grow a penis). When Daniel's therapist in St. Louis realized he intended to complete his impulsive trip, he told him to check in at a clinic where a colleague, Dr. Hirsch, worked.

Dr. Hirsch was called to the clinic waiting room Friday afternoon and saw an obviously schizophrenic young man and an equally confused and distressed father. He saw the patient briefly, during which time the patient verified that this was the *right* Dr. Hirsch at the *right* clinic. An appointment was made for Monday.

In the weeks and months that followed, Dr. Hirsch and the patient worked to reduce the level of psychotic anxiety (using phenothiazines and interpretations based on understanding the patient's dynamics), find a suitable living situation in a halfway house (the father and his new family clearly could not take it), get the patient involved in a day care center, and, in general, stabilize his existence.

Some months later Dr. Hirsch left the clinic, and another therapist (the second of many) took over Daniel's treatment. During his first five years in Los Angeles, the patient had to have three psychiatric hospitalizations (each lasting a few weeks and often coinciding with a visit from mother), but still found a job and was largely self-supporting and self-sufficient. He required a half-hour of psychotherapy every two weeks when his life was relatively unstressful (although the time was increased at periods of stress), and he participated in community, psychiatrically based activities during much of his free time. He will probably need some psychiatric management for life (see Figure 13-4).

Quality of Interpersonal Relationships (Including Previous Therapy). Success in intensive therapy is predicated upon some degree of past success in intimate relationships with others. Not all patients can handle intimacy well: some have not developed sufficient basic trust; some cannot accept a relationship they cannot control; some must use any relationship narcissistically. Equally, some patients react to any therapist as a mother, who must be defied by means of a sequence of pranks and tricks. Others see every therapist as a father, who must be dreaded, obeyed, or defied. Whenever a patient seems to have a particularly striking pattern of creating the same relationship with every partner, the therapist should question whether intensive psychotherapy will be able to uncover the reasons for this destructive pattern or will merely be one more humiliating and costly

Reality

Objectively and
subjectively
stressful

Level of
treatment intervention

Weak;
irruptions from
unconscious
into
consciousness

Conscious ego;
preconscious

Unconscious
personality
structure

Primitive
unconscious
conflicts

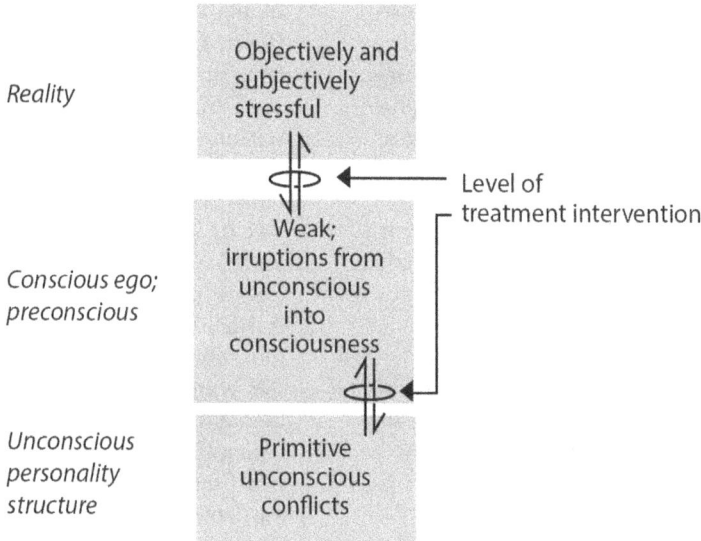

Borderline or psychotic ego defenses make patient vulnerable
to many life situations. *Brief* therapy aimed at resolution
of precipitating stress; *long-term* supportive therapy (often
with medication) needed; appreciation of unconscious dynamics
is an essential part of supplying intelligent support. Length
and frequency of sessions flexible (for instance, increased
at times of crisis), e.g., schizophrenic patient who flew
impulsively to Los Angeles.

Figure 13-4 Daniel.

repetition of the familiar sequence, "adding insight to injury."

The evidence of interpersonal success lies in the outcome of past relationships. This history is the island on which the patient must build in his relationship with the present therapist. Particularly important will be his experience with previous therapists. If the patient thinks that his other therapeutic relationships "aren't worth mentioning" or will not give the names of former therapists, then it can be assumed that things went quite badly. Often the previous therapy is frankly unfinished, and the patient would do best by going back to the former therapist at least to "close the old account." Frequently, an initial consultation for psychotherapy discovers the need to resolve an old transference, and the therapist can help the patient most by helping him end the old psychotherapy in the right way. Then the patient has a decent basis from which to start with someone else.

Of course a previous patient-therapist fit may have been wrong, and the patient may be quite a good candidate for intensive work with the present therapist. The therapist must consult his own feelings: if he feels comfortable with the patient throughout the first hour, there is a strong possibility that they can work together. If, on the other hand, he has doubts, suspicions, vague uneasiness, he should heed them: this may be a patient who cannot handle intimacy with this therapist.

Usually the patient signals early what he will be like in therapy, and the therapist should heed his message. The patient who is intensely narcissistic will ask for some tangible evidence of admiration or approval early in the session, some special favor, and the therapist should notice whether the patient can tolerate refusal. Uncovering therapy is a relatively ungratifying experience; the therapist must often withhold his opinion of what is going on, as well as expressions of admiration and support. If the patient cannot do without these, he cannot endure uncovering therapy.

Still other patients cannot stand the intimacy of fifty minutes a week with the same therapist; paranoid and schizoid patients stand out in this category. Some patients react with painful emotional storms to any suggestion from the therapist of disapproval or disinterest: here, certain hysterical characters and schizophrenic patients stand out. Patients in either of these groups may react to the end of a period of therapy or to a therapist's vacation or illness with psychotic, suicidal, or homicidal behavior. The therapist is protecting the patient and himself by not embarking on intensive psychotherapy.

If transference issues threaten to engulf, not enlighten, the patient, reality-oriented therapy may be the treatment of choice. Or, a therapist who specializes in uncovering work with patients who have certain difficult transferences may be found. (Some therapists subspecialize in work with paranoid, schizoid, hysterical, and schizophrenic patients and seem to know just what to do.)

Finally, visits of limited duration with a different therapist each time (Chapter 18) may be the right approach. This is the least transferential version of reality-oriented therapy, indicated for patients with the most difficulty accepting intimacy, frustration, and dependency.

Presenting Circumstances. The presenting circumstances of the patient who can utilize uncovering psychotherapy must include a baseline stability in his life situation.[13,14] Intensive psychotherapy

is hard work, and it takes concentration and effort. If a patient is sorely beset by reality problems, e.g., job loss, eviction from home, the stress of combat, and so on, he simply does not have the psychic energy available to do the introspective work of uncovering psychotherapy.

One measure of the energy the patient has for intensive therapy is his ability to pay for it (or find a way of having it financed). Here the therapist must help him face the realities squarely. Uncovering therapy always takes months and frequently years if it is to be productive. Insurance coverage for treatment with private practitioners is limited; twice a week at $35 an hour will cost about $3,000 a year. Thus patients undertaking uncovering therapy must be able to plan on staying in the same geographical area for a year, and, if in treatment with a private practitioner, to arrange for the bills to be paid from some combination of personal resources, insurance coverage, or community support, and so on.

In contrast, most reality-oriented therapies do not take so long and do not average so many visits per week. The costs are often underwritten by community agencies, and thus the patient does not have to make so many major commitments when he starts.

Age. The age of patients suitable for uncovering psychotherapy is important in its implications about character structure and ego strength. The developmental level of adolescents can vary widely. Of two 16-year-olds, one shows a childlike, dependent orientation. He perceives himself as relatively helpless, unprepared to grow up and assume adult control over impulses and behavior, and is afraid of independence. This self-perception may reflect his family's feeling that he is ill prepared to leave the nest. He may unconsciously expect adults (including therapists) to be omnipotent and not necessarily friendly. This kind of adolescent fears entry into a therapeutic alliance whose goal is greater self-knowledge leading to a mastery of impulses and behavior, and finally to greater personal independence. Furthermore, his family senses its equilibrium would be upset if the adolescent were to make strides in a "mature" direction, and they might work unwittingly to undo whatever is accomplished in therapy. To make the work proceed at all, the therapist finds it necessary to involve the family in supportive consultations.

A second 16-year-old comes to treatment with a relatively adult ego orientation. Despite characteristic adolescent conflicts about sexuality, assertiveness and aggression, impulse control, fear of relinquishing dependent ties to the family, and so forth, somehow his storms always resolve in the direction of maturity, and his family is basically helpful. This kind of adolescent patient is psychologically much better prepared to enter into the therapeutic alliance required for uncovering psychotherapy.

At best, uncovering psychotherapy with adolescents requires an adaptation of traditional techniques to the patient's specific situation, which, because of the fluidity of character structure, defense mechanisms, coping abilities, and so on, may require session-to-session adaptations on the part of the therapist. For example, an experienced psychiatrist reported that he began to have good results with his adolescents only when he started suggesting to them that he was willing to use the therapeutic hour for a walk to the park.[15]*

At another critical period in development, by the time most people reach the age of 40 their character structures not only are consolidated but have become relatively fixed and are not easily changed. It becomes increasingly more difficult after that age to make significant changes in character structure, even when these seem called for. Nevertheless, a significant proportion of adults over the age of 40 encounter middle-life crises that may propel them into treatment with a commitment to change only occasionally found in younger people. The dramatic changes described by Jung[18] in the individuation process are felt by him to be reserved for the second half of life; his own psychological development after age 40[19] testifies to the potential of this period.

Psychological Mindedness. This term refers to an assessment of the patient's sensitivity and perceptivity to inner, psychological events in himself and others. Some people are intuitive; others are not. Many of the characters in Dostoyevsky's novels expound at length on their own and everyone else's motivations. In Hemingway's works the characters are involved in lives of action, not contemplation. Of the brothers Karamazov, contemplative Aloysha would have been the best candidate for intensive psychotherapy; impulsive Dmitri would have been the worst. Impulsive patients can sometimes talk like psychologically minded people, but they are rarely willing to settle for the slow, hard work of uncovering; they usually argue for dramatic, new approaches if they are interested in psychology.

Intelligence. Psychoanalysis has been termed "the talking cure." In the past it has been assumed that the ability to be articulate was intimately linked with intelligence and that intelligence could be measured accurately by intelligence tests. These are dubious assumptions at best. Intelligence is not always expressed verbally; some highly gifted and creative people find it difficult to express themselves in words, although their painting, music, or mathematics are most impressive. Others may show an impressive wisdom in the business of living and coping with stress, even though they may not be able to describe how they do it.

Formal tests of intelligence are culture-bound and favor those reared in a culture similar to that of those who devised the test. Cultural differences between the therapist and patient often make it

---

*Extensive discussion of the treatment of children and adolescents is beyond the scope of this book. Readers may pursue these issues further in Weiner[16] and Caplan and Lebovici.[17]

difficult for the therapist to appreciate fully the intelligence of a patient from a markedly different background.

For all these reasons, therapists should be cautious about underrating a patient's suitability for uncovering psychotherapy on the basis of intelligence. If the interviewer has doubts, he may do well to have the patient evaluated by a colleague who can work well with inarticulate but otherwise gifted persons or who is closer in cultural background to the patient.

Value Orientation and Culture. The gratifications of uncovering psychotherapy are few at the beginning, once the novelty wears off, and the pains, both emotional and often financial, are many. The payoff is not expected to come for months or years. The goal is usually improvement of the self (rather than, say, improved loyalty to a religious faith). The means include frank self-disclosure and a willingness to be open (rather than, say, the patient's keeping shameful and guilty secrets to himself and maintaining a stiff upper lip in the face of adversity).

Spiegel[20] points out that value orientation and culture operate significantly in how both patients and therapists perceive psychotherapy. Although the predominant American culture favors a future orientation (work hard, strive, and success will come), some subcultures have a present orientation (life's gratifications are few; grab them while you can) or a past orientation (an individual's value in society is tightly connected with continuing important social and religious traditions; to change in a way that renounces those traditions is apostasy).

Traditional uncovering psychotherapy is most congruent with the values of future-oriented persons who look for individual growth through frank revelation even when it is painful, who are willing to delay gratification, and who are willing, at least to some extent, to break with tradition if it stands in the way of their own growth.

For many lower-class Americans there has been little reason to see much virtue in the delay of the few gratifications available. Therefore, if therapy promises to interfere with these gratifications, it is unlikely that the patient will engage in a therapeutic contract. The cost of therapy is one source of such interference. If it does not interfere, e.g., if insurance or the community will pay and the patient will not run up a large bill, then therapy can be considered on its other merits, and the lower-class patient often can invest himself in it.

It is sometimes argued that lower-class Americans do not have a bent for introspective thought and speech. There is much contrary evidence. Words that are quite often different from those used by middle-class therapists for feelings may not be recognized by them as introspective. Equally, therapy has not yet been available to lower-class patients until quite recently, so that its terms and formal concepts may seem unfamiliar to them. Even now therapy is frequently not explained or conducted in a culturally appropriate language, and if this failure of communication occurs, the mystified patient will wisely and understandably mistrust therapy and the intentions of the incomprehensible therapist.

Some Contrasts

The foregoing shows that most uncovering therapy takes time (months, years), that some reality-oriented therapies may be brief, and others may last a lifetime. Most uncovering therapies pay attention to unconscious phenomena, seeking to make them more explicit. Most reality-oriented therapies do not seek to make unconscious phenomena explicit or try to limit their intrusions into consciousness and day-by-day functioning; such therapies operate more at the level of the external and conscious realities of the patient. How these contrasts can be applied to the cases of Allen, Ben, Colin, and Daniel is recapitulated in Figure 13-5.

Figure 13-5 Relationship of stress and personality structure to strategy of therapeutic intervention.

BASIC PROCEDURES IN UNCOVERING AND REALITY-ORIENTED PSYCHOTHERAPIES

The basic procedures that occur most often in uncovering and reality-oriented therapies are listed in Table 13-2.

The Procedures

Advice, Exhortation, Suggestion. Into this category fall advising a patient to get a job, to assert himself more in social situations, and so forth. In insight psychotherapy, in which increased self-awareness is one goal, it may be less productive for the therapist to be drawn into the role of the helpful advice giver than to concentrate with the patient on finding out where his own decision

making tends to fail. In reality-oriented psychotherapy, on the other hand, many patients are simply not intact enough psychologically to make some of their necessary decisions, and thoughtful advice from the therapist may prove quite useful. (This is described in detail in Chapter 18.)

Praise and Criticism. Psychoanalysis has taught therapists to be stinting of praise and criticism in uncovering psychotherapy, although both are employed more frequently in the reality-oriented therapies. The rationale is (1) the therapist becomes an authority who can judge the patient, thus causing him to perform simply to please the therapist, who is now the incarnation of the patient's superego, (sometimes the therapist is referred to as "riding the patient's superego"); and (2) praise becomes a form of narcissistic gratifica-

TABLE 13-2. Basic Procedures in Uncovering and Reality-oriented Psychotherapies

		Extent of Use	
	Procedure	Uncovering Therapies	Reality-oriented Therapies
1.	Advice, exhortation, suggestion	Sparing	Frequent
2.	Praise, criticism	Sparing to moderate	Frequent
3.	Medication	Little	Great
4.	Catharsis	Frequent	Frequent
5.	Therapist initiative in establishing content areas	Little	Great
6.	Relaxation of ego constraints	Considerable	Slight
7.	Analysis of the transference; interpretations aimed at providing deep insights; identification of resistances	Regular	Limited
8.	Discussion of dreams, childhood memories	Regular	Limited
9.	Frequency of visits	1 to 5 per week[*]	1 per week or fewer[*]

[*]Patients in acute crises often need frequent visits, every day or even more frequently, if only for fifteen or thirty minutes. This is true for both uncovering and reality-oriented therapy.

tion for the patient; he comes mainly to be praised by a benevolent father or mother rather than to learn about himself.

Praise can have both a direct and a paradoxical effect. In its direct form, praise is encouragement. When a patient does not need encouragement, or has a neurotic need to please, praise can play into pathology. But when a patient has not had the experience of being pleasing to anybody, the therapist's praise can be as valuable as rain on a dry field; it can allow the patient to grow.

As paradox, praise can have the effect of allowing a valid feeling that is unattractively or annoyingly expressed to be more fully recognized. Often the patient has been expressing emotion in such a way as to elicit the disapproval of the therapist. The therapist's praise undercuts this self-defeating strategy. In one instance a wife continually berated her husband in an annoying, hysterical way; he shrugged off her anger because she permitted him to say to her, the therapist, and anyone else involved, in effect: "Don't pay any attention to what she says; I have a hysterical wife."

Once, as the scene was being replayed in the office, the therapist said to the wife, "You're not attacking him nearly forcefully enough." He had unexpectedly praised her emotion, even though he criticized her way of expressing it. She stopped screaming, and everyone was able for the first time to appreciate the validity of the anger she had been disqualifying with her hysterical style of expression.

Many of the same objections to praise have also been leveled against criticism: the therapist is playing the superego, is being parental. Moreover, there is a tacit assumption that therapists are supposed to be gentle, accepting people who can be too sweet from time to time without being seriously at fault, but must never err toward being too critical without immediately finding out why they are acting out a negative countertransference upon the patient.

Actually, the therapist has a powerful tool in his hands when he is able to criticize a patient who trusts him enough to hear his criticism. Construc-

tive criticism starts in the confrontation phase of psychotherapy and continues through the initiatory phase. If the therapist is going to use criticism, he does best by criticizing behavior that has really been annoying to him and owning the criticism as only his reaction to that behavior. Criticism that implies the therapist is God usually elicits a well-deserved defensive reaction.

Often an adolescent patient who has been unable to hear criticism from his parents and persists in traits that are grossly rude or maladaptive can be helped a great deal by a trusted therapist who is not afraid to tell him he is being obnoxious. Sometimes the therapist is the only person in the patient's environment who *can* criticize him and get away with it. The experience of submitting to someone else's authority can be an extremely valuable one for the patient who is used to controlling others in his environment at all times.

Medication. Patients who are severely anxious or depressed may not have the psychological energy available to them for either psychotherapy or any of life's other responsibilities, and a temporary course of the appropriate tranquilizer or antidepressant may be very useful in tiding them over a rough period. The indications and contraindications for the use of these drugs are detailed in Chapters 25 to 28.

Therapists doing uncovering psychotherapy are usually reluctant to use medication. Mild to modest amounts of anxiety in patients in uncovering psychotherapy may be an indicator that the patient is getting somewhere, that he is beginning to come to grips with unsettling but important issues which have long been buried. Such anxiety can serve both as a signal of the issue and as a spur toward its discovery. Its presence is to be welcomed rather than treated; its origins to be searched for rather than squelched.

In contrast, patients in reality-oriented and supportive psychotherapies may not be able to use anxiety profitably; its presence merely signifies that things are going wrong, not right, and medications may be called for. For chronic schizophrenic patients, long-term administration of phenothiazine drugs is often a necessary part of treatment.

Catharsis. When something has gone wrong in a person's life, it is often very helpful to him to be able to tell someone else about it. If he is in psychotherapy, whether it be uncovering or reality-oriented, the therapist, if he has proven himself an adept and compassionate listener, is a logical person to unburden himself to. Injudicious catharsis, however, is a potential hazard, particularly in patients who have trouble separating the thought from the act, as do some borderline patients with homicidal fantasies and some masochistic depressive patients who uncover feelings toward the end of a session that will be with them all week. With such patients, the therapist may model the repression of destructive affects by *suppressing* the expression of them during the hour. He will set limits, especially in the last part of an hour, on what the patient may express. Clearly, this is a technique at variance with uncovering and is a specialized skill for use only in the treatment of patients who have difficulty repressing.

Therapist Initiative in Establishing Content Areas. In uncovering psychotherapy, in which increased self-awareness is one of the main goals, therapists will often instruct patients to report all thoughts that come to mind, whether they seem important or insignificant, pleasant or anxiety provoking, proper or improper. He leaves the major burden of "producing material" to the patient. Often he lets the patient find his own way of structuring the hour. He occasionally intervenes to make a connection, direct the associations in a particular area, and so forth when a strong hunch or solid knowledge of dynamics suggests that there is some gold to be mined in a particular vein. Interactive therapists who do uncovering therapy leap in only where the patient "lives" affectively (or where he dramatically refuses to live). The cue to interest is patient emotion — strongly expressed or strongly repressed.

In reality-oriented therapies the therapist's task often is more to help the patient improve his day-by-day existence. He may much more often suggest the topics to be talked about; e.g., "How did things go when you visited your mother-in-law last weekend?" Free association can easily be irrevelant, a waste of time to both the therapist and the patient, who drifts to familiar, safe complexes, avoiding deep catharsis. Nevertheless, even in reality-oriented psychotherapy, if a given therapy hour seems to have gotten stuck, it may be useful to ask the patient to report on what is going through his mind to get things moving again.

Relaxation of Ego Constraints. When the patient in uncovering psychotherapy is asked to use free association and is assisted in this by being asked to lie down on a couch, where he cannot be distracted by the sight of the therapist and the therapist's responses to what he is saying, an opportunity for mild regression comes into being. Many of the patient's adult faculties of self-criticism, inner judgments, and so on are relaxed; a state of "willing suspension of disbelief" is called for.

Such regression allows more primitive kinds of thinking and feeling to emerge slowly. Often knowledge of these more primitive modes is crucial to understanding the development and manifestations of the neurotic behavior for which the patient originally entered treatment. As the therapist and patient learn from the patient's reports, the therapist may help the patient to make affective connections between psychological events that had not been previously perceived as related.

At the end of the therapy hour, and in the period between sessions, the patient's adult ego assimilates what has gone on; his critical abilities are implicitly called upon to reassert themselves, and the period of regression ends. Thus the regression has been in the service of the ego: it has allowed the ego access to otherwise hidden stores of information and emotion that can lead to therapeutic growth.

In uncovering therapy, such regression is sometimes painful but often profitable. In work with the marginally adapted, however, it may be a luxury the patient simply cannot afford. Borderline or overtly psychotic patients need all the reality testing they can get. The unstructured situation of being asked to free-associate to a therapist whom they cannot see may weaken already strained ego defenses and allow an eruption of disabling symptoms. In a discussion of treatment of borderline characters, Ralph Greenson[21] notes that with a neurotic patient the therapist may say, "You seem to be reacting to me as if I were your father"; with the borderline patient the therapist must say, "You seem to be reacting to me as if I were your father, but I am not your father," thus adding a needed component of reality testing to a weak ego.

Analysis of the Transference; Interpretations Aimed at Providing Deep Insights; Identification of Resistances. All these procedures are facets of a central body of technique belonging to contemporary psychoanalytic ego psychology, but they find parallels in all uncovering psychotherapies. Each is a way of trying to increase self-awareness, of making conscious the preconscious and unconscious, of bringing that which was out of awareness into awareness. The defenses (defense mechanisms), according to psychoanalysis, are those mental activities that serve to keep conflictual, anxiety-provoking thoughts, feelings, and fantasies out of consciousness. The most common defense mechanisms are repression, denial, and reaction formation. Others include isolation, undoing, intellectualization, suppression, projection, sublimation, and displacement. All are described in elegant, concise detail by Anna Freud.[22] Learning to experience defense mechanisms in action and to develop choice in their development is a major goal of psychoanalytically oriented therapy.

Discussion of Dreams, Childhood Memories. Freud called the dream "the royal road to the unconscious." Dream material can provide an astonishingly direct picture of the affective issue at hand, where free association has repeatedly led away from the central emotion. (Ways in which dream material can be utilized in both uncovering and reality-oriented therapies are presented in Chapter 22.) In general, therapists doing insight therapy will encourage patients to present dream material; in reality-oriented therapies, therapists do not usually encourage, and may even discourage, attention being paid to dreams. If dreams are used, the problem-solving aspect is more likely to be stressed in reality-oriented therapies, and the problem-revealing aspect is often emphasized in uncovering therapy. This is in line with the general principle that the patient in uncovering therapy is best confronted with a neglected problem for his strong ego to resolve, whereas the patient in supportive therapy is best left with a neglected solution for his weak ego to incorporate.

Most neuroses have their origins in childhood. Often an investigation of these origins, and of the related memories of childhood events and fantasies, can be important in uncovering psychotherapy. They are much less important in reality-oriented therapy and are less often sought after.

Frequency of Visits. In all kinds of psychotherapy, current life events and fantasies are important. Therapy occupies only one or a few of the 168 hours of each week; what goes on in the other 164 or 167 is important to know. In dynamic psychotherapy in particular, it is important to know not only what events took place, but what their private and personal meaning was to the patient. Thus the patient who reports a run-in with a boss or lover will then be asked to free-associate about that event to find out what its specific meaning was to him. The patient in uncovering psychotherapy needs time both to report life events and to search after their personal meaning. One hour a week is usually not enough to do both; it may be barely adequate for a report on the external events themselves. Thus patients in uncovering psychotherapy often need two to five sessions a week if they are to have the opportunity to do the necessary work, although instances of productive uncovering psychotherapies with only one session a week are many.

Patients in reality-oriented psychotherapy, in contrast, do not have such needs of introspection imposed upon them by the therapy; one hour a week or less may suffice. Here too exceptions certainly exist. Just as many well-motivated patients work hard on therapy between sessions and improve with an uncovering approach although they meet only once a week, many marginally adapted patients' needs for support demand that they be seen more frequently; they tend to lose their egos if the distance between sessions is too great. Generally, the frequency should enable the patient in uncovering psychotherapy to maintain contact with his unconscious and the patient in reality-oriented psychotherapy to hold onto his ego.

Being in therapy is no insurance that patients will not encounter emotional crises. Indeed, uncovering therapy may not only be an additional stress in and of itself, but it may bring to the surface upsetting and long-buried conflicts and render the patient more vulnerable to feelings of anxiety or depression about life events from which he previously was relatively well-protected by a neurotic defense structure. No matter what kind of therapy a patient is in, if he enters a period of great emotional turmoil, the therapist should see him more often than their usual contract would dictate. Sometimes these extra sessions can be less than the traditional fifty minutes; sometimes they can even be conducted on the telephone (see Chapter 24).

THE GOALS OF PSYCHOTHERAPY

At what point is psychotherapy complete? Where is the therapy going? Throughout therapy the therapist has to continually raise these questions with the patient. As to the question, "What are the symptoms?", the answers belong to the therapeutic process itself. In the first few sessions, the goals of therapy may be quite vague; it is usually impossible for a patient at the outset of therapy to state clearly everything he wants to work on. Indeed, an early goal of therapy should be to establish some idea of goals. Too conscious an emphasis on goals can lead to a kind of premature closure of psychotherapy, with the patient having mouthed a rational goal to his therapist and achieved it, but not expressed the underlying, less well-formulated concern that may have brought him to therapy. It is wise to remember the range of possible stopping points of successful therapy as a kind of guide to what may be an acceptable stopping point for the patient, even if not for the therapist. Jung[23] speaks usefully to this issue as follows:

There is in the analytical process, that is to say in the dialectical discussion between the conscious mind and the unconscious, a development or an advance towards some goal or end the perplexing nature of which had engaged my attention for many years. Psychological treatment may come to an *end* at any stage in the development without one's always or necessarily having the feeling that a *goal* has also been reached. Typical and temporary terminations may occur (1) after receiving a piece of good advice; (2) after making a more or less complete but still satisfactory confession; (3) after having recognized some hitherto unconscious but essential psychic content whose realization gives a new impetus to one's life and activity; (4) after a hard-won separation from the childhood psyche; (5) after having worked out a new and rational mode of adaptation to perhaps difficult or unusual circumstances and surroundings; (6) after the disappearance of painful neurotic symptoms; (7) after some positive turn of fortune such as an examination, engagement, marriage, divorce, change of profession, etc.; (8) after having found one's way back to the church to which one previously belonged, or after a conversion; and finally, (9) after having begun to build up a practical philosophy of life (a "philosophy" in the classical sense of the word).

The Concept of "Cure"

Many psychotherapists have posited one version or another of Bergson's "élan vital," an innate tendency toward life and development and health. It is similar to the body's response to infection or injury: physiological defenses are mobilized to deal with the insult. The physician can assist, but nature heals. Penicillin can assist the body's defenses, but when the defenses do not work, penicillin is of no avail. Psychologically, most persons seek to adjust and overcome psychological insults, and most have the defenses and strengths to make progress. The therapist's job (and the word "therapist" comes from the Greek "theraps," meaning attendant) is to assist, acting as midwife to the patient's strivings toward health. Sullivan[24] says:

> Thus we try to proceed along the general lines of getting some notion of what stands in the way of successful living for the person, quite certain that if we can clear away the obstacles, everything else will take care of itself. So true is that, that in well over twenty-five years – aside from my forgotten mistakes in the first few of them – I have never found myself called upon to "cure" anybody. The patients took care of that, once I had done the necessary brush-cleaning, and so on. It is almost uncanny how things fade out of the picture when the *raison d'être* is revealed. The brute fact is that man is so extraordinarily adaptive that, given any chance of making a reasonably adequate analysis of the situation, he is quite likely to stumble into a series of experiments which will gradually approximate more successful living.

Sullivan makes it sound easier than it is. Doing psychotherapy is hard work, and some therapists find that they cannot devote more than four or five hours a day to it before they feel spent. There are periods of discouragement, of halting progress, of slipping back into the old neurosis in virtually every course of psychotherapy, uncovering or reality-oriented.

Adding this note of caution, then, to Sullivan's statement, and combining it with Jung's, makes it apparent that the notion of ultimate "cure," a blissful renunciation of all stress and challenge and the prospect of an unruffled and tranquil future, the prospective version of an idealized, never-attained "perfect childhood" or "utopia of genitality,"[25] is neither possible nor the realistic promise of therapy. The point, again, is that therapy is a process treating a process. At its least, therapy holds out the prospect of relieving immediate discomfort and enhancing ways of coping with the factors that led up to it. At most it provides the prospect of the individual's utilizing more fully his innate strengths, intelligence, and resilience in dealing with stress, opening up opportunities to choose between self-defeating behaviors and those that can lead to self-fulfillment.

REFERENCES

1. Fromm-Reichmann, Frieda: *Principles of Intensive Psychotherapy,* University of Chicago Press, Chicago. 1950 (paperback).

2. Rogers, Carl R.: "A Theory of Therapy, Personality, and Interpersonal Relationships as Developed in a Client-Centered Framework," in S. M. Koch (ed.), *Psychology: A Study of a Science,* McGraw-Hill, New York, 1959, vol. 3.

3. Haley, Jay: *Strategies of Psychotherapy,* Grune & Stratton, New York, 1963.

4. Watzlawick, Paul: Personal communication, 1971.

5. Gendlin, Eugene T.: *Experiencing and the Creation of Meaning,* Free Press, Glencoe, 1962, p. 1.

6. Ibid.

7. Gendlin, Eugene T.: "A Theory of Personality Change," in P. Worchel and D. Byrne (eds.) *Personality Change,* Wiley, New York, 1964.

8. Glasser, William: *Reality Therapy*, Harper & Row, New York, 1965.

9. Lindemann, Erich: "Symptomatology and Management of Acute Grief," *Am. J. Psychiat.*, vol. 101, September 1944.

10. Gendlin, Eugene T.: "Values and the Process of Experiencing," in A. Mahrer (ed.), *The Goals of Psychotherapy*, Appleton-Century-Crofts, New York, 1966.

11. Fromm-Reichmann: loc. cit.

12. Rosenbaum, C. Peter: *The Meaning of Madness*, Science House, New York, 1970, chap. 14.

13. Kalis, Betty, et al.: "Precipitating Stress as a Focus in Psychotherapy," *Arch. Gen. Psychiat.*, 5:219–226, 1961.

14. Rosenbaum, C. Peter, "Events of Early Therapy and Brief Therapy," *Arch. Gen. Psychiat.*, 10:506–512, 1964.

15. Enelow, Allen J.: Personal communication, 1972.

16. Weiner, J. B.: *Psychological Disturbances in Adolescence*, Wiley-Interscience, New York, 1970.

17. Caplan, G., and S. Lebovici: *Adolescence*, Basic Books, New York, 1969.

18. Jung, C. G.: "A Study in the Process of Individuation," *The Archetypes and the Collective Unconscious*, R. F. C. Hull (trans.), Pantheon, New York, 1959, pp. 290–354.

19. Jung, C. G.: *Memories, Dreams, and Reflections*, Amiela Jaffe (ed.), Richard Winston and Clara Winston (trans.), Pantheon, New York, 1963.

20. Spiegel, John P.: *Transactions: The Interplay between Individual, Family and Society*, Science House, New York, 1971.

21. Greenson, Ralph: Address at American Psychiatric Association convention, San Francisco, May 1970.

22. Freud, Anna: *The Ego and the Mechanisms of Defense*, International Universities Press, New York, 1946.

23. Jung, C. G.: *Psychology and Alchemy, The Collected Works of C. G. Jung*, R. F. C. Hull (trans.), Pantheon Books, New York, 1953, vol. 12, p. 4. Copyright 1953 and © 1968 by Bollingen Foundation, reprinted by permission of Princeton University Press.

24. Sullivan, Harry S.: *The Psychiatric Interview*, Norton, New York, 1954, pp. 238–239.

25. Erikson, Erik H.: *Childhood and Society*, Norton, New York, 1950, p. 266.

JOHN E. BEEBE III, M.D.
C. PETER ROSENBAUM, M.D.

The Use of Dreams in Psychotherapy

In patient's dreams, we meet their natural, unreflected, instinctive reactions. It is in just this play of nature during sleep that some of the most transforming energies are released, as everyone who has gone to sleep depressed and has awakened refreshed after a vivid, remembered dream can testify. Psychotherapy attempts to relate to this unconscious transforming power with conscious insight so that the dream solutions to conflict can be carried over into waking life if they are effective, and criticized or modified where they appear to lead the dreamer into dangerous or unprofitable conflict resolution.

In this chapter we shall illustrate how one young man's psychotherapy was helped by the inclusion of his dreams. Throughout we shall adopt two perspectives: first, that the dream offers an objective statement about the dreamer which he cannot make about himself in any other way; second, that the dream is a tentative, sometimes symbolic, attempt to deliver new information to the dreamer in a form which he can accept. These perspectives reflect many contemporary trends[1-5] in the understanding of dreams, yet leave open the question which the many followers of Freud and of Jung have so often debated,[6] as to whether the motive of dreaming is to disguise or to illuminate the dreamer's ultimate, unconscious intentions. In our view, we can only say that the dream offers the dreamer what his own mind thinks he is ready for. As he looks into his dreams, he may indeed find painful or embarrassing issues expressed in an acceptable, bearable form; or he may encounter just the reverse: familiar thoughts given a shocking, repulsive guise, forcing him to revalue them. In either case, the dream makes of the dreamer's emotions something new, rearranging emotional elements to achieve a new perspective, offering new information.

The task of dream interpretation is first (following Freud) to recognize the important emotional issues contained in the imagery of the dreams, and then (following Jung) to recognize the new statement the dream makes about these issues. The dream is thus a reservoir of information for the psychotherapist, suggesting which themes are pertinent to the therapy and what ways are best to approach these themes. The psychotherapist helps the patient receive the information delivered by his dreams so that it can become part of a conscious repertoire for coping, a working knowledge of the effective and ineffective aspects of the dreamer's own instinctive responses. The attempt at integrating the information that the dream contains -- the dream analysis -- is a pragmatic art, and no two therapists practice it in quite the same way. Dream analysis typifies the psychotherapeutic collaboration, the "working alliance": the two who work together must decide on experiential grounds what is true, and what is of value. Neither can tell what will be valuable until they actually attempt the interpretation.

The emphasis in this chapter will be on what is gained by letting dreams have their say in treatment. Our method will be to let the dreams themselves illustrate our belief that the respectful use of this material helps psychotherapy to become more focused, more thoroughgoing, and more effective.

CLINICAL APPROACHES TO DREAMS

Dreams often rephrase a patient's waking feelings as a tangible sequence of symbolic actions, permitting inferences about the content, the meaning, the purpose, and the value even of transient emotions. Moreover, the feelings expressed during sleep tend to change or extend the emotional attitudes which are present when the dreamer is awake. Thus the dreams serve both to clarify and to supplement the statements which a patient can make about his waking feelings.

Using the dream to shed light on the patient's emotional reactions, the psychotherapist may find evidence of: (1) repetitions of emotional conflicts carried forward from the patient's past; (2) concealed responses to the persons and institutions in the patient's current life (including his surprising reactions to himself); and (3) energy for inner or outer developments in the patient's future. These three ways of relating dreams to events in the dreamer's emotional life reflect the sometimes overlapping contributions of Freud,[7,8] Adler,[9] and Jung.[10,11] Further development and combination of these three basic viewpoints have led to the current psychoanalytic,[12] culturalist,[13] and psychosynthetic[14] ways of working with dreams.

Applications of all three ways of viewing dreams to emotional problem solving in the here and now characterize the "focal-conflict,"[15] existentialist,[16,17] and gestalt[18] approaches to dreams. Contemporary analytical psychologists[19] prefer to determine from the dreams themselves which emotional issues in the dreamer's life the therapy ought to address and to use the dreams as a monitor of the success of the therapy in dealing with these issues; dreams are given a preeminent, guiding role in the treatment, refocusing the work as new themes appear in them.

Methods of Dealing with Dreams

There are several ways of handling dream material. Later in this chapter we shall present a detailed case example in which a modification of a Jungian approach is demonstrated. In a more traditional psychoanalytic approach, the therapist asks the patient for more and contributes less. Although they will vary in the amount of emphasis they give to different steps in interpretation, most therapists employ the following sequence:

1. Get a verbatim report of the entire dream (even therapists who do not often take notes during an hour may well do so here).

2. Ask if further elements of the dream come to mind during the report.

3. Allow the patient to associate *freely* to the dream, letting one thought lead to another, as the dream becomes a stimulus to catharsis.

4. Ask the patient to associate in a *focused* way to the dream, recovering the emotions, nuances, and memories which are connected with each dream element, with special emphasis on those that the therapist's intuition tells him may be important. (In the gestalt approach to dreams, the patient is asked to pretend he "is" the dream element and to describe himself in the first person: e.g., "I am an old house. I have dark rooms and a musty smell, but my front parlor is nice," and so on.) In this important step, the patient should be helped to recapture the experiential richness of each significant dream element. Often even a trivial-seeming element will turn out to have a fund of affective resonance for the patient, if he is allowed to dive back and recover it.

5. Seek for elements of "day residue," split-off thoughts or feelings which preoccupied the patient in the day or days before the dream, and which the dream has chosen to emphasize, satirize, or otherwise respond to.

6. Ask the patient to try to make sense out of the dream, both in terms of its manifest content (i.e., the dream as remembered) and its latent content (i.e., the symbolically expressed ideas which are revealed through the processes of association).

7. Offer the patient some of the therapist's associations to the dream (amplifications of its symbols and ideas about its meaning), to see if any of them strike a responsive chord. (Frequently, further recall will occur at this point, confirming or rejecting the suggestions as to meaning, and any of the preceding steps can be repeated, based on the new material.)

As patients become practiced in working with their dreams, they will automatically provide the associations along with the dream, and will have spent some time by themselves on the interpretation; so that the therapist can concentrate more on sharing his own ideas, based on his knowledge of the patient, and less on procuring associations from the patient. At the beginning, more time is spent asking questions, helping the patient to discover the rich flow of repressed or dissociated emotional life that so often makes its first appearance in his dreams.

In this chapter we shall show how past conflicts, present reactions, and future possibilities all made their appearance in the dreams of a young man, Eric, in once-a-week treatment for eighteen months. The dreams effectively trace Eric's development as he was helped to face the necessity of giving up an adolescent way of relating to his family in order to establish an adult identity. As the patient accomplished his emotional separation from the world of adolescence and began to enter adult life, he found himself experiencing many paradoxical emotions and no little grief. It was his dreams which helped him most to clarify what was happening to him and to trust the process in which he found himself. Through them he found the courage to develop a more mature and satisfying way of relating to his family, freeing his energies for his own life.

Though we will concentrate on Eric's therapy, it should be noted that many of the issues and techniques described apply to work with many patients. There were times when Eric needed support, acceptance, and guidance. There were times when he was confused about his problems and goals and needed help in clarifying them. There were times when he needed greater self-knowledge, needed to be more aware of how his unconscious conflicts influenced his life. There were times when he needed to test new behaviors and ways of dealing with his world, to take the risks of growing into a somewhat different person. Thus his therapy was intended to be, alternately, supportive and ego-oriented, modifying of behavior, and uncovering. His dreams became a major way of helping him in all these modes.

Example 22-1, Eric. Eric was 22 when he entered psychotherapy, a year after graduating from college. He entered feeling ashamed, depressed, and defeated: he had had fantasies of killing himself. A year earlier he had overturned plans to marry a woman of whom his divorced mother had approved and to take a job that his family had set up for him. After ending the engagement he "escaped" to the distant West Coast to pursue the literary ambitions that had been nurtured in his sheltered undergraduate years, leaving behind his mother and a 24-year-old sister who suffered from a chronic respiratory illness.

During the year he had drifted among a group of fraternity friends who had shared creative ambitions, women, and drugs during their college years. Under the spell of the leader of this group, Bert, several other members of the group had also made their way to the West Coast. The year had passed and Eric had accomplished little except to write a few rock songs that had scant prospect of being performed. He was barely supporting himself with a part-time job in a bookstore. At his first interview he told his psychotherapist, "I feel like a golden ass."

Obtaining Dream Material

An early problem for the psychotherapist is finding the right way of asking the patient what his dreams have to say about his predicament. Therapist differ on this point. Some prefer not to ask for dream material but to wait until the patient spontaneously reports dreams. Others explain in the initial interview that they are interested in the patient's dreams as well as in his waking fantasies. Often at this point the therapist will ask the patient if there is any dream which stands out or that he would like to share. Frequently, the patient will say that he does not remember his dreams. This statement can be a test of the therapist's interest. The insecure therapist, none too confident of his ability to work with dream material, may hurry along to other issues at his point in the interview. The experienced therapist will wait, giving the patient time to find a dream. Often this silence will last several minutes, as there is a considerable shift required to share dreams rather than the familiar thoughts of waking consciousness. The therapist may help the patient who is having particular trouble by saying, "Usually there is one dream that stands out, from all the years." At this point, the patient may relate a long-standing dream, often a recurrent dream from childhood.

The therapist's response to this first recounted dream is critical. He must give it attention if he wants his patient to feel he can bring other, current dreams to the psychotherapy sessions. Many therapists offer a simple interpretation at this point. Others make comments which "befriend"[20] the dream, relating to its mood, its elements, and its action with lively interest. The point is to establish that dream material can be talked about comfort-

ably and that the therapeutic effort can benefit if the leads that the dream provides are pursued.

Eric (cont'd.). The image of the golden ass intrigued the therapist, who commented on the vivid picture it gave of Eric's feelings about himself. "There's a book, *The Golden Ass,*" Eric said. "I picked it up at the library the other day."

"I know it," the therapist replied. "Psychologists have written no less than four studies of it, because it contains a tale about the psyche, called 'Amor and Psyche.' "

Pleased by the fact that his therapist seemed to share his interest in literature, Eric ventured to say more about the source of his image: "I had a dream in which I was being led across the stage by a woman. I was the golden ass and she was leading me by a rope around my neck."

"It's interesting that it was a woman," the therapist said. "At the end of *The Golden Ass,* the narrator has a vision of the goddess Isis and is initiated into her cult."

"This woman had a white toga on," the patient reported. "You know, I didn't find out about that book until after I had the dream. I was in the library looking to see if there was such a thing as a golden ass. There was another scene in the dream – a man holding a torch out with people lying dead at his feet. I did find a picture like that in the book!"

Both patient and therapist remarked at the coincidences between the dream and the book, which was in fact a current interest of the therapist. The therapist gave the patient the name of one of the commentaries in case he was interested in following it up.

In this interchange, we see the process of befriending a dream and the kind of collaboration that process engenders. Talking about fantasy material is a kind of play between patient and therapist in which chance associations, coincidence, puns, and inspirations are allowed free reign and the rigorous "scientific" attitude (that might govern the introduction of evidence in a court of law) is correspondingly relaxed. Various names have been proposed for the mode of ego-consciousness required for this sort of play — paralogical, mythopoeic, imaginal — all pointing to the need to relax logic to let the images organize their own spontaneous structures, as they do in myth or poetry. When this activity occurs between two persons, each begins to pick up on the other's imagery and to play with it. Eventually the unconscious itself will continue this activity; the patient's dreams will start to play with the ideas offered by the therapist's reactions in the therapeutic hour (as indeed the therapist's dreams may begin to register the effect of the patient's psyche on his own thinking).

Therapist influence on patient dreams is unavoidable[21]; it has been said that patients of psychoanalysts (Freudians) have Freudian dreams, i.e., dreams rich in the bodily and libidinal symbolism dealt with in that approach; patients of analytical psychologists (Jungians) have Jungian dreams, i.e., dreams rich in archetypal and mythic themes. Therapists vary widely on how much they let themselves consciously influence and interplay with their patients' dreams. The point of following dreams is not to uncover fresh content in a sterile surgical field for clean dissection, but to see how the patient's unconscious handles its contamination by another. In what the patient takes up or rejects, approaches or avoids, the therapist can see most clearly the needy, angry, open, and fearful parts of his patient's psyche. The dream is a monitor of the state of the transference.

At the beginning, the therapist enabled Eric to make a first sharing of fantasy material by following up with resonant interest the first bit of unusual, symbolic imagery that the patient offered in his initial struggle to describe himself. The ensuing discussion led to the discovery of a common interest in a particular book, a classic of fantasy literature. By bringing up the professional nature of his interest in this book, the therapist returned discussion to the realistic task, the psychotherapy, and Eric in turn related the image

to a dream, starting a dialogue in which dream statements were welcomed for what they might add to the therapeutic inquiry. Often both patient and therapist will find much to enjoy in working with fantasy material, and they should let themselves play: paradoxically, playing furthers the work of relating to dreams. (Some patients will find it difficult to play — a fertile point for further therapeutic inquiry.)

Freud, Jung, and Eric's First Dream

Freud and Jung each made unique contributions to the understanding of dreams. Freud was more interested in the way dreams are constructed: looking for evidence of unconscious solutions to conflict, he studied the ways recent life experiences ("day residues") were transformed in the process of dreaming. He attributed these changes to the action of unconscious defenses against libidinal conflicts, stirred by the events of the day. With the help of the patient's free associations, he could use the dream to uncover these conflicts and the defenses erected against them. Jung's contribution lay in exploring the usefulness of the dream transformations. Jung stressed the merits of the dream's symbolic language, as if it were the best way to exchange information about unconscious events with the conscious mind.

Freud was concerned with the translation from manifest content to latent content; Jung was concerned with the manifest content as it revealed a new idea or unexpected statement. One therapist[22] has pointed out that Freud may be said to be concentrating on the root of the tree, where moisture collects and is transmitted, while Jung attends to the crown, where the exchange of oxygen and carbon dioxide occurs; both regions are vital to the health of the tree.

Let us look first at how a psychoanalyst (Freudian) might interpret the dream. (For convenience, we will work with only the first scene.) A psychoanalyst would search for some evidence of the mental mechanisms described by Freud as the "dreamwork." Two of the more important mechanisms are *symbolization* and *condensation*. In symbolization, an idea, thought, or feeling is represented by a symbol. In condensation, two or more thoughts or feelings are represented in a single dream symbol. In waking life, condensation is an important part of wit, puns, and humor, where the expression of a forbidden impulse (usually sexual or aggressive) is merged with a more innocent one, e.g., Groucho Marx telling one of his antagonists, "I'd horsewhip you if I had a horse."

In the past Eric has felt both that he has been led by three women in his life (his mother, his sister, and his former fiancée) and that he has led them on, made asses of them. (This and other attributions of preconscious and unconscious factors in Eric were verified during the course of his treatment, thus permitting these assertions about them in this analysis of his first dream. Had there not been such corroborations, such statements about Eric's feelings would remain unsupported speculation.) Thus, in this dream, the three women are symbolized and condensed into a single woman.

Part of Eric still wishes to be passively "pulled along" by a strong woman, as became evident during the early weeks of treatment, and part of him would resent being "led by the neck" by her. Thus, being pulled along is an ambivalent *wish fulfillment* in the dream. The conscious perception of feeling "led by the neck" had crossed Eric's mind the day before the dream; it constitutes a *day residue* transformed into a dream symbol.

Another mechanism of the dream work is that of *plastic representation*, in which a more or less abstract word, idea, or feeling is represented in a symbolic object. In Eric's case the metaphor of feeling led by the neck appears in visual form. *Reaction formation*, the replacement of a thing by its opposite, is shown in the white toga: it gives an air of purity and exaltation to what Eric perceives as rather a dirty and shabby chapter in his life, one about which he feels quite guiltily depressed. In fact, it was Eric who in a sense has been (mis)leading these women; so this reversal of

role is both a reaction formation and a *displacement* (the shifting of an unacceptable idea or emotion from the appropriate object to a more neutral one); in this case the displacement protects Eric from having to feel he has been leading these women on: in the dream it is they who are leading him on.

Eric reports the dream with some wonder and amazement. In the process there will be some *secondary elaboration;* i.e., he will unwittingly rationalize and make more intelligible the plot and actors in the dream. Only through free association and other attempts at interpretation will the *latent content* — the hidden message he did not want to hear but will need sooner or later to comprehend if therapy is to proceed — emerge from the *manifest content.* Only then will Eric be fully aware of how he has misled the women in his life (for which aggression he is consciously feeling guilty), how he feels the need to be punished (led by the neck, as an ass) for having besmirched the women's image (restored to whiteness as a wish to deny what he had done).

Now let us see how an analytical psychologist (Jungian) might work with the same material. He would work with the manifest content (the golden ass and the woman in the toga) to see what they might yield in new and surprising ideas, as shown in this vignette from that session:

> *Eric (cont'd.).* Indeed, to Eric's depressed frame of mind it came as a surprise that there could be anything golden (valuable) about the asinine way he thought he had been behaving.
>
> New too was this image of woman. In her classic dress she seemed to connote wisdom, spirit, authority. The spiritual aspect was new: he had not seen that in the women he had known; they had tended to meet more his material needs. His mother, a good, practical provider, had always seen to his needs for food, shelter, and clothing. A series of girlfriends in college had met his needs for sex. When his well-meaning mother had begun to arrange every aspect of his future material

existence with his intended bride, he had fled this maternal influence. Yet here he was being led by a woman of another sort — who seemed a positive figure, a spiritual mother, who would influence not his physical, but his psychological development.

To understand this new feminine image in her own terms, an analytical psychologist would use not the method of *association* (by which familiar figures would no doubt turn up) but the method of *amplification.* Here the dream image is compared not with similar images in the life of the dreamer but with similar images in the long life of human fantasy, drawing freely upon comparative symbolism from folklore and mythology. Here the parallels with the Latin fairy tale *The Golden Ass* become important, not just a pleasant coincidence. In that tale, the Ass is an enchanted man, and as so often occurs in such stories, his transformation back into human form is accomplished through the agency of a woman, the Greco-Roman goddess Isis. Isis arranges that the man shall return to the human form in the midst of a procession dedicated to her.

By amplifying Eric's dream, we see a possibility not explicitly stated in the dream itself: Eric could be led out of his asinine condition by the woman in the toga. Only if this possibility fits the feeling and the mood of the dream as remembered by Eric would it be acceptable as a suggestion "of where this dream is leading." But it is often a mistake to withhold such conjectures from patients on the grounds that "the patient didn't know the story when he had the dream," or "that part of the story wasn't in the dream." As moviegoers know, one doesn't always have to have seen a film before to know how it will end, and the unconscious has a remarkable propensity for remembering the endings of the many possible human stories.

To restate the dream, Eric is in an asinine state, but he is submitting to a spiritual mother who he hopes can lead him out of this condition. What could this mean? Since Eric was contemplating

psychotherapy at the time he had this dream and wrestling with the feeling that he could probably not be helped, this dream perhaps conveys the idea that there is something positive in the new dependency he would have to accept were he to enter treatment. A Jungian would say that it is not so much the fulfillment of a wish as a *compensation* for Eric's conscious attitude of despair. It offers to Eric's doubts a classical picture of a process of being helped. At the same time, the dream does not make a moral statement or a promise; it only gives an *objective picture* in symbolic form of what Eric can expect from psychotherapy — a ritual expiation, no more, no less. Whether he can stand to submit, like the ass, to the process of being led is up to him, but this is the rite to which he must submit if he is going to regain his human form (his psychological health). The idea of rite is conveyed not only by the action and cast, but by the setting, the stage.

Jung used the patient's associations to the various dream elements (focused, not free) to *establish the context* for the dream. Here Eric's statement "I feel like a golden ass" seems to provide the context. Thus the dream comes in answer to an implicit question: "What can a talented ass like me expect of psychotherapy?" The answer the dream provides is: a rite of initiation. Although the outcome of the rite is not clear, the imagery strongly suggests Eric's potential for transformation at the hands of another.

Who this other may be is always a problem in interpretation. It is easy to see the woman as the ideal psychotherapist, the spiritual mother. It is somewhat harder to recognize in her a part of Eric. Jung often pointed out that when men try to symbolize the activity of the unconscious, they fall back upon the most potent image of otherness, the opposite sex. Thus for men, the unconscious is often perceived as a woman — a powerful, unknown woman. And indeed, Eric's therapy would involve him in submitting to his unconscious, in listening to his dreams, in accepting the reality of his own emotions. And for patients who are suited for intensive psychotherapy, the unconscious is often the "ideal psychotherapist," showing the patient what he has neglected and now must include in his everyday living if he is not to live against his emotions.

As Eric's dream illustrates, there are three levels in any interpretation.[23] First is what Jung called the *objective level*, at which most Freudian dream interpretation is made: Eric's dream is seen as a statement about his relationship to the women in his life. Second is the *subjective level*, at which Jungian interpretation is often made: the dream is seen as a statement about Eric's relationship to the feminine -- the unconscious emotional life -- within himself. Last is the *transference level*, at which the interpersonal interpretation is made: the dream communicates Eric's intentions in seeking therapy to his potential therapist. The three levels of interpretation all combine to enrich the understanding of the dream.

Of course, the therapist does not attempt a complete interpretation at all three levels with the first dream that is presented to him! Indeed, much of the information on which the interpretations offered here are based was not available to the therapist when the initial dream was offered, especially the intensity of Eric's feeling that he had made an ass of himself, that he had in fact sunk into a dehumanized condition. Only with much hearing of Eric's feelings did the therapist come to know the exact state of despair with which Eric had entered therapy. Gradually he came to see that the ass represented Eric's reality, not just a clever metaphor for it.

A Note of Caution

Therapists associate vividly to their patients' dreams. Listening to a dream is like hearing a short story read aloud: the listener constructs his own images and scene. As he listens the therapist strives to employ his critical faculties in the knowledge that he ultimately wants to understand the dream, making use of his skills in dream interpretation. Many therapists tend to draw from dreams what is revealing of psychopathology and to ignore what is creative or reparative. Often the therapist feels a pressure to "be psychological," ignoring the fun of dreams.

Inexperienced therapists may be awed by how their senior colleagues seem always to get a wealth of information from even a brief dream fragment, not realizing that their senior colleagues are not nearly as likely to report a patient's dream which left them baffled and confused. Yet there are such dreams, many of them. Indeed, it is rarely if ever that a dream can be totally analyzed, that each symbol and nuance can be fully understood. There are many dreams where significant portions remain a mystery despite the best efforts of the patient and the therapist. Sometimes these mysteries are solved weeks and months later (the dream was premonitory in that sense: it was a statement from the unconscious that anticipated developments for which consciousness would be ready only later). It is because of these factors that inexperienced therapists may feel an unjustified pressure to interpret each dream totally, seeking to emulate what they perceive to be the abilities of their experienced colleagues, rather than allowing themselves to remain perplexed and intrigued by those parts of dreams they do not, in fact, understand.

The pressures to look for psychopathology, to be psychological, and to emulate experienced colleagues may lead to premature and simplistic interpretations which drearily restate the obvious, failing to discover anything new. For example, the therapist might have responded to Eric's first dream by saying, "You must feel like you're being led around by women."

Quick interpretation of any variety -- Freudian, Jungian, interpersonal, existential -- can only interfere with the therapeutic process, which always requires a careful discovery of the depth and extent of the patient's feelings. Jung made it his rule to say to himself before venturing an opinion on a dream, "I have no idea what this dream means."[24] Only then could he trust himself to examine the dream, open to the new possibilities a seemingly familiar symbol might offer. It is even harder for the beginner to avoid jumping to conclusions.

Indeed, a single dream has so many possible meanings that it is almost impossible to verify which meaning is correct, even if it seems plausible or acceptable to the dreamer, whose own sense of rightness must always be the final authority. One needs to hear a series of dreams to understand the movement in a given patient's psyche, and we shall continue the case of Eric later in this chapter by offering such a series. In discussing the first dream, the therapist need only make sure that he has created a climate in which the patient will want to share his subsequent dreams; then the initial work will have been more than adequately accomplished.

The Brain, Dreaming, and Remembering

Since the discovery in the 1950s of rapid eye movements and the development of technology for measuring electroencephalographic (EEG) patterns through an entire night of sleep, much valuable information has been collected to the benefit of the psychotherapist who works with dreams. In talking with patients about their dreams, it is particularly helpful to know about the kinds of dreams and their recall. A very useful source of this information is Ann Faraday's *Dream Power.*[25] Much of the basic information can be found in early articles by Dement[26,27] and the more recent elaborations in the books by Hartmann[28] and Medow and Snow.[29]

The key finding has been that there are two states of sleep: sleep in which rapid eye movements do not appear and the EEG patterns (stages II to IV) are slow and synchronized (S); and sleep in which rapid eye movements (REM) do appear and the EEG pattern (stage I) is rapid and desynchronized (D). About 75 percent of the night is spent in non-REM, S sleep, but four or five times a night (at about ninety-minute intervals), the normal subject emerges from this deep level into REM, D sleep, in which he must spend 25 percent of his total sleeping time. In contrast to the S state − which is quiet and restful − the D state is stormy, accompanied by much physiologic

evidence of heightened arousal, including penile erection in men. The D state is often preceded and followed by tossing in the sleep (as if the dreamer were preparing for the curtain to go up), but during the REM period itself, motor paralysis obtains. (Patients sometimes awake still unable to move and are extremely frightened.) Only in the S state can sleep-talking or sleepwalking occur.

There are also two states transitional to sleep: the state of falling asleep (in which *hypnagogic* phenomena are recorded) and the state of awaking from sleep (in which *hypnopompic* phenomena occur). Thus, when a patient reports a "dream," he may be recalling (1) an event during S sleep (a non-REM dream) (2) an event during D sleep (an REM dream), or (3) a hypnagogic or hypnopompic phenomenon (a "dreamlet").[30] Only REM dreams fulfill the definition of "an experience that involves vivid and complex multimodal imagery, a progression of events, and sense of reality."[31] By contrast, non-REM dreams are more like background thoughts, being shorter, less vivid, less visual, less dramatic, less elaborated, less emotional, less active, more plausible, more concerned with current problems, more purely conversational, and more thoughtlike than REM dreams.[32] Dreamlets are strange, hallucinatory visions, often accompanied by unusual sensations. Often they resemble REM dreams, but they are shorter and less dramatic in structure (sometimes resembling a tableau or pageant rather than a play).

Many writers regard only the REM dreams as true dreams. It is in REM dreams that we most often find the distortions which many identify with dreaming. Freud understood these distortions as the effect of censorship upon latent dream thoughts. Jung saw them as evidence for the autonomy of the psyche's symbol-producing faculty, which he saw as possessing an archaic style of language all its own. Rossi[33] has interpreted these distortions as the way new personality structures look when first laid down by protein synthesis during the REM periods.

But it is a mistake to devalue non-REM dreams

just because they are more thoughtlike. Both kinds of dreams play a part in psychotherapy, as the following example shows.

Example 22-2, Alan. Alan, a 28-year-old professional man, had the following typically REM dream in his analysis:

"I was in a classroom with other students, possibly a nursery school. I was absorbed in the positive maternal atmosphere created by the teacher, humming at her desk. I felt at one with the other students, who were all working quietly at their different desks. I didn't actually see anyone in the room, nor did I need to, so contained was I within the pleasant classroom atmosphere. Suddenly an angry male figure, 'The Father,' entered the room, harshly interrupting the comfortable atmosphere with angry words directed toward the motherly teacher.

" 'How could you let this happen?' the father demanded. 'Look at him!'

"I was suddenly acutely conscious of myself and my surroundings. Now I could see that all the other students were wearing red tunics and I a coat of many colors."

In his analytic work, Alan often returned to this dream. It marked the stage of his therapy when he first became aware of his positive mother complex, which had separated him from his father, whose criticism he could not accept – his unresolved Oedipal conflict. Further, in the biblical figure of Joseph, who wore the first coat of many colors, the young man thought he had found a solution to this conflict, which had made it hard for him to adjust to the masculine world of work. Although Joseph was in many ways a mother's son[34] – narcissistic, gifted, eager to please, preoccupied with dreams, concerned with nourishing others, and alienated from his more ordinary brothers – he did succeed in finding a successful masculine identity within the patriarchal biblical world. He became the Pharaoh's right-hand man.

Alan reasoned that he could succeed by staying within his organization, putting his varied talents to the disposal of some higher executive, whose top assistant he could eventually become; the ultimate authority could rest in someone else. For a time, he pursued this role within his own organization with outstanding success. As he carried out assignments faithfully and imaginatively, he was given more to do and was promoted to a job very like the one Joseph had held in Pharaoh's realm.

Then – about two years after the first – came a dream of another type. It followed a day when one of Alan's clients had expressed his keen interest in cosmology – he had even described himself as a cosmologist. The patient mentioned this curious occurrence to his superiors at work, who dismissed the client as a harmless eccentric.

Alan (cont'd.). In this dream, Alan found himself at a dim crossroads, along with three vague, ghostlike men with painfully grinning clown faces who were positioned like characters in a Noh drama. Suddenly, the thought came to him, "Not Joseph, but the cosmologist!"

In working on this peculiar dream (which is a typical non-REM dream), Alan came to recognize that a cosmologist is not a man like Joseph, who works at another's side, but a man like Moses, a lawgiver, who discovers a new order, mapping out the world plan of his particular culture, an authentic father figure.[35] Alan then realized that it was not enough for him to play the dutiful son doing what the "fathers" in his particular organization thought was best, but that he had to map out his own career directions if he were to succeed in professional life and fulfill himself as a man.

The first dream, of the REM type, gave Alan a vivid picture of himself which he could use in reconciling his father's demands with his mother's indulgence, so achieving a first kind of positive identity for himself as a man. The second dream, of the non-REM type, gave him a new idea which he could use at an existential crossroads in his life to give up his overattachment to the earlier solution and develop still further as a man. Both the REM vision and the non-REM revision counted as nodal points in the course of Alan's psychotherapy.

Remembering Dreams. Patients are often guilty or defensive about their ability to remember dreams, as if they were resisting the process of psychotherapy. Actually, as Cohen[36] has pointed out, the recall of dreams is quite influenced by the intensity of the dream images themselves (the more vivid images are better remembered) and by the amount of interruption immediately upon awakening (even a short activity, such as answering a phone, can cause the dream to vanish). Being less vivid, a non-REM dream is particularly hard to remember unless one awakes from a non-REM period and immediately writes it down.

Under laboratory conditions, nearly everyone who is awakened from one of his four or five nightly REM periods reports a vivid dream. Within each of these REM periods, several distinct REM episodes occur: a patient may potentially report ten to twenty episodes just from the REM portion of a single night's sleep.[37] Whether discrete episodes belonging to the same REM period should be regarded as separate dreams or as "acts" of the same dream play is a moot point; usually the patient makes this judgment when he records successive episodes.

The following summary of facts about recall is drawn from Faraday[38] and Cohen,[39] based on research findings. If the subject is allowed to go right back to sleep and is awakened in five minutes, his recall is blurred; if he sleeps for ten minutes before he is awakened again, the dream is usually lost. For a REM dream to be remembered, the subject must waken in the midst of a REM period and stay awake for ten minutes, concentrating on fixing the dream in his mind. Shorter periods of pondering the dream are usually accompanied by forgetting the next morning.

For persons sleeping in their own beds rather than a laboratory, remembering is best if the awakening is sudden — as by a buzzing alarm or telephone — rather than gentle and gradual, as by a clock radio. Awakening should be followed by a ten-minute period of alert inactivity, during which a memory trace is laid down. Distraction by other activities (including turning on the light and searching for a pencil to write the dream down) may significantly impair recall.

There is evidence that dreams which touch upon issues the patient may find embarrassing to talk about with the therapist are not recalled the next morning (though they may be told to a dream experimenter during a night awakening).

The use of drugs or alcohol which suppress REM sleep also blurs the consciousness required for recall; stopping the use of even a small quantity of drugs, such as barbiturates, may enable the patient to remember his dreams.

Usually, people recall only those dreams which occur during the last REM period before awakening, dreams from a difficult night punctuated by many awakenings (as during an illness), and nightmares which awaken the dreamer into a panicked, wide-awake state. Moreover, personality differences separate those who habitually recall their dreams from those who do not. Research has indicated that nonrecallers are trying to look *away* from their dream images during sleep, while recallers are accepting the dream images passively. Nonrecallers usually have a lower tolerance for anxiety. When they do recall dreams, it is usually on nights following days which have been unusually unpleasant.

Frequently, dreams are recalled because the patient is trying to recall his dreams to tell his psychotherapist; autosuggestion given just before going to sleep often works. Scrupulous dream recallers awake during the night after dreaming, quietly scoop the dream fish into the net of a permanent memory trace, and record their impressions in a dream diary. Such conscientious patients may present an abundance of dream material to the psychotherapeutic hour, posing a problem of deciding *which* dream to discuss, as well as the appropriateness of this much emphasis on dream material.

Recording Dreams. It is important to have an accurate record of the patient's dreams. Some therapists have an uncanny recall for dream material; most find that they make substitutions when they try to recall dreams from memory. In a communication so compact, so precise, and so important as a dream, every image counts — like every word of a telegram. It makes a difference whether the patient turned to his right or to his left, whether the girl was wearing red or blue, whether the group consisted of three or of four persons. Often such details become meaningful only months or years after the dream is first mentioned.

Therefore, a good practice is to write the dream down as the patient tells it during the therapeutic hour. This practice, far from interrupting the therapeutic contact, actually reinforces the idea that the dreams will be taken seriously by the therapist and encourages the patient to bring them. The therapist can keep copies of the patient's dreams in a folder. A stenographer's notebook is ideal for recording dreams; associations can be recorded in a parallel column. With practice, the therapist can learn to get the dream reports down nearly verbatim.

Jungian therapists in general ask more frequently for dreams and spend more time on them in therapy than do therapists of other backgrounds. With practice, a Jungian can cover three or four dreams in a session, providing he first fully understands the patient and his conscious predicament. The great bulk of such therapy may be by way of dream analysis, as was true in the case of Eric. In contrast, while Freudians welcome dreams as part of therapy, they do not seek them with such intensity, and if a patient started filling his hours nearly exclusively with dream material, the Freudian analyst might suggest somewhat earlier than the Jungian that he is using dreams as a resistance against looking at waking behavior and thought. Still, a patient in Freudian analysis who failed to bring up any dream material would have this pointed out to him, and Jungians, too, recognize resistance via emphasis on dreams. Much

of the material being presented immediately below represents a Jungian outlook; the emphasis and techniques would be present in less prominent and somewhat moderated form in psychoanalytic and existential therapies.

Many patients will get into the habit of keeping a dream diary. A few will tape-record their dreams, bringing the tapes to the therapeutic hour. Some patients will type out their dreams, unasked, and bring the therapist a copy. While it is not always possible to discuss every dream in a therapeutic hour, the therapist should allow himself time at least to read whatever dreams are brought to him. Often he can allude to such dreams as issues which come up in the therapeutic sessions which seem to have been touched on by the imagery in the dreams. Thus the dreams that have been shared are included, even if not always interpreted in detail.

Only after the patient and therapist are well into a working collaboration should the therapist ask the patient for copies of his dreams, and then only after thought. Many patients do not mind such homework. Others resent it, and the therapy session may become too much like a college class or, as one patient put it, "a responsive reading." Nevertheless, when both patient and therapist keep copies of the dreams, therapy is a truly collaborative effort, with each of the partners assuming a measure of responsibility for the unconscious communication which has grown up between them.

DREAMS IN THE COURSE OF THERAPY

Initial Dreams

Initial dreams are extremely important and should be noted down, no matter what the orientation of the therapist or his practice of concentrating on later dreams in therapy. Initial dreams can predict the entire course of therapy and can identify initial problems, the kinds of emotion which therapy can release, and possible pitfalls the therapist would be wise to anticipate.

In Chapter 19, the dream of the patient on the ocean liner wrecked by a great black whale, with the patient ultimately being rescued, allowed the therapist to ask the patient if he feared getting launched into therapy might stir up severe emotional storms; the patient was able to confirm this and talk further about his fears.

Example 22-3. At his second interview a college student reported this dream to his therapist:

"Last night I dreamed I was coming here for my session today, and at the end of the session I asked you if you thought there was anything *really* the matter with me. You smiled and shook your head 'No,' but above your head there was a neon sign that kept flashing on and off, 'Dementia praecox, dementia praecox!'"

The student knew from his psychology courses that "dementia praecox" was the old name for insanity, and his fear that he would be found mad quickly became apparent as he associated to the dream. The therapist, having observed the student's basically healthy ego functioning, he was able on the one hand to reassure him that he would not go mad and on the other to ask him about thoughts, feelings, and experiences that the patient thought were abnormal, so that they could proceed to work on them.

Initial Dreams and Treatment Choice. Initial dreams can help the therapist decide whether his initial treatment will be primarily uncovering or primarily reality-oriented. Dreams can be both problem-solving and problem-revealing. If the representations of the patient in early dreams are passive, are having things done to them, and especially if these are bad things, such as being attacked by animals, falling into an abyss, entering a foreboding dark room — if the dream somehow gives the therapist the willies — the patient's ego may not be able to tolerate uncovering work at first (though it might well later). If, on the other hand, the patient is active in his dreams and copes

well with adversity, he may well be suited for an uncovering approach, especially if he meets the criteria cited in Chapter 13.

The dream is like a bridge thrown up between the conscious and the unconscious.[40] It can be used to lead the dreamer up or down in whichever direction seems right for his ego to go. In working with patients whose egos are weak, it is best to stay with the manifest sense the dream makes, confining interpretations to the dream's own immediate level of impact. With patients who have stronger egos, a rigorous exploration of the latent dream thoughts is often in order, but even here the dream should be allowed to speak at the manifest level. How these considerations apply to Eric's early treatment is shown in the following vignette:

Eric (cont'd.). The night after his first appointment, Eric recorded this dream:

"I am running on a road, very fast. I think I am being pursued. I have a headlamp attached to my belt and was running down the road just like a car. Pretty soon I had to use a pogo stick and bounce myself along. I crawled under a fence, and I managed to lock myself in a pen right under a freeway overpass."

Here the torch of the man in the first dream standing over the dead people (probably a hypnopompic image) has become a headlamp. Eric's energies had been bent mainly on escaping a marriage and a job that he felt was wrong for him. Running away is eventually a regression, and the childishness of this solution is aptly conveyed by the image of the pogo stick. Eric's associations did not help much with the pen, the low fenced-off place where Eric must endure a period of confinement. At this stage in the therapy, the therapist could only conjecture that this image of confinement meant that Eric could no longer stave off his depression, that he could not run any more without treatment. Indeed, the therapist worried about the "closed world of suicide" in hearing this image.

The dreams showed certain signs of ego strength, including the good headlamp (i.e., his intelligence) and his determination to save himself. Still, the therapist noted how Eric's depression had weakened his ego: the way he was driving himself, like a machine; the way he blundered, self-destructively, into the closed-off pen. Although Eric's intelligence argued for an uncovering approach, his suicidal depression would require considerable realistic support from the therapist. In the end, the therapist decided to combine an uncovering with a reality-oriented approach.

Dreams can also be helpful in supportive psychotherapy where medication is being used. Note that in the following example, it was only after months of treatment that one of the patient's therapists asked for a dream, the initial dream of therapy.

Example 22-4. George, a 55-year-old, chronically depressed plumber, had been seen monthly for refills of his amitryptyline prescription. He complained, almost seeming to enjoy it, about how his wife was always bothering him, but, not being psychologically minded, could not enter into any discussion of how he might be contributing to the situation.

One session, George reported a mildly sarcastic remark his wife had made. The therapist, new to George's case, asked him if he ever dreamed.

George said, "Why, yes. Last night I had a dream about my little dog. I was holding him in my arms, and he was looking up at me ever so tenderly, when suddenly he seemed to droop his head like he was going to die."

The therapist asked George about the dog. It turned out that he loved his pet above all other things because the dog was always sweet and cheerful.

The therapist asked George if this dog might not be his own cheerful disposition, which had faded into despondence after his wife's sarcastic remark. George seemed to like this idea.

At his next monthly session, George related another dream. "The dog was there again, sitting at my feet and looking up at me. As I

watched, its face turned into a vicious wharf rat." George went on to say that he had seen wharf rats in his younger days, working on the harbors "around some people that were hardly better than wharf rats they were so mean." George had once seen a wharf rat leap and bite a man.

Pursuing the lead of the previous month's session, the therapist asked George if he was ever mean, if he ever lashed out. "Well, if you put it that way, doctor, I guess I do. Oh, I don't like that dream. I hate to think my little dog would turn into a wharf rat."

"Yet that's what seems to happen to a good disposition when a person gets mean," the therapist observed.

This was the first picture George had ever had of his mood problem, and he marveled at the insight it gave him. Then, for the first time, George allowed himself to admit that he launched nightly into verbal attacks against his wife, not unlike the content of his monthly sessions. His wife's occasional barbed remarks were her weak defenses against the things he said. "I can be pretty cruel, doctor," George admitted.

The following month, George brought his wife to the medication clinic with him. She turned out to be a quiet, timid woman, somewhat frightened of her husband. She reported that George upset her with his critical remarks, but that lately there had been some improvement. For the first time, she had been curious to see his doctor, and George had been willing to bring her. This contact opened the door to some much-needed couple work.

DREAMS IN THE STAGES OF CONTACT, CONFRONTATION, INITIATION, AND INDIVIDUATION

For the remainder of this chapter we shall concentrate on Eric's dreams during his eighteen-month course of once-a-week psychotherapy. By so doing, we hope both to show how dreams are used in the various stages of the transference described in Chapter 12 and also to present a detailed example of the processes of uncovering, intensive psychotherapy described in Chapters 13 and 19. Material taken directly from therapy hours will be indented; the therapist's internal speculations and more general discussion of theory and technique will be printed with normal margins.

Contact

In the stage of contact, the major task is that therapist and patient feel en rapport, feel that sufficient trust and warmth exist for them to proceed. Eric had come to therapy ambivalently, as do most patients, and he was also trying out an encounter group to see what it would be like. His attitudes about treatment are shown in the following three dreams:

> *Therapy.* Dream: My face was that of a clown's. Then I got shot full of buckshot.
> Dream: My friends from the encounter group had gathered. It seems we are all to see my individual therapist for some reason. As we sat around discussing what we were to do, I felt myself withdrawing. My chair was in a strange position, moved forward to draw a tighter circle. The nurse tried to tell me I could see the psychiatrist either Tuesday or Friday and that I had to make a choice. I thought she had said we were going to meet the doctor today, and I kept repeating it, trying unsuccessfully to remember the time of the appointment. Finally I began to scream and fainted on the floor.
> Dream: I seem to be waiting with my friend Ned outside a grocery store. I can see sailboats preparing for their launch. We're waiting for the wind. Suddenly I notice a beautiful girl, blond with very large breasts, and she is walking off with a friend of mine. Ned tells me that I could have this woman if I wanted her; so when she reappears from the grocery store, I ask her to go to bed with me. At first she

hesitates, then one of her friends shows up too. They strip and get into bed with both Ned and me. She has one orgasm before I do and tries to call it quits, but I tell her that she is wrong and can have more, so we continue.

The first two of these dreams seemed fairly clearly to reflect Eric's fear of entering therapy. At first glance, the third of these dreams had nothing to do with the therapy at all. However, Eric's associations to the grocery store ("a place where you get your supplies") and the sense of anticipation conveyed by the atmosphere of waiting for the launching of the sailboats convinced the therapist that this dream marked the beginning of a positive transference to the therapist.

Before we continue with the interpretation of the third dream, it is well to cite a helpful rule. Often one can understand a dream if one prefaces it with the statement, "It's exactly as if. . . ." Then one simply continues with the dream itself. Thus, this dream of Eric's can be stated, "It's exactly as if I am waiting with my friend Ned outside a grocery store, where I can see sailboats preparing for their launch." The interpretation then becomes largely a process of finding a reference for the "it" in the sentence. In this case, following his intuitive hunch, the therapist decided to see if the dream meant, "Starting to work with you as my therapist, it's exactly as if. . . ." From them on, it was a matter of seeing if this interpretation made sense.

> *Therapy.* The therapist conjectured that Eric might be responding to his own efforts to create a comfortable atmosphere. At the level of their egos, he and Eric could be relaxed, like two friends. Who then was the beautiful woman with big breasts that he was offering to Eric, like a good friend?

Here the therapist had to draw on his knowledge of unconscious symbolism. As we have seen, the unconscious of a man – the pattern and history of his emotional responses – is often personified by a woman. Jung called this figure the "anima,"[41] but Freud, too, had some conception of this figure, although he did not pursue the matter deeply.[42] The therapist recognized that in treatment his own unconscious was as active a participant as his conscious. This figure with big breasts could represent a positive maternal capacity in the therapist, which had also been responded to in the dreams of other patients. (Here, as we see, the therapist's self-knowledge is essential.) Thus Eric was being offered some of the therapist's unconscious — relationship and mothering. At the same time, another copulation was occurring: could that be the therapist making contact with Eric's unconscious?

Indeed, the transference relationship — with its strong overtones of incest — is often symbolized by a sexual activity involving two brother-sister couples.[43] When patient and therapist are man and woman, the "other couple" is the woman's unconscious (masculine) and the man's unconscious (feminine). The four-person sexual act represents the totality of involvement between the consciouses and the unconsciouses of both partners. Such an arrangement — often in a strangely public setting — adequately expresses the peculiarity of transference, which has been described as "the most personal relationship in the most impersonal setting."[44]

What then of the woman having had her orgasm before Eric? This made the therapist think. He was older than Eric and felt himself to have already resolved most of the issues Eric was struggling with emotionally, particularly the separation from home. It would be easy to lose patience, since he had already "come" to the insights Eric had yet to find. In treatment, it would be necessary for him to wait until Eric "came" to such insights on his own. Eric's insistence on this point seemed a good sign to the therapist that an authentic contact had been achieved in the early hours and that Eric would overcome his fear of therapy enough to make necessary demands of the therapist.

As is customary, Eric's therapist made few of these interpretations out loud. Indeed, he was none too sure of them; they were simply what made sense at the time. To the third of these early dreams, the therapist said only, "It seems as if things are just getting started — and whoever she is, she'll have to wait for you." (This left open the question of whether the woman in the dream was a part of the therapist or a part of Eric. If the latter, she might symbolize Eric's impatience.)

Therapy. Later in this hour, Eric confessed that he had had a previous contact with a psychiatrist. The previous year, when he was still at home, Bert had convinced him to lie to get out of the draft. Eric had gone to see a psychiatrist, had pretended — quite falsely — that he was actively homosexual, and had gotten a letter excusing him from the draft. After this experience, Eric felt at once exposed (since he did harbor fears about his potential for homosexuality, which was now a matter of public record) and ashamed (since he had taken a coward's way out). Worse, all this manipulation had been unnecessary: his draft number was too high for him to be called, and he had known that before he had arranged to see the other psychiatrist. Somehow Bert had caused him to doubt his own mind. The therapist strongly suspected that Eric had done all this just to give himself reasons to say he wasn't good enough to marry his fiancée and to break the engagement.

After this confession, Eric put the question to his therapist, "Can you still help me?"

Now the therapist could see why Eric had to persuade the woman in the dream to wait for him. If she did indeed represent the "mother" he hoped to find in therapy, he had good reason to expect that she would lose interest in him, once she "knew" him. Indeed, a part of the therapist was now tempting him to be done quickly with Eric, to be satisfied with this confession as the major part of their work together. The dream, however, indicated that there was "more to come," that he should not let himself be satisfied with just this first bit of understanding.

Therapy. The therapist said, "Well, I think this gives us something to work on, rather than a reason to stop our work. It sounds as if you need to find out why you did such a self-destructive thing."

Much relieved, Eric readily agreed to this search for understanding as a goal for their work. At the next session, he said, "I like you, because you don't always say what I expect you to say." He dropped the encounter group and settled into serious intensive work. The stage of contact had been achieved.

Confrontation

In the stage of confrontation, therapist and patient begin to confront the troublesome issues which have thus far been largely out of awareness. It is here that the therapist can point out sometimes unpleasant facts to the patient, who must now pay attention to them even though he may largely have ignored similar observations made by family and friends in the past. The task for Eric was to confront the things he was doing to himself that contributed to his depression.

Therapy. Dream: I was in a race with other young men. Everyone else had on tennis sneakers; I had on fancy boots that I had bought recently. I was running around the house where I live. After I had gone one and one-quarter laps, I had to get over a barrier, which was a gutter spout. Beyond that was a void into which I hesitated to leap. Moreoever, my shoes were too slick, and so I fell back, and went back to the starting point.

In working with Eric on this dream, the therapist pointed out that in the ancient world, initiation rites, by which young men left the state of childhood and entered the state of full participation in adult life, often involved a race.

"I could use an initiation all right," Eric said.

The one and one-quarter laps was easily enough interpreted: Eric had left home one and a quarter years before. If by leaving home Eric had intended an initiation (which in primitive tribes does indeed begin with a separation from the mother), it looked from this dream as if he had run into a major obstacle which could cause him to fail in his goal.

Somehow, as Eric and his therapist discussed the dream, the slick shoes seemed responsible: if he had had tennis sneakers like the rest, he could have continued the race.

Therapy. The therapist asked Eric about the "fancy boots," which indeed he had worn to the session. They were shiny and conspicuously expensive.

Eric admitted he had paid for them with money his mother had sent him. She often sent him money for clothes, together with letters which pointed out to him how irresponsible he was. In fact, when he had bought these shoes, he had thought to himself, "This is a regression."

The therapist said, "Well, if you want your initiation to work, you'll have to give up depending on your mother for money. Of course, that'll mean facing the unknown – I suppose the risk of ending up in the gutter."

At this point Eric brought forward his great fears of not being able to support himself. Shortly after this session, he was able to increase his earning power with a better-paying job, and he stopped accepting money from home for any of his living expenses. Not long after, he had another dream.

Dream: I was supposed to go to the beach with Bobby Kennedy this day. I had been allowed to invite some friends but didn't. A small Econoline bus – yellow – pulled up and out jumped six uniformed men, apparently guards. One of them was Kennedy disguised so that he wouldn't be shot. I got in and Ethel was sitting on one side. I went to the back of the bus. We got to a very beautiful beach and the waves settled gently on the sand. But then suddenly the tide began to move in and pushed everybody back from the beach almost to the road. A group of men I had noticed to my left were playing volleyball on high ground, so I nonchalantly joined them. I noticed they were playing quite sloppily. I asked the driver, who couldn't hit the ball uphill, if I could please serve for him. He replied that it was his serve. After a while I seated myself on a rock and was approached by a graying, middle-aged man who asked me if I would like to take a ride in his Stutz Bearcat, the Spade model, making a stop for tea or a drink. I asked him where we would stop for a drink, and he replied, "My place, of course." I replied, "No, thanks," that I wasn't like that and he would probably have trouble if we went.

This dream followed a letter from his mother in which she implored him to show some responsibility and come home to her. Here she was playing on a quite vulnerable spot in Eric, his idealism. Indeed, during the period he had been most caught in playing the savior to his mother and sister (the man who would recoup the family fortunes), Robert Kennedy had been his ideal. Ethel Kennedy was a woman of about his mother's age.

Here, in a nutshell, was Eric's identity problem. Until he had forced his way out of the part with some distinctly unheroic acts, he had sought to become a man by playing the part of his mother's hero, living out her idea of what a man should be, rather than finding his own. To the degree that he still felt guilty about leaving her, her ideas of what was right for him still had possession of him, like the bus in which he was a passenger. This was her trip.

Indeed, in her letters, his mother made all this quite explicit, in the guise of concern for his security and her own. (Hence the disguise. And, as Jung points out, a woman's opinions are often symbolized by a crowd of male figures.)

Although his mother's wishes for him had their beautiful, idealistic side (symbolized by the seduc-

tive beach), the fact remained that living out her intuitions (yellow, the color of the bus, is often a symbol of intuition) of what he might be could only be an unconscious solution to his problem. Indeed, if he allowed himself to return now to trying to be what she wanted, he would only engulf his own fragile identity in the tide and undertow of his divorced mother's needs, aptly symbolized by the sea. This regression could not be.

Yet entry into the conventional masculine world was closed to him. Neither the inept volleyball player nor the homosexual playboy could offer him much worth having in the way of masculine support. Their images led the therapist to ask Eric about his father.

As it turned out, Eric's father (the son of a rich, indulgent mother) had long before succumbed to his own mother complex. He had become alcoholic, and though he had overcome this problem while married to Eric's mother, he had remained ineffectual, becoming a petty manipulator in the business world after leaving the marriage when Eric was thirteen. Throughout Eric's college years, Eric and his sister had grown accustomed to being offered inappropriate, seductive gifts at vacation times, while regular support money was withheld or erratically given. Thus the volleyball player and the seductive older man were two sides of Eric's father (at least as he saw him, still in part through his mother's eyes).

Thus, there was no man in the family to show Eric the way to identity. To the therapist, there was something both poignant and reassuring about Eric's sitting on that rock. Often a rock symbolizes one's innermost determined sense of self, and despite the inability of either mother or father to help Eric to an identity that was his own, he did appear to have this rock.

"It felt good under me," Eric observed.

It was clear that a conventional solution -- identification with his father's values -- would not be possible for Eric. If he were to find his way, it would have to be along individual lines. The next dream was the first to suggest what these might be:

Therapy. Dream: I was standing with a group of men at the top of a hollow, looking down into a cavernous hole. All seemed afraid to approach it. I was lowered into the hole and was looking around. I ran across a very soft spot of soil. I dropped to my knees and started digging. As I dug deep I struck some symmetrical-looking stones. I called the others and the excavation began. As they were excavating, a few people from the team decided to scour the walls in search of any other markings. Two openings were found; one on either side. One group enters one cave and I the other. My side is cafeteria-like; we discover glasses, silverware and some dishes, while the other team discovers beautiful pottery and stoneware and some artifacts mostly in very good condition. Meanwhile, the team leaders are marking our findings. The symmetrical stones are finally uncovered, and it seems that these stones form letters from the scripts of the Holy Grail. There are clues on how to discover it.

In working on this dream, the therapist felt that the "cavernous hole" represented the patient's depression – which in turn reflected the hole left in his life by the loss of his father in early adolescence. Yet in going into this problem (as indeed the therapy had been doing), the basis for a solution to it seemed to emerge. At this point it seemed no more than a fantasy, a wish, or a hint, but the "letters of the Holy Grail" seemed like archetypes of writing itself, going back to that time before Gutenberg, when printed letters were indeed rare and precious, guarded by priests. Could not this mean that Eric's future did indeed lie in his interest in writing? Of some interest to the therapist was that not only these precious letters were uncovered, but also a practical means of support – the cafeteria.

The therapist pointed out to Eric that the dream indication was extremely positive for his at least

trying to make a go of his writing. At this point, Eric began to work regularly on a piece of writing which was to engage him for much of the next stage of his therapy.

Initiation

In the stage of initiation, the patient must try out new behaviors and new ways of experiencing things if he is to escape from a neurotic web of limitations which interfere with his abilities to master his own life. It is akin to the role of adolescence in different cultures: in leaving childhood behind, various experiments in living, some culturally encouraged and some frowned upon, some successful and some unsuccessful, must be undertaken.

During this period of Eric's therapy, much of his energy was spent working on a piece of writing for publication. This involved him in doing much research, indeed in the very period of the Grail legends. He found himself increasingly saying no to members of his college group who wanted to stay with him, to girlfriends who threatened to interrupt his work, and to his mother and sister, who had begun calling him, urging him to come home.

A series of dreams reflected these changes.

Dream: My mother is lying on her deathbed. Her face is badly marred. Part of it is bandaged. Her lips are yellow with pus from a fever. She gives me a lamp and makes me kiss her. I give her a check for $10.

In this dream, what is dying is Eric's identification with his mother (in dreams, often one's affect toward a person is represented as that person). Or, in other words, he is getting over his mother complex. The $10 was not hard to figure out: Eric's parents had divorced exactly ten years before he had this dream; the money represented the years he had given to being her man. The recognition of the time he has given her enables him to be brutally unsentimental: he has given her enough, and he can set himself free.

Dream: My father was playing golf on a golf course with two women. I came in out of the woods and made a foursome. I walked on the green. I wasn't playing (I hadn't all day). I caught up with him. He sank his putt, looked up and said, "Oh, hi, have you decided to join us? C'mon to the next tee."

We went up to the next tee. Two women bickering – family squabble. "Look at these people," father said. "Aren't they funny? We're past our games." I said, "I want to communicate with you as a real person. We're playing this game!"

In this dream, Eric was able to confront his father directly with his particular style of seduction. Now "out of the woods" himself, i.e., less depressed, Eric was beginning to face some unpleasant family issues squarely. The father would often set his mother and sister quarreling by strategic phone calls which drove Eric's sister into hysterics. Then Eric would be called upon by one of the women, also by phone, to intervene. To his inquiry, his father would say over the telephone, "You know how hysterical women are." Eric had always felt helpless in the face of such maneuvering. Now he was beginning to refuse to "play the game"; he needed the energy for his own tasks.

At this point, the family began fighting back hard (as is inevitable when one member breaks out of a long-established patter , even if to the ultimate benefit of all concer..ed). Many difficult-to-turn-down requests were made of him, all having the same basic message: be the way you used to be. The therapist was frequently called upon to support Eric in standing up to these requests. Here is how Eric's dreams monitored this period.

Dream: Being chased, sought after, shot at, killed. Somebody at point-blank range putting bullet in neck. I know who it is. When I wake up it's a man, but I can't remember who." (In other dreams it is one or two men; in yet another, a gang of men.)

Dream: Kept trying to get away from a gang of men in an old Buick. Twice they killed me. The third time I got away, ran back to my place, finding my old clothing in drawers; from the time that I lived at home.

In describing the bullet that went through his neck, Eric noted that its path was through the mouth and out his neck, "along the vocal tract," as he put it. Indeed, a long-standing symptom was his stuttering, which tended to clear up as he began successfully to resist his family's pressure to conform with aspects of their way of communicating in which he could not believe.

The old Buick was the family car. All these dreams seemed to offer the threat of regression, of a return to old ways of doing things, of being pursued by old habits of communicating which had landed him in a depressed state. In fact, they came at a time when he was doing well at giving up these old ways, which may indicate that the habit-patterns had now become anxieties rather than behaviors.

After this sequence of dreams, Eric's anxiety began to become less, as is indicated by the following two dreams:

Dream: Swimming in water, afraid. Looked down in the water, saw a snake. It turned out to be just a little black snake and didn't hurt me.

Dream: In a pit with poisonous and other kinds of snakes, including cobras, rattlers, green snakes, copperheads and diamond backs, but this time there was no fear. I danced around, light on my feet, and walked out again.

These two dreams represent the mastery of fear which can be expected when an understanding of one's own emotions occurs. Snake dreams generally represent primordial instincts: the unknown or unconscious itself. To be unafraid of the snake is to be unafraid of one's own instincts. At about this time, Eric no longer was stuttering, no longer feared that he would kill himself, and was not terrified by his occasional homosexual impulses.

He was on good terms with the animal in himself. As if to emphasize the point, he had the following dream:

> Dream: A killer gorilla is on the loose and is killing single women. I'm visiting my parents when I hear about the murders. I guess who he will strike next – my old girlfriend. So I quickly go to see her. But when I lift her head to give her some water, it turns out to be my mother. I tell her I'll protect her, and the killer (who is a huge man) walks in. He says he will sit there until she marries him. A king comes in and hides behind a pillar to observe. He finally leaves distraught.
>
> Next there is a curious scene. All the clowns pour out and circle the stadium before the release of the lion. They welcome him and let him run around. Next the king's court procession in whiteface is released to march around. This time my old girlfriend is playing the queen. She goes into the bathroom to change headdresses when I notice behind the door a gorilla climbing over the stall coming after me.
>
> I run into a men's room and lock the door behind me, but the window is too small to escape from; so I go back and try and save my girl. As I try to convince her of the danger, the gorilla breaks in with a drawn knife and says he is going to kill me.
>
> Suddenly the curtains dividing the rooms are drawn and the procession of judgment dressed in black enter, and they take away the knife. We disrobe the gorilla, who is now small and black, and tell him we will take him to a mental hospital. He gives me his stamps and tells me to sell them for money to buy cigarettes for him. We trail past many ancient stone buildings to a beach where there is a crowd. My friends have gone with me. They discover that the killer is a homosexual and ask me what to do with him. I shrug and walk away.

In this dream we see the four-act structure that Jung noted in many dreams, as a dramatic process of conflict resolution proceeds. In the first act,

there is *exposition* of the problem – the dream begins with a return to an old way of coping, a visit home. There, an uncivilized element, a bit of untamed instinct, threatens the status quo. Naïvely, Eric attempts to function as hero and protector to his "girl," who turns out to be none other than his mother, a second sign that this is a regression, not mature coping. Later, the untamed element turns out to be homosexuality; it appears so threatening at first because Eric is afraid of it.

At a personal level, the distraught king who leaves the scene is a repetition of his father, who offered him so little identity support. At an archetypal level, this the the typical problem of the man who becomes his mother's son-lover. He is abandoned by the truly masculine world of the fathers.

In the second act, there is *development* as he makes an effort to cope with the problem by releasing various defenses – humor (the clowns), courage (the lion), and dignity (the king's court procession) – all in the service of shoring up the heroic mode.

In the third act, a *culmination* to his efforts to function as a hero is reached: the men's room window (i.e., this masculine viewpoint) is too small to allow escape, and his mother is strangely refractory to rescue.

Heroism is a dismal failure, and his anxiety is at its peak. Finally, in the fourth act, a *solution* is reached, but by means of a new element, the procession of judgment, which represents Eric's capacity for appraising his problems. By submitting the difficulty to feeling-inquiry, he discovers that his once irrational fear is really a human problem, for which there can be no sure heroic answer, only the uncertainties of treatment (the mental hospital).

Eric's shrug suggests the insignificance of this issue to the larger scheme of his life, but he does not find a definitive solution in this dream, nor did he in his therapy. He simply walks away from the problem. Yet, as Jung observed, this is the common path of much conflict resolution: the basic problems of life are not solved, they are outgrown. The major part of Eric's initiation was complete. He was now ready to become his own man.

Individuation

In this stage of treatment, therapy and the therapist diminish in their importance. The patient is more autonomous, more able to make his own decisions and to carve out a lifestyle which will be congruent with his own abilities and interests. Indeed, the patient may come to resent the constant introspection which therapy demands, as if his new identity were a millipede which never dared walk before treatment; now that therapy has given it its coordination and rhythm, the patient fears that too much inspection of how movement came about might once again result in paralysis. How Eric moves toward autonomy is shown in the following vignettes.

> Dream: I had hiked a great distance with a friend. We came to a ridge. On one side was a river and two cities. One metropolis and another suburb on the side of the river. The river had a lot of sailboats, was very beautiful-looking except for the skyline. They were building and building new high rises out into the river, huge monoliths. We met what looked to be a goat boy in the mountain. He took us to the top of another ridge where we could see that the river extended into a valley which was lush and green. I asked him why the valley wasn't used for agriculture and he just shrugged, said it was full of swamps and was no good. We climbed down, and I rested by the road. As I lay there, a lamb came and rested his head on my chest. I caressed it, and it licked me. A tourist came along and wanted to know about the sheep. I couldn't tell her much. She wanted to show me the city from an observation booth. I told her how it had once been beautiful but now they were filling it with monolithic buildings. I then showed the tour buses the right road to take to get to the

city, and I also started walking toward it. I tried rowing across the river to get to it, but a whirlpool dragged my boat under and almost me with it, but I managed to swim back to shore where I was safe.

For Eric this dream represented an overview of his life. The friend, he felt sure, was his therapist. The "goat boy" was a part of himself — the natural man, whom he had come to enjoy now that he was not so afraid of his family and of himself. The undeveloped marsh he saw as his own creativity, and the goat boy's shrug worried him here: he still had to fight against his laziness. The metropolis looked very much like the city where he had grown up, and to which the dream made it clear he would not be returning. The more he thought about this dream, the more clear it became that he would have to develop the undeveloped territory in himself if he were ever to amount to anything.

At about this time, he showed his piece of writing, now completed, to his therapist. It showed promise, but it ran out of steam. The lazy shrug which the goat boy had given to the undeveloped marsh was showing in the undeveloped work. After careful deliberation, the therapist confronted Eric with what he felt to be the weakness in his work. This was a painful time for them both, because both knew that only Eric could carry his therapy forward from this point on.

Then came the dream which seemed to bring home to Eric the reality of all he had been through. At the time that he had it, Eric had been in therapy just a year.

> Dream: I walked into a room where my cousin Pam was reading a postcard. She had just begun to read when I walked in. I flopped myself on the floor right away so as not to disturb her. I think the letter was about someone returning home. I looked around this room and saw all my relatives and my family, yet I greeted no one. Suddenly this gathering turned into a wedding reception and dinner

was served. There were many tables, but not everyone was anxious to sit down. There were scattered people seated at the red tables, here and there, but most of the people just stood and looked at the waiters who scurried between the tables.

At this point I greeted my father, threw my arms about his neck and began to weep, although I tried hard not to show any emotion. I did the same for my mother and sister, hugging them at the same time. I had to leave them, for I was in pursuit of three robbers. I took to horseback and roamed the countryside. I caught up with them in a barn. Suddenly I heard gunfire, I tied nooses around the necks of the robbers and pulled them back to the wedding as quickly as possible. By the time I got there, dead bodies were strewn everywhere. All my family had been killed, and there was a stunned cardinal father giving the last rites and planting flowers by the dead bodies. I knew then the robbers had been decoys to lure me away so that the event, which I thought I could have prevented, could take place.

For Eric, this dream was the turning point of his therapy. The three robbers, he felt, were his breaking the engagement, turning down the job, and trying to evade the draft. In his guilt over these things he left home, to redeem himself, he thought, for an eventual return. But as this dream put it so eloquently, these things were only decoys: life had really meant for him to leave home; he was one of those who have to break from the parental mold, and there was no way now to go home again: psychologically speaking, his parents were dead.

This dream was followed by another, in which he assumed more direct responsibility for the changes in consciousness which had occured.

Dream: I dreamt I killed Robert Kennedy and was jumping over fences to get away from pursuing police. As I jumped over the fence I dropped a red pen on the ground and would

pick it up and proceed. Finally, after running through a few intersections, a girl in a car was waiting to pick me up. I decided to drive but couldn't get the window to latch. The police were everywhere, but no one seemed to bother us as we drove away with the window finally latched.

In this dream, Eric has finally terminated his role as mother's hero, and although the police pursue him (a symbol of his mother's attempts to use conventional pressures to get him to return to her), he gets away with a woman (i.e., an emotional life) having nothing to do with his mother. We notice, too, that he gets over the barrier that he could not pass in the early dream of the race. Surely the red pen is a symbol of his writing, in which his feeling of manhood is rooted (the pen being also a phallic symbol). The latching of the window represents his hard-won achievement of ego-integrity against the criticisms of his mother, as indeed he had resumed writing after the honest but wounding criticisms of the therapist.

As is usual in therapy, this dream was a bit ahead of the actual developments in his life, but it was accurate in predicting a potential for freedom from anxiety where his parents were concerned. The next dream shows the advantage of this achievement:

Dream: Digging into the ground and finding all the money I could want.

Money in dreams is often a symbol of energy, and indeed at this point in his therapy, Eric began to have real energy for his life. He began another piece of writing, developed many new social contacts, and began to think about his next steps, which involved using these contacts to get his writing published.

At this juncture, Eric had a dream which made him think again about this way of starting a career.

Dream: I called a number to try and reach Albert Einstein because I had recently been to a course where I heard his lectures and read everything he wrote. I called, but Margaret

Mead answered and said that everyone wanted to speak with him, but I couldn't. I awoke, acutely disappointed.

Here his old problem of not being able to reach the father and being stuck with the mother is presented in a different light – as the unavailable independent thinker versus the available authority on socialization, in a hilarious invidious comparison. The temptation for Eric at this point was to concentrate on getting the work he had already done accepted rather than develop his original ideas further, which meant more hard and lonely work, in poverty. The dream made him realize that approval alone was not enough for him, and he determined to stick out the painful process of learning to do something original and good. This decision was marked by a follow-up dream in which he did meet Albert Einstein in a bus station. As he put it in associating to this dream, the bus is a "common carrier," handling everybody. Many patients discover that their own individuality appears in the most ordinary contexts, rather than in prestigious places. Eric discovered that he had to give up his concern with importance in order to get in touch with his own personal genius.

At this point, the basic guidelines for Eric's further development had been laid down. He knew his goal – to become a good creative writer. He knew he had to work hard, and he had learned to watch out for the temptations of immediate prestige. His dreams had been so helpful that he found himself turning more and more to them for inspiration. And then he had the following dream:

Dream: I was in a light canoe, rowing through a thick underbrush along a deep creek. Hundreds of birds of all varieties – popinjays, sparrows, bobwhites, etc. – and some small animals – rabbits, squirrels, etc. – lived along the creek's banks. As I passed, some of the animals fled, others remained. As I reached the end of the creek, it seemed that it turned into a tunnel ending where a great number of birds had gathered, grounded. As I went to pass through the opening into the great river, an

owl and a lion jumped up to block my approach. As I reached up to drive the owl away, he bit my finger and I was forced to retreat.

Working on this dream, Eric's therapist was reminded of Jung's many warnings about the dangers of overavid exploration of the inner world. Jung found that many of his patients, after painful probing of their "personal" unconscious material, would come to enjoy the process of self-exploration and would start to assimilate material from the wider, deeper source of emotion he called the collective unconscious. Jung often warned that this process was not for the young, who could too easily use it it to avoid establishing themselves in life.

This dream is a good example of how the dreams themselves monitor the dangers of uncovering: had it come at the start of therapy, it might have been a warning not to move into dream material. Coming at this point, it represented a natural limit to the amount of work Eric should do on himself in therapy at this time. It was as if Eric's own instincts, represented by the animals, could sense the danger, and with great authority prevent him from going further with his introversion. He was forced to accept this healthy resistance and curb his curiosity. At this point, both Eric and his therapist realized that psychotherapy was coming to an end, and they began to think toward termination.

A particular issue was Eric's first visit home, now that he had found his identity. The therapist urged him to wait for the right time to make this return, to wait for some sign from his family that they could meet him where he now was. At first, it seemed to Eric that there never would be a right time. Marking this waiting period was the following dream.

Dream: I had to transport cadavers from an abandoned house somewhere on another planet to earth. The cadavers were anti-matter and so the settings had to be perfect in order for the bodies to be shipped without blowing up the transporter. I had two machines – the second of which was the more accurate as to what settings should work. I seemed totally apprehensive and was unable to procure the correct readings.

Here the problem of relating the events which occur in "the reality of the psyche" to the realities of everyday life is acutely presented. For Eric, the "cadavers," i.e., the deaths of his old ways of relating to the various members of his family, were absolutely real – but these changes had occurred on another plane. Now he had to return to visit his family carrying the knowledge of the changes he had undergone in therapy.

At this point, that scene in his initial dream in which a man was holding a torch over some dead bodies became clear to the therapist. It was clear to the therapist that Eric would have to carry consciousness for all the members of his family about the changes that had occurred. The rest of the family, not having been in psychotherapy, could not be expected to understand them.

The two machines, for Eric, were his therapist's intuition and his own: the therapist's, he felt, was more accurate. He took the advice and despite a scheduled vacation from work elected to wait until a real sign came from his family.

Not long after, this sign came. His sister decided to move from home and get an apartment of her own. She had become much less hysterical, and many of her respiratory symptoms had cleared up. This seemed directly related to Eric's refusal to act as a go-between in her battles with their father. His mother issued an invitation for him to join them in marking her move away from home. His father even offered to pay his way.

This visit went smoothly. Eric showed his mother a finished piece of writing that deeply impressed her: she could accept that he was serious in pursuing this goal. He returned to his therapist with plans to leave treatment in order to go to another city to pursue the technical studies he would need for the specialized writing that was his bent. Eric agreed to keep in touch with the therapist through informal contacts, just to assure his gains.

The night after his final session, Eric had the following dream:

> Dream: I was driving an old family car. I went to see Bert, the leader of my college group, who had given me the original advice to lie to the first psychiatrist, to escape the draft. Bert got in the car with me, but I wouldn't let him drive the car. The final image was of a parking space in the new city for which I was headed.

Having worked through the termination with his therapist, Eric was ready to try out his hard-won individuation in his personal life. Having learned to stand up to his mother and father, he now could even stand up to a once all-powerful peer. As he put it in telling this dream to his therapist at an informal contact several months later, "I seemed to have separated our natures; I was strong enough to say no."

COMMENT

Much of psychotherapy proceeds in the dark. The therapist and patient struggle to understand each other as issues of therapy are brought out, tested, resisted, and worked through. In many other chapters of this book, we describe the conscious techniques by which this process may be facilitated. In this chapter, we hold up the mirror of dreams to the conscious work of therapy. Dreams catch the reflection of the meaning of the therapy to the life of the patient.

REFERENCES

1. Mackenzie, Norman: *Dreams and Dreaming,* Aldus Books, London, 1965.

2. Becker, Raymond de: *The Understanding of Dreams,* Michael Heron (trans.), Hawthorn, New York, 1968.

3. Kramer, Milton (ed.), with Roy M. Whitman, Bill J. Baldridge, and Paul Ornstein: *Dream Psychology and the New Biology of Dreaming*, Charles C Thomas, Springfield, Ill., 1969.

4. Jones, Richard M.: *The New Psychology of Dreaming*, Grune & Stratton, New York, 1970.

5. Faraday, Ann: *Dream Power*, Hodder, London, 1972.

6. Mackenzie: op. cit., chap. 7, "The Dream Debate," pp. 176–207.

7. Freud, Sigmund: *The Interpretation of Dreams*, James Strachey (trans.), Basic Books, New York, 1959.

8. Freud, Sigmund: *On Dreams*, James Strachey (trans.), Norton, New York, 1952 (paperback).

9. Shulman, Bernard: "An Adlerian View," with discussion by Kurt A. Adler, in Milton Kramer (ed.), op cit., chap. 5, pp. 117–140.

10. Jung, C. G.: "General Aspects of Dream Psychology," in *The Structure and Dynamics of the Psyche*, vol. 8, in *The Collected Works of C. G. Jung*, Pantheon, New York, 1960, pp. 237–280.

11. Jung, C. G.: "The Practical Use of Dream Analysis," in *The Practice of Psychotherapy*, vol. 16, 2d ed., in *The Collected Works of C. G. Jung*, Pantheon, New York, 1966.

12. Altman, Leon L.: *The Dream in Psychoanalysis*, International Universities Press, New York, 1969.

13. Bonime, Walter: *The Clinical Use of Dreams*, Basic Books, New York, 1962.

14. Rossi, Ernest Lawrence: *Dreams and the Growth of Personality*, Pergamon, New York, 1972.

15. French, Thomas M., and Erika Fromm: *Dream Interpretation: A New Approach*, Basic Books, New York, 1972.

16. Boss, Medard: *The Analysis of Dreams*, Ryder, London, 1957.

17. Caligor, Leopold, and Rollo May: *Dreams and Symbols: Man's Unconscious Language*, Basic Books, New York, 1968.

18. Perls, Frederick S.: *Gestalt Therapy Verbatim*, Real People Press, Lafayette, Calif., 1969.

19. Whitmont, Edward C.: *The Symbolic Quest*, G. P. Putnam's for the C. G. Jung Foundation for Analytic Psychology, New York, 1969.

20. Hillman, James: *Insearch: Psychology and Religion*, Scribner's, New York, 1967.

21. Sampson, Harold: "Discussion," to Bill Domhoff's "Home Dreams Versus Laboratory Dreams," Milton Kramer (ed.), op. cit., chap. 10, p. 221.

22. Osterman, Elizabeth: Personal communication.

23. Kirsch, Thomas B.: Personal communication.

24. Jung, C. G.: "On the Nature of Dreams," in *The Structure and Dynamics of the Psyche*, vol. 8, op. cit., p. 283.

25. Faraday: loc. cit.

26. Dement, William C.: "The Psychophysiology of Dreaming," in G. E. von Grunebaum and Roger Caillois (eds.), *The Dream and Human Societies*, University of California Press, Berkeley, 1966, chap. 4.

27. Dement, William: "Psychophysiology of Sleep and Dreams," in S. Arieti (ed.), *American Handbook of Psychiatry*, Basic Books, New York, 1966, vol. 3, pp. 290–332.

28. Hartmann, Ernest (ed.): *Sleep and Dreaming*, Little, Brown, Boston, 1970.

29. Medow, L., and L. Snow (eds.): *The Psychodynamic Implications of the Physiologic Studies on Dreams*, Charles C Thomas, Springfield, Ill., 1970.

30. Faraday: op. cit., p. 51.

31. Dement: "The Psychophysiology of Dreaming," op. cit., p. 98.

32. Faraday: op. cit., pp. 41–42.

33. Rossi: loc. cit.

34. Henderson, Joseph L., and Maud Oakes: *The Wisdom of the Serpent*, George Braziller, New York, 1963, pp. 20–22.

35. Perry, John Weir: *Lord of the Four Quarters,* Collier Books, Macmillan, New York, 1970, pp. 18–23 (paperback).

36. Cohen, David B.: "To Sleep, Perchance to Recall a Dream: Repression Is Not the Demon Who Conceals and Hoards Our Forgotten Dreams," *Psychology Today,* pp. 50–54, May 1974.

37. Dement: "The Psychophysiology of Dreaming," op. cit., p. 99.

38. Faraday: op. cit., chap. 3, "Why We Forget Our Dreams," pp. 52–67.

39. Cohen: loc. cit.

40. Alex, William: "Dreams, the Unconscious, and Analytical Therapy," published by the C. G. Jung Institute of San Francisco, 1971, p. 1.

41. Jung, C. G.: "Concerning the Archetypes, with Special Reference to the Anima Concept," in *The Archetypes and the Collective Unconscious,* vol. 9, part 1 of *The Collected Works of C. G. Jung,* Pantheon, New York, 1959.

42. Grinstein, Alexander: *On Sigmund Freud's Dreams,* Wayne State University Press, Detroit, 1968, chap. 17, pp. 392–422.

43. Jung, C. G.: "The Psychology of the Transference," in *The Practice of Psychotherapy,* vol. 16, 2d ed., in *The Collected Works of C. G. Jung,* Pantheon, New York, 1966, p. 227.

44. Whitney, Elizabeth: Personal communication.

PERMISSIONS

www.ingramcontent.com/pod-product-compliance
Lightning Source LLC
Chambersburg PA
CBHW080233270326
41926CB00020B/4214